The Psychology of Lifestyle

Impro… s of reduci… ver, despit… ant differe… and obesit…

The … in revers… the comm… can inform … alth promoti… d to enable pe… ours that impa… sex and drug … pter contains int… note lifestyle char…

This uniqu… and practical gras… ts of lifestyle change… nals committed to h…

Kathryn Thirlaw… t the University of Wal… chol-ogist and currentl… e for health professional…

Dominic Upton is He… iver-sity of Worcester. He is also a Chartered Health Psychologist.

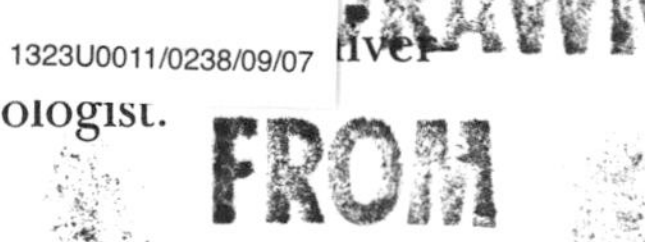

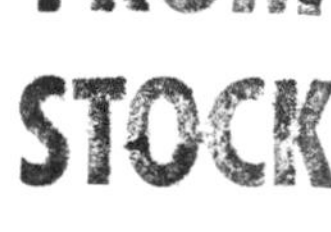

The Psychology of Lifestyle

Promoting healthy behaviour

Kathryn Thirlaway and Dominic Upton

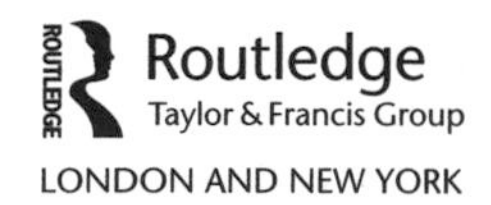

LONDON AND NEW YORK

First published 2009
by Routledge
2 Park Square, Milton Park, Abingdon, Oxon OX14 4RN

Simultaneously published in the USA and Canada
by Routledge
270 Madison Avenue, New York, NY 10016

Routledge is an imprint of the Taylor & Francis Group, an informa business

Typeset in Baskerville by Saxon Graphics Ltd, Derby
Printed and bound in Great Britain by
Antony Rowe, Chippenham, Wiltshire

British Library Cataloguing in Publication Data
A catalogue record for this book is available from the British Library

Library of Congress Cataloging-in-Publication-Data
Thirlaway, Kathryn
The psychology of lifestyle : promoting healthy behaviour /
Kathryn Thirlaway and Dominic Upton
p. ; cm.
Includes bibliographical references.
1. Health promotion—Great Britain. 2. Health behavior—Great Britain. 3. Lifestyles—Health aspects—Great Britain. I. Upton, Dominic. II. Title.
[DNLM: 1. Health Behavior—Great Britain. 2. Health Promotion—methods—Great Britain. 3. Life Style—Great Britain. W 85 T446p 2008]
RA427.8.T45 2008
362.10941—dc22 2008018011

ISBN 10: 0-415-41661-2 (hbk)
ISBN 10: 0-415-41662-0 (pbk)

ISBN 13: 978-0-415-41661-0 (hbk)
ISBN 13: 978-0-415-41662-7 (pbk)

For Mark without whom I would achieve nothing and for Megan, Anna, Hetty and Keir whose lifestyles have undoubtedly been compromised by the writing of this book (KT).

For those who have influenced my lifestyle for good or for worse: my parents and now Penney, Francesca, Rosie and Gabriel (DU).

Contents

Acknowledgements

This project has been a major undertaking for both of us and has involved the reading and reviewing of a considerable number of research and review papers. These articles have been published not only in psychology journals but also in the wider literature including those drawn from health care, medicine, sociology, philosophy and governmental policy documents. We have tried to encompass the literature from both an academic and a practitioner basis. Obviously we thank the researchers, clinicians and policy makers for all this work and the contributions they have made to the current knowledge base.

On a more personal level, several key colleagues have acted as researchers and reviewers for us and have contributed their time, effort and opinions with vigour and a frankness that was as refreshing as it was useful. Particular mention should go to Holly Andrews, Erica Thomas, Rebecca Ingram and Julia Mathias (for DU) and Debbie Clayton, Tina Alwyn, Jacqueline Campbell, Anna Sweeney, Jenny Daw, Helen Campling, Mark Palmer and Megan Thirlaway (for KT).

Many thanks also to the team at Routledge for helping us through this project. We also thank those involved in the production of this text – the designers and production editors for enhancing the text with some excellent features, which we hope has provided guidance, direction and added value to all readers.

We must offer thanks and acknowledgements to those who have provided support for us both at work and at home. Particular thanks must go to Sue Thomas, who unfailingly provided priceless peace of mind. We also thank our colleagues (for KT) at the University of Wales Institute, Cardiff (UWIC) and (for DU) at the University of Worcester for their help, advice, friendship and practical guidance.

Finally, we would also like to thank our family and friends for bringing us sustenance and calming us down during our manic periods when we could think of nothing else other than 'the book', especially during the final 'push' when our lifestyle became less than optimal, as did our health.

Introduction

Background to this book

In 2006 the then prime minister, Tony Blair, expressed the view that 'lifestyle diseases' were one of the major challenges facing the National Health Service (NHS). During Tony Blair's time as prime minister considerable attention was given to these diseases, whether this be within academia, social policy or the media. Prior to this high level nudge, we had already recognised the importance of psychology in the development of the so-called lifestyle diseases and were discussing the development of a 'Lifestyle Psychology' degree. Further research and discussion with colleagues led us to believe that there was a market for a book on lifestyle psychology and we began a dialogue with the publisher from which this text has resulted.

Illnesses associated with a poor lifestyle are becoming ever more prominent and there is increasing recognition that these are having a considerable impact on both an individual's and the population as a whole's health. Lifestyle diseases are not evenly distributed across the nation; the influence of social class, gender and ethnicity should not be overlooked. Moreover, there are differences between the individual countries of the United Kingdom, with certain behaviours and health and illnesses more prominent in some areas compared to others. Finally, there are psychological variables which may be described as either 'risk' factors or 'protective' factors. Some of these social and demographic factors have been integrated with the psychological factors to create psychological models to predict behaviours and develop theoretically based interventions. All of these factors are highlighted in this text. We have not simply concentrated on individual factors as we consider Tony Blair's perspective on these behaviours – 'they are the result of millions of individual decisions, at millions of points in time' – to be simplistic. The social environment has a clear and well documented impact.

But what is lifestyle psychology? We discuss this at length Chapter 1, but as a working definition we consider lifestyle psychology to be the study of the antecedents, consequences and interactions of lifestyle behaviours including: eating, drinking alcohol, smoking, taking drugs, physical activity and sexual practices. We see the role of psychology in lifestyle as of significant, if not primary, importance. We see the role of lifestyle in health and in illness as predominating and likely to become ever more important to the NHS in the coming decades. Indeed, the Foresight report described the 'obesity epidemic' as a problem comparable to climate change (McPherson et al. 2007). How these issues are going to be addressed is worthy of debate and range from the theoretically driven to the more light-hearted. Lifestyle is an issue that every commentator feels confident to express an opinion about. For example, the stigmatisation of obese people (albeit in, one would assume, a humorous article) is not uncommon: 'Most obesity is a consequence of stupidity and indolence and not of some genetic affliction. It is a lifestyle choice which people would be less inclined to adopt if they knew we all hated them for it' (Liddle 2008). We review some of the more serious and theoretically driven approaches in this text, debate their value and discuss the potential ways forward in promoting lifestyle change.

Structure of this book

We discussed the structure of this book for some time. Indeed, initially we could not come to a final conclusion and the structure of the text has evolved over the writing process to its current state. At the outset, we knew the content (or thought we did), we knew how we wanted to present the material, we knew the order of the material and we sketched the structure. So what was the cause of our consternation? What did we spend so much time discussing? We appreciated at the outset that there was a possibility of considerable repetition within this text: many of the behaviours discussed are underpinned by similar psychological variables and have been investigated within similar theoretical modes. After writing the first couple of chapters we recognised this and rejigged the book to include the chapter on theoretical approaches. We hope that this has removed considerable overlap. We also recognised that there was the possibility of omitting important material but we hope we have avoided this and have attempted to address the key lifestyle behaviours and the key psychological factors.

We would like to stress, however, that this is not a book about smoking or obesity or social cognition models or social marketing *alone*. It is a book that attempts to cover a range of topics from both perspectives in an integrating framework. Hence, there are sections on social marketing, for example, that some may consider skimpy and there are psychological factors and models that could have been included in many more chapters than currently presented. We have done this on purpose – we have not written a book that is dedicated to any one behaviour or any one approach. There are good books on psychological models (e.g. Conner and Norman 2005), on smoking (e.g. Lapointe 2008), on obesity (e.g. Leach 2006) and so on. We cannot obviously compete with these texts for the specific behaviours or models. However, we present an overview with a thematic connection between the chapters which we hope readers will find useful and thought provoking.

We should also discuss why we have selected these topics for inclusion. On the one hand we could have simply discussed those mentioned by Tony Blair in his 2006 speech: 'obesity, smoking, alcohol abuse, . . ., sexually transmitted disease', but we recognised that this did not cover the complete range of behaviours we wanted to discuss. We initially included sleep as a lifestyle behaviour and thought that it was of key importance with the emergence (or in reality continued presence) of the 24-hour society and the increasing proportion of individuals involved in shift work. However, we came to realise that this did not fit with the other behaviours described in this text so we abandoned this chapter. We then reviewed those behaviours which have the most significant impact on health and went for the chapters presented in this volume. This was subsequently supported by information we found on websites from the four UK countries. They had labelled the behaviours we ultimately included in this text as lifestyle behaviours and we were happy to go with these behaviours. Following our introduction to this chapter we have presented nine substantial chapters in this book dealing with key issues in lifestyle psychology.

Theories of change

In this chapter we describe a number of key psychological theories that are of relevance to the topic of lifestyle and lifestyle change. It is by no means intended to be a comprehensive evaluation of all relevant theories; that would be a book in itself. Theories that are commonly utilised across all lifestyle behaviours are included; which means that some, for instance those used consistently with one behaviour but not with others, are omitted. The aim of the chapter is, first, to give an outline of each theory so that its value in relation to lifestyle behaviours can be properly evaluated, second, to analyse the similarities and differences between the various theories, and finally to draw attention to key common factors across the theories described and discussed.

Eating

In this chapter we explore the so-called 'obesity epidemic' and the 'obesogenic environment' that have been highlighted within the media to such an extent recently. The problems in providing a clear message of a 'healthy diet' are stressed, as are the issues surrounding the social environment impact on diet. The governmental approaches to the 'epidemic' will be outlined and the role of psychological models in the development of appropriate interventions will be stressed.

Physical activity

In this chapter we consider the predominance of sedentary lifestyles in the population. Physical activity is the output side of the input–output energy equation and so is a key factor in the rising levels of obesity. The role of the obesogenic environment and how psychological interventions can work in such adverse environmental conditions is explored.

Drinking

Drinking is a popular component of many aspects of leisure in Britain. Drinking has adverse consequences for social and physical well-being. The changing nature of drinking patterns in the UK and in particular in women is described and discussed. Government policies to establish healthy drinking patterns in young people and promote healthy drinking in adults are outlined and the role of psychological interventions to support healthy drinking and deter deleterious drinking will be evaluated.

Smoking

The health consequences of smoking are well established and well known throughout the population. However, approximately a quarter of the UK population still smoke and this has a significant impact on the individual and country's health. Given the significant impact that smoking has on the health of the nation, there has been extensive research into smoking and much of this has a psychological nature. In this chapter these factors are identified and how they have been incorporated into both public health and clinical interventions.

Sex

The safe sex message is still being promoted in order to reduce the spread of sexually transmitted diseases. Sexual behaviours are not simply a consequence of physiological drives, but there are social, emotional and cultural (to name but three) variables that influence our drives and intentions. Within these broader influences the psychological factors have to be appreciated and the developed models evaluated. The success of these social cognition models used to predict safe sex practices and how appropriate interventions can be best developed are explored.

Illicit drug use

Illicit drug use is perhaps different from the other lifestyle behaviours explored in this text. It is a relatively rare behaviour but it has a clear impact on the community and the country at large. Furthermore, when exploring government material and recent academic texts, many include this as a lifestyle choice (although we acknowledge the debate around the use of the C-word). It is also important to recognise that illicit drug use can be considered as a subcategory of smoking and alcohol abuse. Finally, the interventions designed to reduce illicit drug taking employ psychological approaches which are relevant and essential to other lifestyle behaviours.

Evaluating lifestyle psychology

In this chapter we will consider the evidence to support the existence of lifestyles rather than the discrete practice of a set of behaviours. The key psychological themes that have emerged from the exploration of each of the lifestyle behaviours will be discussed and evaluated. Potential new avenues of research for improving the likelihood of behavioural change will be considered. Finally, the chapter will consider the value of more comprehensive models that include socio-demographic and environmental factors as key components rather than as confounding variables.

Strategies for the twenty-first century

In this final chapter the strands from all the previous chapters will be drawn together in order to present concise review of where we are now in our understanding of, and success in, promoting lifestyle change. Within the context of primary care and prevention a set of generic strategies for effective promotion of lifestyle change will be presented. Finally, research priorities for the future are identified.

We hope that you will enjoy, and be both interested in and stimulated by this text.

1 Conceptualising lifestyle psychology

There are people who strictly deprive themselves of each and every eatable, drinkable, and smokable which has in any way acquired a shady reputation. They pay this price for health. And health is all they get for it.

Mark Twain

At the end of this chapter you will:

- have a working definition of lifestyle diseases and lifestyle behaviours
- understand the development of a lifestyle model of disease
- be aware of the problems with measuring lifestyle behaviours
- recognise the multiple influences on lifestyle choice.

The decision to write a text on lifestyle psychology reflects an appreciation of the importance of the government and policy makers' use of the term lifestyle to refer to diseases where behaviour plays a part in the aetiology of the condition. In a speech in 2006, the then prime minister of Great Britain, Tony Blair, called for 'lifestyle change' to relieve the pressure on the National Health Service (BBC News 2006). The prime minister suggested that 'failure to address bad lifestyles was putting an "increasing strain" on the health service'. The centrality of the message, the role of lifestyle in health, and the role of psychology in promoting and improving lifestyle will form the focus of this text.

The term 'lifestyle diseases' is now commonly used and implies that not only are there a number of diseases that have in common a behavioural influence in their development, but also that there are behaviours that collectively contribute to a 'lifestyle'. Furthermore, the use of the term lifestyle implies related rather than discrete behaviours (Dean et al. 1995). One of the challenges for this text is to evaluate the nature of the relationship between lifestyle behaviours and the implications for lifestyle change. Lifestyle diseases and lifestyle behaviours are commonly referred to in the media, government documents and academic papers and are intuitively understood by this broad range of audiences although there is no consensus about which diseases and consequently which behaviours can come under the umbrella term of lifestyle. As early as the 1980s the World Health Organisation (WHO) had recognised the emergence of a concept of lifestyle and offered the following definition:

> Lifestyles are patterns of (behavioural) choices from the alternatives that are available to people according to their socio-economic circumstances and the ease with which they are able to choose certain ones over others.
>
> (WHO 1986: 118)

This early definition of 'lifestyle' recognises the contextual element of choice and how choice may be limited by factors out of the control of the individual but does not specify which behaviours are considered to be key in terms of maintaining health and preventing disease. Indeed the WHO states: 'it is one of the WHO's responsibilities to ensure that the lifestyle concept is not used as a blanket explanation in which the victim is always blamed' (WHO 1986: 118).

Nevertheless, despite this clear message that behavioural change cannot be left to the individual to achieve but must be addressed at societal and policy level, the paper concludes by commenting that: 'We have reached the age of responsibility' (WHO 1986: 124). In this way the notion that chronic diseases can be avoided and that we, both at an individual and at a societal level, are responsible are clearly linked to the use of the term lifestyle.

Dean et al. (1995) describe lifestyle as a sociocultural phenomenon. They argue that patterns of behaviour interact with the situational context to create a lifestyle. Cultural values and beliefs shape behavioural practices which are either constrained or encouraged by specific socio-economic conditions. Both of these authors hold a view of lifestyle as a pattern of behaviours (WHO 1986; Dean et al. 1995).

Lifestyle diseases

Doyle (2001) suggests that the six major lifestyle diseases are coronary heart disease, stroke, lung cancer, colon cancer, diabetes and chronic obstructive pulmonary disease. The rationale for their inclusion is that they 'trace mainly to imprudent living' (Doyle 2001). While Lloyd and Foster (2006) and Wanless (2004) agree with Doyle (2001) in his choice of those diseases which can be given the title of lifestyle diseases, other authors would widen the group. For instance, Bugel (2003) additionally included cancers in general and osteoporosis as examples of lifestyle diseases.

One of the problems with attempting to arrive at a conclusion about what constitutes a lifestyle disease is the myriad of definitions under which diseases are categorised. For instance, the Department of Health (1999b) uses the umbrella term of cardiovascular diseases (CVD) to refer to angina, heart attack, stroke, heart murmur, irregular heart rhythm, 'other heart trouble', reported high blood pressure or diabetes. Other publications delineate between coronary heart disease, cerebrovascular disease (stroke) and diabetes (Welsh Assembly Government 2005). It is possible to conclude that cardiovascular diseases as defined by the Department of Health (1999b), some respiratory disorders and some cancers have a behavioural component to their aetiology and are eligible to be called lifestyle diseases.

Interestingly, few authors would include sexually transmitted diseases under the lifestyle umbrella, although they could be argued to be entirely under behavioural control, with none of the genetic component that plays a part in aetiology of the six major lifestyle diseases as identified by Doyle (2001). Sexually transmitted diseases are more usually defined as infectious diseases (e.g. ONS 2007), an important distinction for clinicians but perhaps less so for primary care and community based practitioners with a remit of disease prevention through behavioural change.

In between an 'imprudent lifestyle' (Doyle 2001) and the development of a chronic life-threatening or life-foreshortening condition lie a number of precursors of disease. High cholesterol, high blood pressure and obesity are risk factors for the development of a number of the aforementioned lifestyle diseases. The distinction between these precursors, the diseases they predict and the behaviours that are associated with them is often blurred. They are often presented as diseases per se and interventions prescribed by the medical profession. The Department of Health (1999a) categorises high blood pressure as a cardiovascular disease. Obesity is frequently referred to using disease parameters. The phrase 'obesity epidemic' (Gard and Wright 2005) is one that has been widely used and characterises obesity as a disease. Consequently, obesity can be considered a lifestyle disease by some authors whereas others categorise it as lifestyle behaviour (Doyle 2001).

Lifestyle behaviours

The behaviours that are usually cited as being involved in the aetiology of lifestyle diseases are poor diet, lack of physical activity, cigarette smoking (Blaxter 1990; Doyle 2001) and, increasingly, excess drinking (Blaxter 1990; Burke et al. 1997). The taking of illegal drugs is also lifestyle behaviour with health consequences. Reducing illegal drug taking seldom appears in general government health targets (National Assembly for Wales 2000), although many specific policy documents address this issue, and this may well be because, while often high profile, drug takers constitute a minority of the population (ONS 2007).

Sexual practices are also often described as health and/or lifestyle behaviours by public health professionals (Wardle and Steptoe 2005) and are considered a key health issue by policy makers (National Assembly for Wales 2000). Despite not being directly linked to what clinicians refer to as lifestyle diseases, sexual practices nevertheless are still considered by most public health practitioners to be an aspect of lifestyle worthy of both concern and intervention (Wardle and Steptoe 2005). Furthermore, sexual practices are a clear cause of preventable and treatable diseases.

Accidents are another key cause of preventable deaths (Department of Health 1999b) that have a behavioural component, road traffic accidents being the most common. Many individual, local community and national government interventions are set in place to avoid them (Department of Health 1999b). In contrast to interventions for healthy eating, drinking and so on, many of the interventions to prevent accidents involve legislation, perhaps because many accidents involve third parties. While people may be advised to eat more fruit and vegetables, they are required by law to wear a seatbelt in the United Kingdom. Individuals can be banned from driving if they are found to be driving dangerously and are compelled to take a driving test before getting behind a wheel. New houses and extensions to old houses are legally required to include smoke alarms. Consequently, avoidance of accidents is far less of a voluntary lifestyle choice in the United Kingdom than healthy eating, physical activity, drinking, smoking and sexual habits. Accidents often require medical treatment and can cause disability but do not usually cause the development of disease. Consequently, accidents and accident prevention fall outside of the remit of this text with its focus on chronic disease and volitional behaviours.

In consequence it is argued that health-related lifestyles can be defined as behavioural choices made by individuals about eating, physical activity, drinking alcohol, smoking tobacco, taking drugs and sexual practices. Lifestyle psychology can then be defined as the study of the antecedents, consequences and interactions of lifestyle behaviours, including eating, drinking alcohol, smoking, taking drugs, physical activity and sexual practices.

Collecting together a set of behaviours that contribute to the aetiology of lifestyle diseases does not justify a subdiscipline of lifestyle psychology. Bad weather and individual driving skills both contribute to road accidents but nobody would argue that bad weather and driving skills are related in any way other than their ability to influence accidents. However, it is possible to put together a cohesive argument that lifestyle behaviours share more than their ability to influence a range of chronic diseases. First, lifestyle behaviours have multiple functions; they are not simply or even primarily health focused. Lifestyle behaviours can be mood enhancing; they can be used as a coping strategy; they are often pleasurable; and they play an important function in the development and maintenance of social relationships. Second, lifestyle behaviours are all under some degree of volitional control, although the amount of control individuals have over their lifestyle choices is contentious and likely to vary widely from context to context. Third, lifestyle behaviours are all chronic rather than acute behaviours. Usually individuals will practise regular patterns of these behaviours and their future behaviour will be best predicted by the choices they have made in the past. Finally, lifestyle behaviours have the majority of their positive consequences in the present and the majority of their negative outcomes in the future. Any lifestyle behavioural change intervention consequently requires individuals to be future orientated. Consequently, it is possible to argue that lifestyle behaviours, although each unique, share a set of common factors that unify them and indicates that common theoretical principles may underpin the aetiology and progression of these behaviours.

The rise of lifestyle models of disease

It is commonly accepted in medical, psychological and sociological texts on Western medicine that a 'medical or biomedical model of disease' has been, and remains still, the underlying principle behind practice (e.g. Scambler 2003). In essence a medical model is individualist and reductionist assuming that all disease can be traced to specific causal mechanisms within the person (Turner 1987, cited in Hansen and Easthope 2007). The traditional medical model derives from germ theory which postulates that each disease has a single and specific cause. This model dominated medical research up to and including much of the twentieth century ensuring that research was focused on the laboratory rather than the community and the test-tube rather than the individual (Najman 1980). The medical model can support a perceived dichotomy between disease and illness: disease being the domain of the health professional and illness the domain of patients, families and, increasingly, social scientists (Hansen and Easthope 2007).

While it is legitimate to argue that a medical model of disease is dominant in Western medical practice, other models of disease coexist and, increasingly, challenge current orthodoxy, influencing health and health care. Environmental, genetic, psychological and lifestyle models of disease all operate within medicine (Hansen and Easthope 2007). One of the key unifying themes between these alternative models of disease is one of prevention rather than cure. This could be viewed as a threat to the medical profession and commercial companies that make a living from curing disease. Prevention can offer commercial prospects as well, although perhaps not for the same players.

Genetic models of disease are similar to germ-theory-based traditional medical models of disease in that the causation of disease is considered to be internal. Although current responses to identified genetic risk are social and essentially preventative, for instance as genetic counselling to inform family planning, research is actively pursuing curative solutions (Collins et al. 2003).

Environmental and lifestyle models of disease differ considerably from medical and genetic models because their explanations for disease are based in social rather than biological processes. Environmental theories of disease focus on factors such as poor foodstuffs, environmental hormones, solar radiation, pollution, medicines, chemicals, substandard housing, sanitation, population density and the biological environment (Chavarria 1989; Hume-Hall 1990; Foster 1995; all cited in Hansen and Easthope 2007). These factors are usually associated with the workings of governments or major corporations and outside of the control of individuals. Environmental models stress societal and political responsibility. They focus on factors that are potentially modifiable in the long term, given political will. However, an overarching political commitment to reducing socio-economic inequalities by investing in infrastructure has not been forthcoming in the years since the Black report of 1980 (Berridge 2002; Shaw et al. 2005) first offered irrefutable evidence that health is linked to socio-economic circumstances.

Lifestyle models emphasise the role of individual choice in health-related behaviour and focus on factors such as physical activity and alcohol consumption. Lifestyle models stress personal responsibility. They focus on factors considered to be modifiable in the short term that have primarily long-term consequences; in this way they are orientated towards the future, with an emphasis on maintaining health and preventing disease. As such it is the most positive disease model with potential for individuals to take control of their own health. An increasing acceptance of a lifestyle model of disease creates pressure for a change in funding emphasis away from curative practices toward health promotion and public health.

Lifestyle models of disease are not new but during the nineteenth and twentieth centuries were subsumed in the battle to control infectious diseases that dogged developing industrial societies. During the twentieth century infectious diseases declined, and a history of how this occurred can be found in the classic text of McKeown (1979), and chronic diseases with behavioural and social determinants have increased, partly as a function of our ageing population and partly as a result of our changing lifestyles. It is these changing demographic and disease parameters that have primarily instigated the rise of the lifestyle model of disease. However, epidemiology, the development of a risk society, health care economies and consumerism have also contributed to a changing emphasis in health and health care.

Epidemiology is the study of the distribution and determinants of disease occurrence and outcomes in humans (Hansen and Easthope 2007) and traditionally investigated the spread of infectious diseases. Epidemiology played a central role in the reduction of infectious diseases and consequently has moved on to consider non-infectious diseases.

Epidemiologists work with a probalistic conception of causation; that is to say they deal with risk and risk factors (Rothman 1998, cited in Hansen and Easthope 2007). Epidemiologists interested in chronic disease usually adopt a web of causality approach which considers chronic disease to be the result of a complex interaction of variables. Generally, social factors such as socio-economic inequality, living conditions and employment are considered too distant and non-specific to be included in epidemiological analyses (Remennick 1998, cited in Hansen and Easthope 2007) so epidemiologists have focused on more proximate causes of disease such as lack of exercise, smoking, diet or environmental hazards (McKinlay 1993, 1994, cited in Hansen and Easthope 2007). Epidemiology has been criticised for such reductionist methodologies. These criticisms are based in a belief that lifestyle behaviours are not the fundamental cause of disease but are a mechanism through which social inequalities influence disease. However, recent research on the relationship between lifestyle behaviours and socio-economic status indicates that the relationship is far from clear and detrimental lifestyle choices do not solely arise out of disadvantage (Department of Health 2003; Welsh Assembly Government 2005; Scottish Executive 2005; Department of Health, Social Services and Public Safety 2001). Furthermore, lifestyle behaviours have clear physiologically supportable links to disease and epidemiologically identified links between behaviour and disease can direct genetic, pharmacological and physiological research down promising avenues. For instance, breast cancer has been found to be linked to diet but not to smoking behaviour.

Epidemiology deals with risk factors and in this way contributes to what Beck (1990) identifies as the 'risk society'. Beck (1990) describes modern society as one where perceptions of risk are heightened and the identification of risk and management of risk has become a major concern at all levels of society. Lifestyle 'risks' are just another category of risks that we must manage.

A lifestyle approach fits well with the modern emphasis on rationality. Social actions can be rationalised in terms of a cost/benefit approach. An economic rational approach sees preventive programmes that emphasise the role of the individual rather than the state as having the potential to reduce health care costs in the future. Nevertheless, few preventive programmes provide any cost/benefit analysis in their evaluations (National Institute for Health and Clinical Excellence (NICE) 2006b). An environmental approach to health care improvement may also reduce health care costs in the future but would require more economic intervention from the state. Modern society is increasingly individualistic and so an approach that sees health as an individual's responsibility is in line with current political thinking and ideology. Giddens (1991) argues that stemming from individual responsibility comes the idea of health as a project to be worked on. This notion of health as a project enables our consumerist society to reconceptualise health as a commodity that we can buy. While traditional medical drug companies peddling cures may view lifestyle models of disease as a threat to their income a new generation of 'health and fitness' companies make a good living out of selling diets, vitamins, fitness, alternative therapies, clothes to exercise in and so on.

Despite well-voiced concerns about a medical model of disease that places its primary emphasis on cure rather than prevention a changing focus to prevention through lifestyle change has not pleased all public health practitioners. The epidemiological focus on specific behavioural factors rather than underlying social causes enables governments who would prefer not to take responsibility for the health of the nation to argue that lifestyle behaviours are an individual's responsibility. To those in favour of political action at the roots of social problems to reduce health inequalities, lifestyle explanations of disease are viewed as oppositional. Indeed, early responses to epidemiological evidence of behaviourally caused disease did focus on knowledge-based health promotion campaigns that left the individual to resolve any behavioural flaws.

In response to the arguments that a risk factor health education lifestyle approach is flawed, public health policy makers at all levels have made position statements about expanding the medical definition of lifestyle to take into account the social nature of lifestyle behaviour (Ashton and Seymour 1988; Bruce 1991; Armstong 1983, cited in Hansen and Easthope 2007). 'New public health', as it has been coined, purports to replace individual behavioural modification achieved through education in favour of enhancing people's life skills and creating supportive environments (Ashton and Seymour 1988; McPearson 1992, cited in Hansen and Easthope 2007). New public health operates with a biopsychosocial understanding of health which requires education and lifestyle modification to be part of general public policy, the work place and education, not restricted to health promotional campaigns (O'Connor and Parker 1995, cited in Hansen and Easthope 2007). The lifestyle model of disease rather than being individualistic can at its best enable individuals to take control of their health and to influence policy to enable them to do so. A good example of this is the Welsh Assembly Government's decision in 2007 to make swimming free for children in all municipal pools in Wales.

If we are to move away from a health promotion approach to lifestyle behaviour towards developing people's 'life skills' then a sound basis in lifestyle psychology will be necessary. To move from knowledge to ability to change behaviour requires a psychological approach. We need to work with people within their current socio-economic resources while pressurising governments to provide the resources to enable change.

Measuring lifestyle behaviours

The measurement of lifestyle behaviours is fundamental to studying lifestyle behaviours and their consequences and to evaluating interventions aimed at changing behaviour. Consequently, there is a need for effective measurement tools. Measuring any type of behaviour creates a number of challenges for psychologists. Instruments need to be valid, reliable, practical, non-reactive (that is to say they should not alter the behaviour they seek to measure) and have the appropriate degree of specificity (Buckworth and Dishman 2002). Few methods of measurement meet all these requirements. For none of the lifestyle behaviours identified by this text is there a single accepted 'gold standard' measurement tool.

Methods of behavioural assessment can be categorised as observational, self report or physiological. Observational and self-report methods are often not validated effectively, whereas physiological methods are often valid but impractical or unacceptable to the study population. Self-report questionnaires are the most commonly utilised method of assessment particularly in large scale experiments, community or population surveys (DoH 2003; Welsh Assembly Government 2007; Scottish Executive 2005; Department of Health, Social Services and Public Safety 2001). Observation or physiological assessments are more common in smaller scale experimental studies and individual assessment, but the utilisation of different methods varies enormously between different behaviours and will be discussed in more depth in individual chapters.

There are a number of self-report methods available to health professionals: interviewing, diaries and recall questionnaires. The choice of method depends on the nature of the problem, the clinical or research perspective. While it is impossible in this text to review all methods available (other texts such as Marks and Yardley 2004; Webb et al. 2005 present suitable overviews), specific methods employed for assessing behaviour will be presented in the appropriate chapters.

The variation in methods available to measure lifestyle behaviours creates problems in interpreting research and survey data. First, researchers differ in what they choose to measure and second, even if they choose to measure the same aspect of behaviour, they can differ widely in the method they choose to collect their data and the way they choose to present their findings. Throughout the research literature on lifestyle behaviours, different methods of measurement confuse and hinder direct comparisons. On the positive side, consensus achieved by using a range of instruments is more robust than consensus achieved with one tool.

Socio-demographic influences on health and lifestyle

As recognised by the World Health Organisation (1986) lifestyle is more than simply an individual choice. The way we live has economic and cultural dimensions (Blaxter 1990). Indeed the adoption of the term 'lifestyle change' reflects the importance of socio-demographic factors in health behaviour change rather better than the term 'health promotion'.

Ethnicity, sex, age and socio-economic circumstances and cultural groups all interplay to influence the way we choose to behave (Blaxter 1990). The evidence for socio-demographic influences on lifestyle choices is irrefutable (DoH 1999b; Department of Health 2003; Scottish Executive 2005; Welsh Assembly Government 2005; Department of Health, Social Services and Public Safety 2001).

The UK government and more recently the devolved institutions of England, Wales, Scotland and Northern Ireland have been collecting demographic mortality and morbidity data for some time, enabling comparisons between the health of different demographic and socio-economic groups. More recently data on physical activity, eating habits, drinking and smoking have also been included. In these national surveys, as well as in the wider health behaviour literature, data has been primarily collected by self-report questionnaire, although the English and Scottish surveys include physiological data collected by nurses for a proportion of their samples. Each of these UK institutions have commissioned surveys on a continuing basis to enable comparisons between behaviours over time and to monitor health targets. The demographic data collected includes sex, age and socio-economic class in each survey. The summary documents for each survey do not consider ethnicity, although data about ethnic minorities has been collected in other government surveys and the Health Survey for England (DoH 2003) had ethnic minorities as its focus in certain sections. While these surveys do ask different questions using different methodologies, there is enough in common between the surveys to enable a comparison between data from different nations. This enables an extra socio-demographic dimension to be evaluated that was not possible before the instigation of devolved assemblies.

The Health Survey for England is a series of annual surveys about the health of people living in private households in England. It was commissioned by the Department of Health to provide information about various aspects of people's health. A number of core topics are covered every year and each year's survey has a particular focus on a disease, condition or population group. Similarly, in Wales the Welsh Health Survey is an annual survey commissioned by the National Assembly for Wales so that trends in health and behaviour can be established. However, a changing disease, condition or population group focus is not in the remit of this survey. The Scottish Health Survey was commissioned in 1995 by what is now the Scottish Executive Health Department and the 2003 survey is the third in this series of surveys. It too has a static focus with no change in emphasis from year to year. The 2001 Northern Ireland Health and Social Wellbeing Survey is the second commissioned by the Department of Health, Social Services and Public Safety.

All of these national surveys involved a large sample of the population living in the country at the time. The surveys in England and in Wales were the largest, interviewing 14,836 adults and 3,717 children and

14,300 adults and 3,100 children respectively. The Scottish Health Survey interviewed 8,148 adults and 3,324 children. The Northern Ireland Survey was the smallest, interviewing 5,205 adults and not including children in its remit.

The remit and focus of each survey is slightly different although they all ask questions on smoking, drinking and physical activity. Interestingly, the Northern Ireland survey did not consider diet but included a far more in-depth assessment of sexual health than that attempted in the other three national surveys.

Each survey uses different methods to collect and present data. Smoking behaviour has the most consistent self-report methods of all the lifestyle surveys, making comparisons between time points and populations straightforward and valid. Similarly, although asking a very varied range of questions about physical activity overall, all four surveys reported the percentage of people achieving the government guidelines of 30 minutes of physical activity five or more days a week. Measurement of drinking behaviour between the four surveys was so various that a comparable question on the percentage exceeding the government daily drinking guidelines was possible in only three of the four surveys. Similarly, measures of diet were comparable in only three of the four surveys. Nevertheless, the surveys do provide points of comparison for diet, smoking, physical activity and drinking behaviours in the four countries of the UK.

Gender differences in lifestyle

Both biological sex and gender are related to health and health outcomes but it is generally accepted that it is gender rather than biological sex that influences lifestyle choices. Indeed, the gender influence on health is primarily mediated through lifestyle choices. Many studies confuse the terms sex and gender. Sex is the biological underpinning – our genetic make-up. Gender, on the other hand, is more socially constructed – it is more concerned with how we think and behave (Burr 1998). Hence when talking about sex we will talk about males and females or man or woman. Alternatively, when we talk about gender we talk about masculine or feminine. Thus, it is possible to be a 'masculine' female (i.e. a woman that acts in a 'typically' masculine manner) and similarly it would be possible to be a 'feminine' male (i.e. a man that acts in a typically 'feminine' manner). Obviously the definition and description of what is typically feminine or masculine is difficult and varies from culture to culture. Few texts or papers acknowledge the delineation between gender and sex effects and actually the terms are used interchangeably (Burr 1998).

A woman born in 2007 has a life expectancy of 84 years, a man only 77 years (ONS 2007). Men and women also have different morbidity rates. For example, women are less likely to suffer from cardiovascular disease and more likely to suffer from breast cancer than men (Department of Health 2003). Prostate cancer is a solely male disease as women do not have a prostate gland. Male and female differences in morbidity and mortality are influenced by biological sex and also by gender and gender role casting (Annandale and Hunt 2000). The difference in male and female mortality rates is diminishing and this is generally held to be due to changing gender roles in Western societies rather than to biological sex, although early menarche may play a part in the prevalence of some female hormonally linked cancers. Unfortunately, not all of these gender adaptations are positive and some of these changes in gender expectations have resulted in women adopting unhealthy, traditionally male lifestyle behaviours (Emslie et al. 2002). The influence of gender over health is mediated through the lifestyle choices that men and women make. The implications of gender roles for the various lifestyle behaviours will be developed and discussed in the relevant chapters.

Age differences in lifestyle choices

Age is different from every other demographic variable in that the majority of us will experience belonging to all categories of age: infancy, childhood, adolscence, adulthood and old age. Sex and ethnicity are difficult to alter and the majority do not attempt it. Socio-economic circumstances can change for an individual but it is not inevitable nor indeed probable (Giddens 2006). Nevertheless, despite the fact that presumably we must all hope to become older, older people experience considerable discrimination (Scambler 2003) which has implications for their health and well-being and for their lifestyle choices. There are clear differences in health and health outcomes between different age categories and unlike sex/gender differences a large factor will be physiological changes over the lifespan rather than cultural expectations about age-related behaviour. Nevertheless, cultural expectations of how people of different ages should behave do play a role both in the way that, for example, teenage mothers approach their pregnancies and older people participate in exercise and sport. Hence, it is important to explore the impact of the cultural influences of age on lifestyle and health and this will be addressed in each of the lifestyle behaviour chapters.

Socio-economic differences in lifestyle choices

Socio-economic is a broad term encompassing many variables and is assessed using a range of different factors: social class, income, work, housing, physical and social environments have all been found to influence our health directly and also indirectly through their influence on lifestyle choices (Doyle 2001). The definition of social class has been provided by the seminal Black Report (Townsend and Davidson 1982) which first clearly stated the link between health and social class in modern society. This definition is the one used whenever social class is referred to in this text:

> Segments of the population sharing broadly similar types and levels of resources, with broadly similar styles of living and (for some sociologists) some shared perception of their collective condition.
>
> (Townsend and Davidson 1982: 39)

In essence, different classes have differential power to access material resources: homes, cars, white goods, electronic goods and so on (Giddens 2006). However, as Blaxter (1990) demonstrates in her analysis of the health and lifestyle survey of 9003 adults living in England, Wales and Scotland, socio-economic differentials in health are actually more complex than they first appear. Evaluating local environment using the conceptualisation of Craig (1985) illustrates the complexities of the relationship between health and social class. Craig (1985) delineates between local environments by describing them as one of the following: high status, rural/resort, industrial, city, local authority, inner and central London. For example, the relationship between health and social class was stronger in industrial areas than in more favourable areas (high status, rural/resort) suggesting that socio-economic and environmental disadvantages have a multiplicative effect. However, sex confounds the relationship and the benefits of a favourable local environment were less for women. In other words, the class difference in health was not mitigated by living in a favourable area for women in the way that it was for men. Blaxter (1990) offers the explanation that women's health may be influenced more by 'class' factors and less by 'environmental' factors. Other authors have proposed different methods of categorising local environment. For instance Jones et al. (2007) suggest that five variables are important: deprivation, availability and access, urban form, aesthetics and quality and, finally, supportiveness. One popular way of describing the role of the environment in behavioural choice is to refer to obesogenic environments. The common use of the term obesogenic environment reflects the widening acceptance of the role of factors external to the individual in the development of obesity. Swinburn et al. (1999) in a similar fashion to Craig (1985) recognise the role of both macroenvironments (e.g. education and health systems, government policy and mainstream societal attitudes and beliefs) and microenvironments (school, workplace, home and neighbourhood). Less important in this text than attempting explanations for the subtle interplay between various socio-economic, other demographic factors, health and lifestyle choices is the recognition that such subtleties exist. Any one socio-economic or demographic factor's influence over an individual's lifestyle choice can be intensified or mitigated by another.

Explanations for behavioural choices are contentious and politically sensitive. Townsend and Davidson (1982) recognised that there were a number of explanations for differing levels of health in different sections of society. The key most plausible explanations are a behavioural explanation or a materialist explanation. Simply, a behavioural explanation suggests that most of the class differences in health can be explained by the choices that people make. A materialist explanation suggests that most of the class differences in health can be explained by the environmental circumstances that individuals find themselves in. At first sight these explanations would seem to argue different causes of disease but actually the distinction is more subtle. To use late onset diabetes as an example, a behavioural explanation would argue that a proportion of the class difference in diabetes morbidity can be explained by what individuals choose to eat. A materialist explanation does not attempt to propose that diet is not a major cause of late onset diabetes but questions the degree of choice that individuals actually have about the food that they eat. Another way of framing the dichotomy is in terms of individual or collective responsibility. In the first case the right for individuals to do as they wish with their own lives is emphasised; in the second, the inability of individuals to exert control over their environment and consequently ways of living is invoked (Blaxter 1990). At first sight a discipline of lifestyle psychology would appear to operate within behaviourist or individualistic explanations for lifestyle choices. However, adoption of the term lifestyle is a deliberate attempt by these authors to recognise the role of socio-environmental factors in decisions individuals make about behaviours that impinge on their health. The challenge for lifestyle psychology is to identify how to enable individuals to effect positive change within the socio-economic parameters that constrain them. In other words, recognising that social and environmental circumstances are an integral aspect of lifestyle choice does not rule out the possibility of effective behavioural change within those parameters. It seems clear that blanket style approaches to lifestyle change are unlikely to be successful and lifestyle interventions must be tailored to the unique situations in which individuals find themselves.

Modern lifestyles

People have been overeating, drinking to excess and making other negative lifestyle choices for centuries and yet the current dialogue in policy documents and the media suggests that this is a recent and modern problem (Department of Health, Physical Activity, Health Improvement and Prevention 2004; Mulvihill et al. 2005; HM Government 2007; Jones et al. 2007). Certainly, more people live long enough to experience the chronic conditions associated with old age as the death toll associated with infectious diseases has declined. However, there is considerable evidence that, in addition, people take less exercise (Department of Health, Physical

Activity, Health Improvement and Prevention 2004), drink more alcohol (HM Government 2007), are less safe in their sexual practices (e.g. Centers for Disease Control (CDC) 2007a), are more likely to take illegal drugs (ONS 2007) and eat poorer diets (Reilly and Dorosty 1999; Fox and Hillsdon 2007) than they did in previous generations. Smoking is the only lifestyle behaviour where incidence is declining, although a considerable minority of the population continue to smoke (ONS 2007). It is important to try to understand why unhealthy lifestyles have become so widespread, particularly since Western societies seem to be exporting these deleterious practices to developing nations (WHO 1986).

The lifestyle of a whole society will change with modernisation and with social change. This is evident from the different patterns of lifestyle choices in countries at different stages of modernisation and with different cultural norms (WHO 1986). Modern life involves far less physical effort than it did in previous generations (Department of Health, Physical Activity, Health Improvement and Prevention 2004; Fox and Hillsdon 2007). Paid work is more likely to be sedentary, housework is less demanding and far fewer people are physically active in the process of travelling. There is no evidence that people are less active in their leisure time than they were in previous generations but because the majority of physical activity is now leisure, people's total physical activity has declined (Department of Health, Physical Activity, Health Improvement and Prevention 2004). The rise of fast food outlets, high calorie snacks and ready prepared meals and the declining cost of such items all contribute to the poor diet reported by many individuals (Myslobodsky 2003). Alcohol is considerably cheaper, relatively, than it has been in previous generations and is more readily available (Babor et al. 2003; Plant and Plant 2006). Cultural acceptance of heavy drinking remains a stable facet of British life and, while it used to be unacceptable for young women to drink heavily, changing gender expectations are making it more acceptable for young women to match young men in their excessive drinking (Plant and Plant 2006). It is in terms of sexual behaviour that cultural expectations have probably changed the most dramatically with sex outside of marriage and children out of wedlock no longer holding as significant a taboo as in previous generations (e.g. Schubotz et al. 2003). Nevertheless, a more liberal attitude towards sex has also enabled better education and communication about safe sex, enabling some women to control their sexual destinies and consequently putatively protect themselves from sexual infection and pregnancy. Whether this 'freedom' and greater responsibility has resulted in better health with control over infection and pregnancy is a matter of political debate, however.

Lifestyles in daily life

Lifestyles are enacted in, and constrained by, daily life. Most people's lives involve four aspects: sleeping, travelling, working and caring, and leisure (Buckworth and Dishman 2002). It is impossible to describe a typical 24 hours for someone working in the UK. The complexities of modern life in terms of work patterns and outside responsibilities mean that the 9 to 5 day is not applicable to many people living and working in Britain. However, if you consider an average night's sleep to be about 8 hours, the average working day to be 8 hours and an average journey to and from work to be an hour, then there are about 7 hours left a day for leisure and/or caring and household responsibilities. Clearly, many people will take longer to travel to work, sleep for longer or less, have greater or fewer responsibilities outside of work but many people will have some time each day that is not taken up with travelling, work, caring or sleeping. Many people do not work an 8-hour day. People in the UK work some of the longest hours in Europe and also many people work fewer but longer days each week, e.g. police officers and nurses. Shift work is commonplace and is well recognised as being deleterious for health and lifestyle choices (Folkard et al. 2005). Probably one of the major changes in daily living in the UK has been the huge increase in parents with childcare responsibilities who also work (ONS 2007). This has implications for the household responsibilities that could have been carried out during the day but that now need attention outside of working hours. Given that the physically active nature of housework and shopping has diminished substantially (Department of Health, Physical Activity, Health Improvement and Prevention 2004), and there has been a reduction in time available for physically active pursuits then it is not surprising that the change in the pattern of a 'normal' day has consequences on both lifestyle and health.

The work we do, the way we travel and our leisure activities will all influence the lifestyle choices we make. Socio-economic factors often dictate the work we do, the way we travel, our leisure activity and, in this way, this directs our lifestyle choices. Choices about eating, drinking, smoking or physical activity are possible, although not for everyone in every context, during work, travel and leisure.

Sleeping

Sleep is really the only aspect of a person's daily life when no lifestyle choices, other than sleeping itself, take place. However, when, where and how well people sleep will influence the lifestyle choices they make and will in turn be influenced by the lifestyle choices made.

Travelling

While we are travelling we could be physically active, we could eat or smoke. However, smoking has recently been banned in all public places, including public transport vehicles, in the UK. This is the first major piece of legislation that pertains to volitional lifestyle behaviour for many years. Private cars are not subject to the legislation so it is possible that the ban may encourage people to use their cars if they wish to smoke on a journey. The impact of the smoking ban needs to be evaluated across all possible outcomes, not simply population smoking rates.

For the majority of people the trip to work, school or college is the most frequent journey. A minority of people take the opportunity to walk or cycle to their place of work or study but the majority will drive or use public transport for the majority of their journey. Since the late 1970s regular travel by foot or by bicycle has declined by 26 per cent (Department of Health, Physical Activity, Health Improvement and Prevention 2004). Factors postulated to contribute to the decline of regular travel by foot or bicycle include perceived and actual safety; the provision of facilities to segregate conflicting road users and the proximity of local shops or workplace (Jones et al. 2007).

Working, caring and other responsibilities

Working and caring, for children, disabled or elderly family members, are the primary occupations for most people and the majority of jobs these days are predominantly sedentary (Department of Health, Physical Activity, Health Improvement and Prevention 2004). At work most people will eat at least one meal and the quality of available food may influence the food choices made by people. Jeffery et al. (2006) found no relationship between the proximity of fast food outlets to the workplace and eating in such places. However, less work has been done on on-site food provision in the workplace, although the healthy workplace initiatives in Scotland (e.g. www.shaw.uk.com) and Wales (e.g. The Corporate Standard – http://new.wales.gov.uk/topics/health/improvement/healthatwork/corporate-standard/?lang=en) are making inroads into such provision.

The majority of work on on-site provision of food has been carried out with children. It has been suggested that unhealthy food choices have dominated school food sales but the impact of new nutritional standards introduced in schools in September 2006 is yet to be evaluated (Jones et al. 2007; see also Chapter 3 on eating).

While people are not usually allowed to drink alcohol while at work the workplace culture of drinking has been found to be significantly related to both drinking in the work context and non-work-related drinking (Delaney and Ames 1995; Barrientos-Gutierrez et al. 2007). The establishment of healthy drinking norms in the workplace may have beneficial effects for drinking both with work colleagues and more widely.

Leisure activities

Patterns of leisure activity have changed dramatically with the onset of television and subsequently video, DVD, computers and computer games. The relationship between time spent in such sedentary activities and both level of obesity and time spent in physically active pursuits has been the subject of much concern, particularly in children (Department of Health, Physical Activity, Health Improvement and Prevention 2004). The number of health clubs and gyms has proliferated and a small increase in the proportion of people taking physical activity has been reported (Department of Health, Physical Activity, Health Improvement and Prevention 2004). However, overall physical activity levels are still declining due to the reduction in necessary physical activity, in particular travel. Similarly, a proliferation of 'low fat' healthy option foods are available and cookery programmes are popular on the television but it would seem that watching cookery programmes rather than cooking are popular leisure pursuits! Other popular leisure activities such as going to the cinema are associated with unhealthy food availability and large portion sizes. Similarly, studies have highlighted the increase in portion sizes of meals served in restaurants (Nielsen and Popkin 2003). Hence, leisure activities themselves can lead to an increase in unhealthy lifestyles.

Conclusion

This introductory chapter has highlighted the concept of lifestyle and the influence of various demographic factors on this. We aim to consider whether the focus of the prime minister, the government, the policy maker, the civil servant and the health care professional on lifestyle is warranted. Furthermore, how can the 'increasing strain' on the health service, as Tony Blair described it in 2006, be addressed by psychologists and health professionals?

The following chapters explore individual lifestyle behaviour in detail: how it is defined, measured and recorded. The epidemiology of the behaviour and the consequences of that behaviour will subsequently be explored. Finally, each chapter will consider how health care professionals can use psychology to influence individuals, groups and communities to improve their lifestyle and their consequent health. The penultimate and final chapters of this book will evaluate the usefulness of a psychological approach to lifestyle and lifestyle change. They will consider whether there is enough evidence of general psychological principles underlying the practice of all the lifestyle behaviours to justify the term lifestyle psychology. In the final chapter a strategy for improving lifestyle in the UK will be proposed.

Summary points

- Major lifestyle diseases are coronary heart disease, stroke, lung cancer, colon cancer, diabetes and chronic obstructive pulmonary disease.
- Health-related lifestyles can be defined as behavioural choices about eating, physical activity, drinking alcohol, smoking tobacco, taking drugs and sexual practices that individuals make.
- Lifestyle psychology can be defined as the study of the antecedents, consequences and interactions of lifestyle behaviours including: eating, drinking alcohol, smoking tobacco, taking drugs, physical activity and sexual practices.
- Changing demographic and disease parameters, epidemiology, the development of a risk society, health care economies and consumerism have all played a role in the risk of the lifestyle model of disease.
- For none of the lifestyle behaviours identified by this text is there a single accepted 'gold standard' measurement tool. It is common, particularly in large population studies, to utilise self-report measurement techniques.
- Social and environmental circumstances are an integral aspect of lifestyle choice.

2 Theories of change

> He who loves practice without theory is like the sailor who boards ship without a rudder and compass and never knows where he may cast.
>
> Leonardo da Vinci

At the end of this chapter you will:

- understand the importance of social cognition models in lifestyle psychology
- appreciate the importance of the concept of risk
- explore the basics of the fear-drive model and its implication for health promotion campaigns
- evaluate the health belief model, protection motivation theory and theory of planned behaviour
- realise the importance of social cognition theory
- appreciate the importance of stage theories in behaviour change
- understand the role of such models in the prediction of behaviour and in behaviour change.

In this chapter we introduce the key social cognition theories and concepts employed by health psychologists and health professionals to predict, explain and increasingly to underpin interventions to change health behaviours (Conner 1993). Good theory is the key pin of evidence-based practice (NICE 2006b). Best practice is most likely to emerge from theory-based interventions that in turn inform and improve theory. Hillsdon et al. (2005) in their review of the literature found that interventions to change physical activity based on theories of behavioural change were associated with longer-term behavioural change than interventions with no such theoretical underpinning. Theoretical models can help identify important variables and furthermore tell us something about the relative effects of different variables (Conner 1993). One chapter cannot hope to cover all potentially relevant social cognition theories, however, the aim of this chapter is to provide a working understanding of those theories most usually applied to lifestyle behaviours.

Social cognitive approaches to health behaviour change

A social cognitive approach argues that social behaviour is best understood as: 'a function of people's perception of reality, rather than as a function of an objective description of the stimulus environment' (Conner and Norman 2005: 5). Conner and Norman (2005) refer to a 'perception of reality', a phrase that is firmly based in the present. In the context of lifestyle behaviours, 'reality' may not be the most appropriate term. The aim of recent government policy has been to reduce the incidence of lifestyle diseases in the future by getting people to change their behaviour now:

> Everybody should try to look after themselves better, by not smoking, taking more exercise, eating and drinking sensibly.
>
> (DoH 1999b: vii)

Policy is not focused on perceptions of current reality but on perceptions of possible futures. This is fundamentally different to getting individuals who are currently ill to alter their behaviour. To achieve behavioural change in well individuals, the government, health professionals and the population as a whole require a way of visualising the future, in other words a 'perception of risk'. The concept of risk has been embraced by experts and risks have been objectified and expressed as numerical representations of the future for all types of behaviours in relation to many types of disease.

The British Medical Association recognises that risk impacts on every aspect of health (Skolbekken 1995). However, there is a considerable evidence that lay people struggle to understand numeric probability expressions and no agreement about which numerical representations of perceived risk are best understood (Windschitl and Wells 1996; Lobb et al. 2003; Michie et al. 2005; Weinstein et al. 2007). As we will see in this chapter, underpinning all social cognition models is a perception of risk (Brewer et al. 2007; Brown and Morley 2007). Different models use different terms but fundamentally whether described as severity, vulnerability or outcome expectations all these factors from different models are referring to a perception of risk; specifically 'the probability that harm will occur if no preventative action is taken' (Weinstein et al. 2007: 146). Therefore, it is pertinent to start this chapter with a brief introduction to the concept of risk.

Risk perception

Risk in its broadest definition includes both positive and negative outcomes and classically involves objective evaluations of the magnitude of losses and gains (Fischoff et al. 2000b). Risk has been integral to all aspects of government policy in departments as diverse as the Department of Environment, Food and Rural affairs and the Justice Ministry. In 2002 the Cabinet Office Strategy Unit described risk as: 'Uncertainty of outcome, whether positive opportunity or negative threat, of actions and events. It is a combination of likelihood and impact, including perceived importance' (Cabinet Office Strategy Unit 2002: 7). However, the National Consumer Council (2002: 1), suggests that 'consumers typically see "risk" as a situation that is likely to be unusual – that has significant potential for damage'.

While uncertain outcomes can be positive or negative, risk in its lay conception has been argued to be predominantly associated with negative outcomes (Joffe 2003). However, interestingly, lay understanding of the bipolar nature of risk has been reported. Thirlaway and Heggs (2005) report that some individuals responded to a communication about the negative risks of drinking alcohol by presenting the positive risks, for example the protective benefits of alcohol for the heart; supporting the utilisation of a bipolar definition of risk (Cabinet Office Strategy Unit 2002). Goldberg et al. (2002) similarly report the importance of positive risks in behavioural decision making. However, for the purposes of health behavioural change a negative concept of risk is usually adopted. Furthermore, risk in the field of health is often utilised to generate a fear response. As the majority of health behaviours have multiple effects; influencing physiological and psychological function in a number of positive and negative ways, the bipolar definition provided by the Cabinet Office Strategy Unit (2002) may be most appropriate in the field of lifestyle change.

Risk perception and the related field of decision making have been dominated by cognitive psychology and by the central tenet that there is an objective and accurate risk perception as conceptualised by 'experts'. Based on this notion of an accurate perception of risk the dominating theme of research in this area has been lay error and the reasons for lay error (Thirlaway and Heggs 2005). Lay error can be defined as any perception of risk that is different to the expert-held perception.

Within the field of perceptions of risk from health behaviours under volitional control optimistic bias has received a lot of attention as a cause of lay error (Weinstein 1984; Weinstein and Klein 1996; Brown and Morley 2007). Other identified biases are that individuals are influenced by availability of information (Fischoff et al. 2000a); that they are insensitive to the rate at which risk increases with repeated exposures (Connolly et al. 2000); that they are influenced by their personal experiences of the risk (Shiloh and Saxe 1989) and they are influenced by how the risk is framed (Tversky and Kahneman 1981). These factors, and others, can be viewed as sources of error in the process of risk perception. Indeed, Joffe (2003) has argued that the key tenet of a broad spectrum of cognitively based risk perception models is that most people, although naturally risk averse, miscalculate their risk due to cognitive deficits. For instance, Slovic (2000) reported that numerous studies found the majority of people exhibit unrealistic optimism in relation to a range of risks.

The argument that lay perceptions of risk are inadequate is increasingly being recognised as an over-simplification of a complex issue (Thirlaway and Heggs 2005). First, expert risk calculations include a degree of subjectivity and consequently experts can get it wrong, particularly about new risks (Harrabin et al. 2003). What is accepted as fact in one generation is sometimes rejected in the next, and of course such changes can occur quicker than this. Furthermore, risks are usually reported in isolation whereas in reality the impact of any health behaviour is seldom unitary. Health behaviours usually have multiple effects, some positive and some negative. Again, this points to a bidirectional definition of risk being the most appropriate for lifestyle psychology.

A further problem with the cognitive approach to risk perception is that the analytical component has been the only valued aspect of a process which also utilises, to a lesser or greater degree, intuition and emotion. Slovic (2000) states that:

> Although risk perception was originally viewed as a form of deliberate, analytic information processing, over time we have come to recognise how highly dependent it is upon intuitive and experiential thinking, guided by emotional and affective processes.
>
> (Slovic 2000: xxxi)

Other researchers have addressed the issue of affect in risk perception. Weinstein et al. (2007) have argued that perceived vulnerability, which can be conceptualised as a cognitive-affective state, might be a better predictor of behaviour than perceived probability which is an entirely cognitive judgement. Loewenstein et al. (2001) have argued that people do not always use a rational cognitive strategy to make decisions about risky situations. They propose the 'risk-as-feelings' hypothesis which highlights the role of emotions experienced at the moment of decision making. Furthermore, they argue that emotional reactions to risky situations can often diverge from cognitive assessments of the same situation. If division occurs emotional reactions usually override cognitive reactions and drive behaviour. One reason for the domination of emotional responses over cognitive assessment is that emotional responses are rapid and rational analyses usually take time (Loewenstein et al. 2001).

Many researchers investigating the role of emotion in risk perception conceptualise it as inferior to analytical responses. Indeed it is often dismissed as a source of lay error (Joffe 2003). Emotion has been conceptualised as a heuristic, a mental shortcut, whereby people access their pool of positive and negative feelings towards an issue to guide judgement (Oatley 1996). The emotion most usually associated with risk is anxiety (Joffe 2003). Dismissing anxiety as a biasing factor in 'accurate' risk perception is problematic. Anxiety is the intermediate goal of many risk communications, particularly public health communications. The primary goal is preventative behaviour but anxiety is considered an essential initiating motivation. Many health promotions are based on this fear drive hypothesis (Janis 1968, cited in Boer and Seydel 1996). They continue to be so despite little evidence that they succeed, and some evidence that if you produce excessively frightening messages you may reduce preventative behaviour (Boer and Seydel 1996).

The cognitive emphasis in risk analysis also fails to account for the social nature of risk, focusing as it does on the intra-personal rather than the interpersonal. Risk by its very nature is a social construction and social, cultural and political ideas will guide not only people's judgement of risks, but also those risks that scientists investigate and those which the media choose to report. This can clearly be seen in the recent media interest in obesity and diet in children. Relatively recently Harrabin et al. (2003) were berating the British media for their obsession with dramatic risks outside of individual volitional control, such as SARS, which in actuality confer little increased risk to the general population. Harrabin et al. (2003) reported low coverage of less sensational risks such as poor diet and rising obesity. However, the social climate has changed, for a variety of reasons, and diet and obesity have been high profile media stories throughout 2005 and 2006 (Saguy and Almeling 2005, cited in Campos et al. 2006a).

In lifestyle psychology the important risk issue is the impact that risk perceptions have on uptake of preventative strategies. Cognitive research into risk perceptions using hypothetical lifestyle risk scenarios conclude that errors in processing of risk information results in inappropriate decision making (Joffe 2003). Evidence from population surveys of self-reported lifestyle behaviours supports this hypothesis; for example, people do not take enough exercise, they drink too much, they drive too fast. In general, the public fail to adopt the preventative behaviours recommended by the Department of Health (1999b). One conclusion, drawn by the government (DoH 1999b), is that lay risk perceptions must be challenged by more effective risk communications. However, lifestyle decisions are influenced by a number of other psycho-social factors as well as risk perception. Evidence from studies where the relationship between risk perception and the associated preventative behaviour is clearer suggest that accurate risk perceptions are not essential for appropriate decision making. Evans et al. (1994) found that the majority of women (59 per cent) attending a breast cancer family history clinic could not recall the objective risk figure provided by the clinician. Nevertheless, 96 per cent of women attended annually for mammography. Here is a challenge to the widely accepted tenet that an accurate perception of risk is necessary for appropriate behavioural change. Indeed, Leventhal et al. (1999) have argued that risk perception may have little impact on health behaviour.

Brewer et al. (2007) have argued that the importance of risk perceptions will vary across behaviours. They argue that risk perceptions are probably less important for behaviours such as exercise and diet that have a wide range of both health and non-health consequences. We have argued that the term lifestyle is useful to denote those health behaviours that also have non-health outcomes. As such, lifestyle behaviours may be conceptually different from other health behaviours in terms of the influence that risk perceptions play in their expression. However, Brewer et al. (2007) caution that the plethora of cross-sectional and correlational studies are likely to underestimate the influence of risk perception on behaviour. They found that the few prospective studies on vaccination (a solely health behaviour not a lifestyle behaviour) included in their meta-analysis yielded larger effect sizes than did the cross-sectional studies. It is beyond the scope of this text to discuss the methodological issues that make cross-sectional studies problematic when measuring risk perception but this is well elucidated by Brewer et al. (2007).

Public analyses of risk do not follow the analytical processes valued by experts. Nevertheless, risk communication is an integral part of modern healthcare and as such it is in line with modern concerns of informed consent and litigation. It is also often high on news agendas having news values such as negativity and continuity. Furthermore, it offers opportunities for sensationalism, personal interest and celebrity-linked stories and expert commentary. Consequently, health risk information is prominent in many media outlets: books, magazines, newspapers, radio and television news programmes and documentaries. Representations of risk are unlikely to go away. At the start of this section on risk perception it was argued that risk perception (and with this comes a notion of an accurate risk perception) is an essential component of any theory of behavioural change. However, while a risk perception may be a necessary for behavioural change it is unlikely to be sufficient to consistently effect a change. Health promotion has focused on risk communication for the past decades with little impact on lifestyle choices. In many instances people now have appropriate risk perceptions with little evidence of behavioural change (Lawton and Conner 2007). Indeed, Murgraff et al. (1999) have suggested that only when a subject is introduced to a new unknown threat does the perception of this risk influence uptake of a preventative strategy. Risk perception is clearly not always, and arguably not often, sufficient to promote the levels of behavioural change that the government would like. We now need to focus on identifying the other factors that contribute to a change in behaviour. The social cognition models presented below offer a number of factors for consideration as moderating variables in the behavioural change process.

Fear-drive model

The fear-drive model is generally considered outdated in academic health psychology (Norman et al. 2005) but it is worth considering as it remains a central, if unacknowledged, tenet of many health promotion campaigns. It is closely related to the negative concept of risk as understood by both lay and many expert populations.

The fear-drive model principally proposes that fear is an unpleasant emotion and people are motivated to try to reduce their state of fear. Health promotion has taken this notion and applied it to communication. If a communication evokes fear or anxiety then the fear drive model suggests that the recipient will be motivated to reduce this unpleasant emotive state. If the communication also contains behavioural advice, either implicitly or explicitly, then individuals may follow this advice. If following the behavioural advice leads to a reduction in fear then the probability of performing the behaviour in the future is enhanced. However, if following the behaviour does not lead to a reduction in fear then other ways of reducing fear may be employed.

A key and immediately obvious problem with this proposal for lifestyle behaviour is that the effects of lifestyle change are not immediate and are not certain. Only a long way down the line can we be certain that we have avoided the threat, be it heart disease or lung cancer. Consequently, other defences against anxiety are likely to be employed. A risk objectifies a potentially dangerous future, but any anxiety it evokes is immediate. Consequently, for many people their focus will be to reduce their anxiety, it may be less effortful and more immediate to adopt strategies other than behavioural change, such as denial.

Fear is intuitively appealing as a means of promoting behavioural change but the role it plays in initiating behavioural change is not clear cut or consistent (Janis 1968; Bandura 1998; Nabi 2002; Plotnikoff and Higginbotham 2002). However, this has been effectively denied (one of the strategies adopted equally successfully by the recipients of health fear communications) by health professionals for over half a century. There is little evidence to support the initially proposed inverted U-shaped relationship between fear arousal and acceptance of a recommended action (Sutton 1982). The Inverted U hypothesis postulated that fear induces both facilitation (acceptance of ways to reduce danger) and interference (a critical evaluation of recommended advice). Initially facilitation increases faster than interference but at a certain optimal level interference starts to increase faster than facilitation and likelihood of following recommended advice drops. Sutton (1982) subsequently proposed that the evidence was better for a linear relationship between fear arousal and acceptance of action but it is equally difficult to find support for a linear relationship. Rigby et al. (1989) reported that the Australian 'Grim Reaper' campaign raised anxiety and awareness of HIV and AIDS but failed to increase knowledge or facilitate a change in behaviour. However, any simple relationship between action and negative emotion, be it anxiety or fear, has been rejected by many theorists (Milne et al. 2000) and in the 1970s Rogers developed the protection motivation theory (Rogers 1975) in an attempt to provide conceptual clarity about the place of fear appeals in health promotion (Norman et al. 2005). In fact, almost all social cognition models could be conceptualised as adaptations of the fear-drive hypothesis while incorporating other variables.

Heath belief model

The heath belief model (HBM) was one of the first and remains one of the best known social cognition models (Rosenstock 1974; Harrison et al. 1992) developed in order to predict preventative health behaviours including lifestyle behaviours (Portnoy 1980; Li et al. 2003). The HBM suggests that your belief in a personal threat together with your belief in the effectiveness of the proposed preventative behaviour will predict the likelihood of that behaviour (Figure 2.1). Belief in a personal threat is proposed to arise from perceptions of susceptibility and severity, while a cost–benefit type analysis results in a belief in the effectiveness of the ameliorating behaviour (Figure 2.1). In essence this is an extension of the fear-drive model (although it is seldom recognised as such) but it delineates theoretically between the threat (fear inducing) and the evaluation of the proposed behavioural solution. This model also goes further than the fear-drive model by distinguishing the various components of a threat or a risk into susceptibility and severity.

The model suggests that the likelihood of a behaviour occurring is related to these four core beliefs (Figure 2.1). However, since its inception a number of additional concepts have been added to the model in an attempt to improve its predictiveness. 'Cues to action' was initially added to reflect the role of personal experiences or health promotional events on the likelihood of action. In some versions of the model health motivation has been included to reflect an individuals readiness to be concerned about that health matter in question. Latterly Rosenstock et al. (1988) suggested the inclusion of perceived behavioural control. Perceived behavioural control is a broad concept including both self-efficacy and environmental impediments (Ajzen 1998). It is included to respond to the increasing evidence of the importance of efficacy in behavioural change (Milne et al. 2000). This results in a model with a potential of seven factors

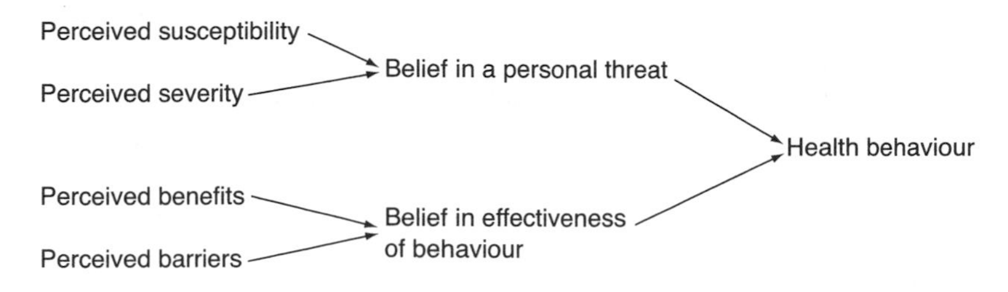

Figure 2.1 Health belief model
(Adapted from Becker et al. 1977, cited in Biddle and Mutrie 1991)

rather than four, however the various proposed factors are not consistently adopted. For example Ali (2002) measures 'belief in a threat' and 'cues to action' from the model but not 'belief in the effectiveness' of the action. Harrison et al. (1992) excluded articles that did not measure the four dimensions of the original HBM: susceptibility, severity, benefits and barriers (Figure 2.1), therefore 55 studies purporting to be based on the HBM were not eligible for their review.

The HBM model has not been operationalised to the extent that the relationship between all components of the model have been statistically described (Abraham and Sheeran 2005). Nevertheless, some relationships have been considered. Intuitively it would seem that the two aspects of threat should be considered as multiplicative rather than additive. If you do not consider yourself at all susceptible to a condition then your belief in a personal threat will remain zero regardless of the severity of the threat. However, there is little evidence to support this proposal (Abraham and Sheeran 2005). The effectiveness of the behaviour can be considered to be additive. It is a straight forward cost–benefit analysis, costs are represented as barriers in the model (Figure 2.1). None of the postulated barriers to behaviour exclude the simultaneous recognition of the benefits.

Two quantitative reviews of research based on the HBM (Harrison et al. 1992; Janz and Becker 1984) include preventative, sick role and clinic utilisation behaviours in their analyses, making separate considerations of the value of the model for lifestyle behaviours difficult. However, the main conclusion from the more methodologically robust of the two reviews (Harrison et al. 1992) suggests that while all the four core constructs of susceptibility, severity, benefits and barriers correlate significantly with health behaviour they only account for a rather small amount of the total variance in behaviour (between 1.5 and 4 per cent). Such small effects are unlikely therefore to contribute a great deal to the promotion of health behaviour change. There is considerable concern about the theoretical construction of susceptibility and severity into an overarching concept of belief in a personal threat. The notion of a personal threat has been argued to be more complex than a simple multiplication of susceptibility and severity. Similarly, the conceptualisation of effectiveness of behaviour as a cost–benefit analysis fails to consider that while barriers are often concrete and based in the present (lack of time, distance to leisure centre, cost of fruit) benefits are less clear cut, less certain and based in the future (Lawton and Conner 2007). Barriers therefore may well need more weighting in a model which predicts behaviour now and benefits in the future. Conner and Norman (2005) found few studies considered the concepts of cues to action, health motivation or perceived behavioural control. Perceived behavioural control has been well studied, however, in other models (Luszczynska and Schwarzer 2005). The lack of research into these variables from later versions of the HBM may be due to the failure of the model to sufficiently operationalise these variables. As Harrison et al. (1992) point out, to be a valid model weights and interaction terms that show how the components work together should be developed. There needs to be agreement about which components are part of the model and all studies need to be consistent in how they operationalise these variables.

Protection motivation theory

The protection motivation theory (PMT) is often presented as the successor to the fear-drive model (Norman et al. 2005), although most of the traditional behavioural change models can be conceptualised as adaptations of the fear-drive model. Any model that includes an element of risk perception is potentially including a fear appeal. The PMT postulates that sources of information (i.e. fear appeals) initiate two independent appraisal processes: threat appraisal (risk) and coping appraisal (effectiveness of behaviour) (Figure 2.2).

Threat appraisal focuses on the source of the threat and factors that increase or decrease likelihood of maladaptive behaviours (presumably this is any response different to the one encouraged by the health promotion, although this is harder to establish in risk communications where an explicit behavioural change is not offered). Norman et al. (2005) offer avoidance, denial and wishful thinking as potential maladaptive processes. Milne et al. (2000) also include fatalism and hopelessness as potential maladaptive strategies. Intrinsic rewards (for instance, pleasure) and extrinsic rewards (for instance, social approval) are conceptualised as factors that may increase maladaptive behaviours. Severity and vulnerability are seen here as potential inhibitors of maladaptive adaptive processes.

Coping appraisal focuses on the coping strategies available to deal with the threat and the factors that increase or decrease the likelihood of the preferred strategy. The belief in the efficacy of the proposed behavioural change and the self-efficacy of the individual contemplating the change

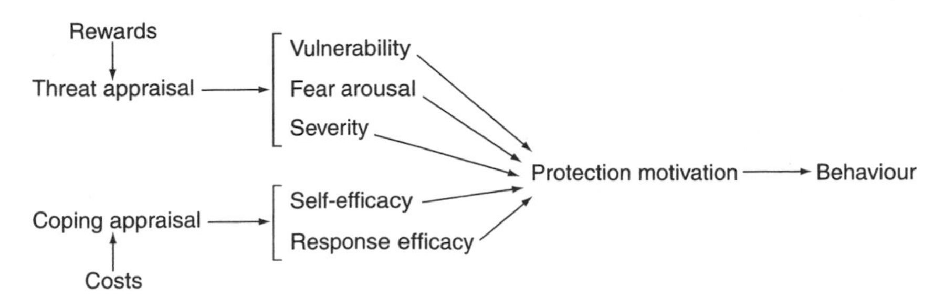

Figure 2.2 Protection motivation theory
(Adapted from Plotnikoff and Higginbotham 1998)

are postulated to increase the likelihood of the response. Self-efficacy can be defined as the degree to which an individual believes they can successfully engage in a behaviour in a particular situation with known outcomes. Costs are those factors that inhibit behavioural change. Costs can be external, such as lack of facilities or resources, or internal such as physiological cravings or withdrawal symptoms. Costs reduce the likelihood of the desired response.

The intention to perform a recommended or preferred behaviour, protection motivation as it is called in the model, is a positive function of perceptions of severity, vulnerability (or perceived personal threat as it is represented in the HBM), response efficacy (effectiveness of behaviour as it is represented in the HBM) and self-efficacy. Protection motivation is also a negative function of perceptions of rewards associated with maladaptive processes and response costs of adaptive behaviours (or barriers as the HBM describes them). The two-pronged approach of threat appraisal and coping appraisal can be interpreted as implying that perceptions of severity and vulnerability should outweigh rewards of maladaptive processes and that perceptions of response efficacy and self-efficacy should outweigh response costs of adaptive behaviour before any protection motivation is initiated (Figure 2.2). However, most studies of the model simply consider the additive effects of these variables. Protection motivation has been described as a variable that 'arouses, sustains and directs activity' (Rogers 1975: 98). Protection motivation is postulated to precede the deliberate adoption of any health behaviour.

Originally a multiplicative function of severity, vulnerability and response efficacy was postulated (Rogers 1975). The original version of PMT assumed that protection motivation would not be initiated if the value of any of these three components were zero. This is an intuitively appealing proposal but as there was no empirical evidence to support such a conjecture Rogers (1983) proposed a simpler additive model which is utilised in most analyses. Furthermore, most applications focus on five variables and do not attempt to measure the rewards of the maladaptive behaviour. Milne et al. (2000) in their meta-analysis of research based on the PMT reported only one study which attempted to include rewards. The argument made for ignoring the 'rewards' aspect of the model has been that the conceptual distinction between the reward value of a risk behaviour and the cost of a preventative measure is hard to operationalise (Abraham et al. 1994).

Evaluations of the protection motivation theory usually take one of two strategies. One strategy is to manipulate components of the model in a persuasive communication and then measure subsequent effects on protection motivation and/or behaviour. Two meta-analyses by Floyd et al. (2000) and Milne et al. (2000) of studies of this type both conclude that coping appraisal variables provide stronger predictions of protection motivation and/or behaviour than do threat appraisal variables. Although all components of the model had some predictive value the coping components and particularly self-efficacy produced the largest effect sizes (Floyd et al. 2000; Milne et al. 2000). The studies included in these meta-analyses of PMT look at how well the variables in the model predict both intention and behaviour. Milne et al. (2000) found twenty-one studies that related PMT components to intentions and eight that related the theory to actual behaviour. The PMT is consistently a better predictor of intention to behaviour than of actual behaviour.

A second strategy is to use the protection motivation theory in a more traditional manner to predict health behaviour. In many such studies self-efficacy has consistently either been the only or the best predictor of intention to behaviour and/or actual behaviour in a range of studies looking at diet (Plotnikoff and Higginbotham 1998), exercise (Plotnikoff and Higginbotham 2002), drinking (Murgraff et al. 1999) and safe sex (Greening et al. 2001).

Self-efficacy is the most promising predictive component of the protection motivation theory for intention to behave, concurrent behaviour and future behaviour, although its ability to predict behaviour is the least well evidenced (Murgraff et al. 1999). Self-efficacy is the key difference between the fear-drive model on which this model is based and the health belief model with which it shares many variables. Later models of the HBM have suggested the inclusion of perceived behavioural control which Conner (1993) has argued is conceptually similar to self-efficacy. Ajzen (1988) considers perceived behavioural control to be a broader concept than self-efficacy as it includes both intrinsic control (self-efficacy) and extrinsic control (environmental impediments).

Theory of planned behaviour

One of the identified problems with both the protection motivation theory and the health belief model is that they assume that the behaviour under consideration is solely a health behaviour. While behaviours like vaccination or applying sun screen could justifiably be argued to be behaviours carried out solely for health reasons, lifestyle behaviours have both health and non-health functions. A more general theory such as the theory of planned behaviour may therefore be more useful. The theory of planned behaviour (TPB) was developed from the theory of reasoned action (TRA) and is different only in that it includes perceived behavioural control. Ajzen (1998) included this concept to improve on the predictive power of the TRA. It enables people who have a positive attitude and supportive social situations but perhaps low self-efficacy for the action or no time for the action to be predicted non-compliant with the desirable action. The original TRA would predict compliance. Hagger et al. (2002) reviewed the predictive validity of both the theory of reasoned action and the theory of planned behaviour in a meta-analysis of 72 studies and concluded that the TPB is superior to the TRA. Perceived behavioural control is a more sophisticated concept than the barrier concept from the HBM as it enables the same factor to be a barrier for one individual and not for another depending on how they perceive the situation. It is also a broader concept including as it does both extrinsic and intrinsic influences on behavioural control (Figure 2.3).

Intention to behave is conceptually similar to the variable protection motivation from the PMT. Both the PMT and TPB concur that a motivating intention must exist before any deliberate behaviour occurs. Intention to behave is postulated to be a linear regression function of attitudes, subjective norms and perceived behavioural control. The amount of weight assigned to each variable is assumed to vary for different behaviours and different situations (Conner and Sparks 2005).

Aspects of the TPB are conceptually similar to both the HBM and the PMT. Only the components of social norm can be argued to be unique to the TPB. However, the social norm component of the TPB is also the least predictive component of the model (Godin and Kok 1996; Hagger et al. 2002; Conner and Sparks 2005).

Godin and Kok (1996) reviewed the TPB in 56 health behaviour studies; 44 of these studies investigated a lifestyle behaviour. Of the 56

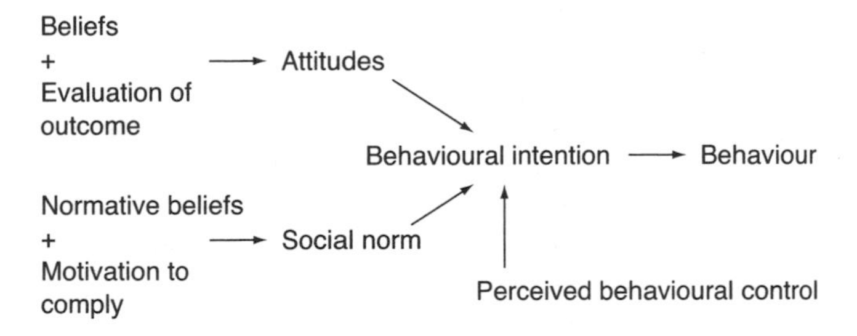

Figure 2.3 Theory of planned behaviour
(Adapted from Ajzen 1988, cited in Biddle and Mutrie 1991)

studies included in the review, only 26 provided data on the prediction of behaviour as well as the prediction of intention to behave. Godin and Kok (1996) concluded that in the domain of health about one-third of the variation in behaviour can be explained by the combined effect of intention and perceived behavioural control (Figure 2.3). They also conclude that the type of behaviour was clearly linked to the strength of the relationship between intention and behaviour because the correlation between the two concepts was far stronger in some behaviours than in others. Godin and Kok (1996) found that social norm was the least predictive component of the model and argued that this may be to do with poor operationalisation of this construct. There is support for this argument from studies of smoking in high school students where modelling behaviour has been found to be a significant predictor of smoking behaviour (Grube et al. 1986; De Vries et al. 1995 cited in Godin and Kok 1996). It may be the concept of social norm needs to be expanded to include: 'perceptions of others' behaviour' and 'pressure from significant others' to improve its predictive power. However, Sheeran and Taylor (1999) report in their meta-analysis of the TPB and intention to use condoms that social norms were equally as important as perceived behavioural control and attitudes in predicting intention to use condoms. As using a condom is a particularly social activity involving two people, the importance of social norms for this particular behaviour is understandable.

In Hagger et al.'s (2002) meta-analysis of the TPB and physical activity they found that that the TPB was a better predictor of both intention to behave and behaviour than the TRA. The inclusion of a measure of perceived behavioural control increased the amount of variation in intention that the model could explain from 37.27 per cent to 44.5 per cent and increased the amount of explained variation in behaviour from 26.04 per cent to 27.41 per cent. Hagger et al. (2002) went on to include the additional variables of self-efficacy and past behaviour finally arriving at an expanded model (Figure 2.4) which explained 60.18 per cent of the variation in intention to behave and 46.71 per cent of the variation in behaviour. The role of past behaviour is of particular interest. The inclusion of past behaviour adds considerable predictive power to the model yet is not acknowledged in the majority of social cognition models. Furthermore, social cognition models assume that attitudes and intentions influence behaviour but not that behaviour may influence attitudes and intention. If, as evidence suggests, the relationship between behaviour, attitudes and intentions is two-way, then the effects of intentions on behaviour and attitudes on intentions may be inaccurately high in studies that do not control for or include past behaviour in their analysis (Hagger et al. 2002).

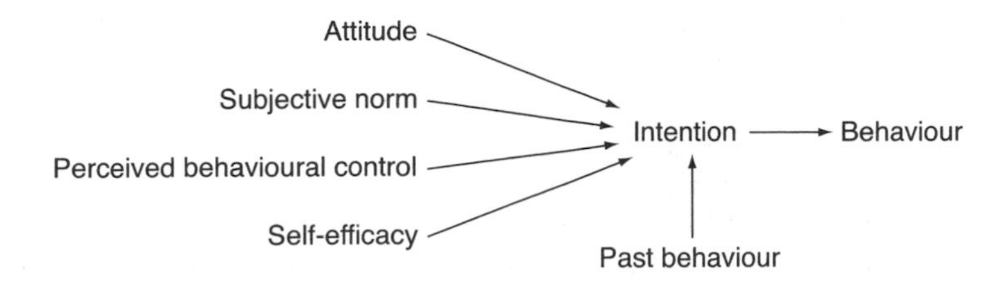

Figure 2.4 Hagger et al.'s expanded version of the theory of planned behaviour (Hagger et al. 2002)

Social cognition theory

The health belief model, protection motivation theory and theory of planned behaviour all include a number of similar constructs (Ajzen 1998). Having similar constructs with different names can imply a range of different determinants of health behaviour and a level of complexity that does not actually exist. Bandura (1998) has expressed concern that the proliferation of health behaviour models has lead to researchers picking and mixing constructs from various theories, rather than utilising and developing a unified perspective. Social cognition theory (SCT) is an attempt by Bandura (1998) to provide an 'overarching framework' and to clarify theoretical thinking within social cognition (Ajzen 1998: 737). Consequently, the underlying social cognitive principle of actions being regulated by rational thought is maintained. Social cognition theory includes all the constructs from the previously mentioned models but elaborates them further. Instead of beliefs about behavioural consequences as there are in the health belief model it identifies physical, social and self-evaluative outcome expectations (Figure 2.5). Perhaps most importantly instead of a single factor of perceived behavioural control, it distinguishes between self-efficacy and environmental impediments (Ajzen 1998).

Self-efficacy is the belief that one can carry out specific behaviours in specified situations (Bandura 1997). Self-efficacy has been extensively studied (Bandura 1997, 1998; Lannotti et al. 2006) within the context of this theory, where it takes a central place (Figure 2.5). Self-efficacy has been argued to be enhanced by personal accomplishment or mastery, vicarious experience or verbal persuasion (Walker 2001). Self-efficacy is not unrealistic optimism as it is based on experience (Luszczynska and Schwarzer 2005). Self-efficacy is similar to the broader construct of self-esteem but can be distinguished by three aspects: self-efficacy implies a personal attribution; it is prospective, referring to future behaviours and finally it is an operative construct in that the cognition is proximal to the behaviour (Luszczynska and Schwarzer 2005). Self-efficacy is one of the best predictors of behavioural change whereas self-esteem has been found to be a poor predictor of behavioural change (Ajzen 1998). Ajzen (1988, 1998) has consistently argued that behaviour-specific constructs fare better than generalised dispositions in predicting behaviour. The success of self-efficacy and the failure of self-esteem in predicting a range of behaviours adds considerable weight to this principle of compatibility.

Outcome expectancies are another central construct of social cognition theory (Figure 2.5). Physical outcome expectancies maybe discomfort while exercising or hunger while eating healthily. Social outcome expectancies are similar to the social norm component of the TPB in that they anticipate the responses of family, friends and colleagues. Self-evaluative outcome expectancies refer to potential experiences of being proud or satisfied of achieving goals (Bandura 1998). Most of the factors included in the HBM, the PMT and TPB correspond to one or other outcome expectation.

Goals in SCT can be distal and proximal. Intention to behave or protection motivation are most similar to proximal goals (Bandura 1998). Ajzen (1988) has argued convincingly that the more specific the goal or intention the more likely the subsequent action. Outcome expectancies are involved in the setting of goals. A decisional balance of anticipated positive and negative outcomes results in the setting or not setting of a goal. Self-efficacy is then crucial to translate the goal into action. The model recognises that socio-structural factors will influence goal setting. Implementation intentions are another emerging field of work, that addresses how goals can be realised (Sheeran et al. 2007). An individual is unlikely to set a goal of swimming twice a week if there is not an accessible swimming pool. However, the model recognises that self-efficacy will influence how an individual perceives environmental situations as potential opportunities or impediments. Consequently, self-efficacy can act directly and indirectly on behavioural change (Figure 2.5).

Perceived self-efficacy has been found to be the major instigating force in both intentions to change lifestyle behaviours and actual behavioural change (Shaw et al. 1992; Bandura 1998; Plotnikoff and Higginbotham

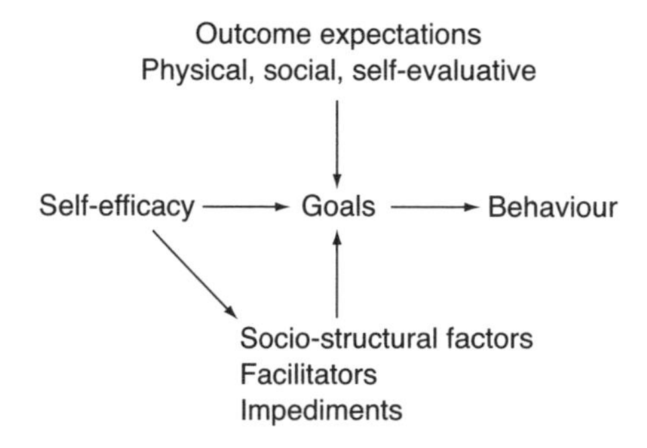

Figure 2.5 Social cognition theory
(Adapted from Luszczynska and Schwarzer 2005)

1998, 2002; Murgraff et al. 1999; Greening et al. 2001; Rodgers et al. 2002; Rovniak et al. 2002; Williams et al. 2007). Outcome expectancies, goals and perceived impediments have also been found to be predictive in some studies (Luszczynska and Schwarzer 2005). When the whole model is utilised, Rovniak et al. (2002) found it predicted 55 per cent of the variation in physical activity in their study of physical activity in university students, with self-efficacy being the most predictive construct in the model.

Stage theories of behavioural change

Stage theories have become increasing popular in recent years (Sutton 2005). Many theorists have argued that different cognitions may be important at different stages in promoting health behaviour. Some recognition of this is evident in the SCT which argues that outcome expectancies are important in setting goals, whereas self-efficacy is important for ensuring the goal is translated into action. There are a number of stage theories, for instance the precaution adoption process model (Weinstein and Sandman 1992) and the health behaviour goal model (Maes and Gebhardt 2000). However, the most well known and well researched is the transtheoretical model (Prochaska and DiClemente 1983).

According to all stage theories a person can move through a series of stages in the process of behavioural change (Figure 2.6). The hypothetical model in Figure 2.6 represents the basic structure of all stage theories. The roman numerals represent stages, of which there can be more than three. The letters represent the variables that are held to influence the stage transitions. Different factors are important at different stages, although the theory allows for some overlap. This is a basic structure of a stage theory in contrast to a continuum theory such as the theory of planned behaviour, when the likelihood of someone performing the behaviour is a linear function of the strength of the intention to do so, the stronger the intention the more likely the behaviour. A purist stage theory contests that each stage is qualitatively different to the next (Bandura 1998). Weinstein et al. (1998) argue that stage models should satisfy four principles:

- stages should be mutually exclusive and qualitatively different categories
- the stages should be sequential
- each individual within a stage should be experiencing similar barriers to making a change
- people in different stages should be experiencing different barriers to making a change.

The transtheoretical model (TTM) is the dominant stage model in health behavioural change (Sutton 2005). It is often referred to as the stages of change model reflecting the well-described backbone of the model.

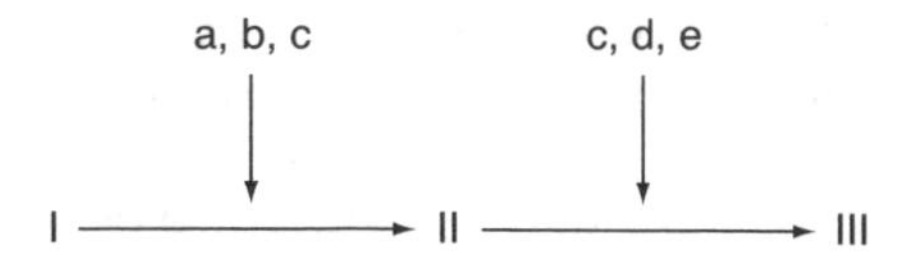

Figure 2.6 A hypothetical three-stage model

However, it is actually a collaboration of several constructs. These constructs are: the stages of change, decisional balance, self-efficacy and processes of change. The model is an attempt to integrate constructs from different theories of behaviour change into a single coherent model (Sutton 2005). Consequently, in its aim of rationalising conceptual thinking in the area under one framework it is similar to SCT. However, frequently, researchers focus on the single construct 'stages of change' (Sutton 2005; see also Bandura 1998). In the full model the construct 'stages of change' provides the basis organising principle, which postulates that people move through stages in order, although they may relapse from action or maintenance to an earlier stage. The three other constructs are then postulated to influence the transition from one stage to the next. Decisional balance, although derived from Janis and Mann's (1977) model of decision making, represents the for and against components that are present in most theories of health behaviour. Factors such as perceived severity, or perceived vulnerability (health belief model), social norms and barriers are relevant here. Self-efficacy has been introduced as the key component of social cognition theory earlier. Processes of change are the experiental and behavioural processes that people engage in to progress through the stages.

In summary the TTM describes health behaviour adoption and maintainance as a process that occurs through a series of behaviourally and motivationally defined stages (Table 2.1).

Table 2.1 The stages of change, conceptualised using alcohol as the health behaviour

Stages of change	*Behavioural and motivational characteristics*
Pre-contemplation	Individuals are drinking and have no intention of stopping in the next six months
Contemplation	Individuals are drinking but they intend to stop in the next six months
Preparation	Individuals are drinking less and intend to stop in the next six months
Action	Individuals have stopped drinking to excess within the past six months. The perceived benefits are greater than the perceived costs. This is the least stable stage
Maintenance	Individuals have been non-drinkers for over six months and risk of relapse is small

The TTM is seldom tested in its entirety (Sutton 2005), which is undoubtedly due to its complexity and its failure to conceptualise the role of all of the constructs. While the stages of change clearly distinguish between individuals in terms of their movement along the road to behavioural change, where the other constructs fit into this stage framework is less clear. Many researchers have taken the conceptually appealing stages of change and used it to distinguish between individuals in order to investigate the utility of their own particularly favoured intervention.

Evaluating the utility of such a complex model as the TTM is a difficult challenge. Cross-sectional studies have classified individuals into stages and then compared them on one or more of the other constructs from the model: decisional balance, processes of change or self-efficacy. Stage theories of change would predict differences in these measures at different stages (Herzog and Blagg 2007). However, the evidence from Rosen's (2000) meta-analysis of cross-sectional studies did not provide strong support for distinct stages with different cognitive processes utilised at different transitions. For example; when Herzog and Blagg (2007) looked at the motivational characteristics of pre-contemplating and contemplating smokers as categorised by the stages of change algorithm they found no common characteristics among people in the pre-contemplation stage. Conversely Marshall and Biddle (2001) in their meta-analysis of the TTM and exercise behaviour did find clear differences in the measures between stages, particularly in the pros component of the decisional balance construct and in experiential processes. They found a steep increase between pre-contemplation and contemplation in the self report of these variables no increase between contemplation and preparation and a further increase between preparation and action. Marshall and Biddle (2001) interpret their findings as supportive of the TTM. However, other researchers have argued that simply finding some differences is not necessarily supportive of the TTM if the model would not have predicted the utilisation of the constructs in this pattern. To a certain extent it depends if you view the behavioural process as a cause or a consequence of a stage transition. It is clear to see how a behavioural process such as self-efficacy could be the cause of a transition but also self-efficacy may increase as the consequence of a transition. If you expect self-efficacy to enable the translation from preparation to action you might predict high self-efficacy at this transition but no subsequent increase. However, if you view self-efficacy as being in some way dependent on experience, as has been suggested (Bandura 1998), then self-efficacy may be predicted to increase from action to maintenance as the experience of success increases self-efficacy for behaviour. The same kinds of arguments can be made for the other behavioural constructs postulated to intervene in stage transitions. Consequently, interpreting whether the data supports a stage theory of behaviour is fraught with difficulties.

It is similarly difficult to interpret the data from longitudinal studies of the TTM. Most longitudinal studies of the TTM report that those in contemplation at baseline were more likely to be in preparation at follow up than those in pre-contemplation and similarly those in preparation were more likely to be action than those in contemplation and so on through the stages. This has been interpreted as a 'stage effect' (Sutton 2005). However, if you were to take a continuous variable and categorise it you could create the same effect. If the stages are simply arbitrary delineations of a continuous variable then it is a pseudo-stage effect (Bandura 1998). If we were to take a population and divide them into those aged under 25 and those aged over 25 we could demonstrate that young people drink more than older people. However, people do not dramatically reduce their drinking once they reach 25, rather drinking rates decline gradually through the lifespan. The arbitrary categorisation of age could create a pseudo impression of the relationship between age and drinking. Bandura (1998) argues that the stages in the TTM are pseudo stages because instead of being qualitatively different, the first two stages (Table 2.1) are differences in degrees of intention and the subsequent stages are graduations of the behaviour the theory purports to explain. The action and maintenance stages are arbitrary subdivisions of duration of behaviour. It is not clear what process occurs at six months that means an individual is now in maintenance rather than action. Without a clearly identified transformational change, the behaviour could be spilt anywhere along the time continuum (Bandura 1998). Herzog (2007) found that smokers did not think about cessation plans in terms of fixed time-frames.

Perhaps the best way of testing stage theories is experimentally. Stage matched interventions should be more effective than stage mismatched interventions. Similarly, to research on other social cognition models experimental designs are the least frequent. However, the evidence from the few studies which have attempted to match interventions to stages has found little to support the stage model predictions (Quinlan and McCaul 2000; Sutton 2005).

Regardless of the method of analysis there appears to be little empirical evidence for the existent of discrete stages that could not equally well be explained as categorisation of a continuum (Sutton 2005; Herzog 2007; Herzog and Blagg 2007; Williams et al. 2007). However, the notion of matched interventions should not be discarded with the concept of discrete stages but the way interventions are individualised needs to be researched. It seems likely that the best interventions will be matched to the particular psychosocial determinants operating for any individual (Bandura 1998).

The transtheoretical model is so called because it utilises a wide range of theories. However, despite the interventions proposed to initiate behaviour change at various stages, without specifying the specific determinants or mechanisms of change it could actually be described as atheoretical (Bandura 1998). For example, categorising an individual as pre-contemplative is descriptive. We do not know why they are not contemplating a change of behaviour. The explanations for their pre-contemplation may be lack of information about the risk, lack of self-efficacy about the necessary change, or dislike of the proposed change. The determinants fall into the categories of risk perception, self-efficacy and outcome expectations, each requiring a different strategy to initiate behavioural change. It is plausible that an individual with no idea that smoking was dangerous, may learn of the risks and never smoke again. A stage theory of change could not provide an adequate explanation for such an event whereas other social cognition models could.

The stage model has been presented as a dynamic process model but at best it can describe set points in a process but makes no attempt to describe the processes involved in moving towards behaviour change (Bandura 1998).

Strengths and weakness of social cognition models of behavioural change

The social cognition models described above have guided and directed research in the field of health behaviour since the early 1960s (Prentice-Dunn and Rogers 1986). They have been used to predict, explain and increasingly to underpin interventions to change health behaviours. In this way they have provided a framework for an impressive body of work in the field. Increasingly, practitioners are recognising the important of theory in underpinning their interventions. The National Institute for Health and Clinical Excellence (NICE) has gone a long way towards encouraging evidence practice in the field of behavioural change by highlighting that theoretically based interventions are more effective (Hillsdon et al. 2005). While the value of the various theories for each individual lifestyle behaviour will be discussed in subsequent chapters, general issues with the use of social cognition models to predict lifestyle behaviours will be reviewed here.

Social cognition models and research into the predictive power of their components have clearly demonstrated that although a perception of risk may be necessary for behavioural change it is rarely sufficient. This is filtered through into practise with health practitioners now recognising that informing their clients of the need for lifestyle change is not enough, regardless of how high the risk. The emergence of motivational counselling, based on the TTM, and the increasing interest in psychological theories of behavioural change demonstrate how psychological theorising has influenced practice. The influence of social cognition models culminated recently in the publication of competencies for health trainers (Skills for Health 2007). Health trainers are a new role developed by the Department of Health in England to encourage lifestyle change in the population. The competencies required to be a health trainer are firmly based in social cognition theory and recognise the importance of enabling individuals to change their behaviour, emphasing self-efficacy and goal setting.

Stage theories introduce the concept of behaviour as a process. One of the great strengths of the TTM is that it introduces a concept of maintenance, which is theoretically similar to adherence. Previously social cognition models have conceptualised behavioural change as an acute event. While this may be appropriate for behaviours such as vaccination, lifestyle behaviours involve an ongoing process. Once change has been initiated it must be maintained. It is arguable whether the behavioural process can be conceptualised as discrete stages but recognising it as an ongoing process rather than a discrete event is a major step forward in conceptual thinking.

The social cognition model states the most plainly what all the models imply; behavioural change involves a thoughtful evaluation of the pros and cons of behavioural change. The models introduced above have been described as expectancy-value and expected utility theories (Weinstein et al. 2007) or as rational choice theories (Balbach et al. 2006). Less than thoughtful evaluative processes or heuristic shortcuts to behavioural decisions are not accounted for. Similarly the emotive, instinctive or habitual influences over behaviour are not recognised. Furthermore, the issue of volitional control is not consistently addressed in these models. All these models converge on intention as the key determinant of behaviour but this makes the assumption of volitional control. Some models include a component such as 'perceived behavioural control' that is recognised to act both indirectly on behaviour through intention but also directly on behaviour to account for the non-volitional components of some behaviours.

Social cognition models do not consider process, they simply describe factors postulated to be involved in the decision to change behaviour. Some models consider whether these factors are additive or multiplicative (Abraham and Sheeran 2005). If a factor has a multiplicative affect it is particularly important for health promotion. If personal vulnerability is a multiplicative factor and an individual perceives themselves as invulnerable then no amount of intervention to change perceptions of other factors will be effective. However, the limited evidence on the multiplicative relationship between components would suggest that intuitatively multiplicative components such as perceived vulnerability do not function in this way (Rogers 1983). The process by which individuals evaluate the various components of the model is not considered by social cognition models because the assumption is that individuals engage in rational decision making. Stage theories recognise that behaviour is a process but still does not consider the processes involved in influencing behaviour, as the assumption of rational decision making is still maintained.

While all social cognition models can be found to statistically predict behavioural change the actual amount of variation in behaviour they can account for is hard to assess. Some have argued that effect sizes are small (Harrison et al. 1992; Denny-Smith et al. 2006) whereas others argue that they predict behaviour successfully (Conner 1993; Hagger et al. 2002; Rovniak et al. 2002).

All the social cognition models evaluated here converge on the idea that intention is the key determinant of behaviour. Any theory that assumes rational decision making could not avoid a concept of conscious intention. In consequence, some studies evaluate the effect of an intervention on intention without directly measuring actual behavioural change (Sheeran and Taylor 1999; Milne et al. 2000). In one meta-analysis of research on protection motivation theory nearly half the studies used intention rather than behaviour as the outcome measure (Floyd et al. 2000). McClenahan et al. (2007) state that the aim of their study was to test the utility and efficiency of the theory of planned behaviour and the health belief model in 'predicting Testicular Self Examination behaviour'. However, in the study they do not make a direct measure of behaviour, utilising intention and self-reported past behaviour as indirect measures of behaviour. Using past behaviour as an indirect measure of behaviour is problematic as past behaviour is recognised as an influencing factor on future behaviour (Hagger et al. 2002). It is undoubtedly difficult to directly measure any behaviour and particularly difficult to measure such a personal behaviour as self-examination of the testicles. It makes sense to use intention to behave, if it is a reliable predictor of behaviour, as both the theory of planned behaviour and the health belief model imply.

Correlational studies show that intentions are reliably associated with behaviour (Webb and Sheeran 2006). Webb and Sheeran (2006) report that meta-analyses of correlational studies indicate that intentions on average account for 28 per cent of the variation in behaviour, which is described as a large effect on behaviour according to standard estimates of effect size (Cohen 1992). However, there are problems with the use of correlational studies to estimate the effect of intention on behaviour. There are two main issues with correlational studies. First, they assume intention causes behaviour but causation cannot be elucidated from a correlational design. Behaviour may predict intention and Bem's (1972) theory of self-perception makes a compelling argument for this initially counter-intuitive causal route. There well may be instances when people infer what they intend to do from what they have recently done. Second, correlational studies simply report associations between two factors but the relationship may be due to an unmeasured third factor. For example, there is a correlation between eating ice cream and drowning. However, it is clear that eating ice cream does not cause drowning. In this instance the causal factor is 'being at the beach' which is associated with both the eating of ice cream and swimming in the sea, which in turn is associated with an increased risk of drowning. In other instances the existence of a third 'true' causal factor may not be so apparent and the correlation wrongly accepted at face value.

If we want to know the impact of intention on behaviour we need to change intention and measure whether there are subsequent changes in behaviour. In other words we need an experimental study design. Webb and Sheeran (2006) carried out a meta-analysis of 45 experimental studies of the relationship between intention and behaviour. They concluded that although a medium-to-large change intention results in a small-to-medium change in behaviour, the effect size is far smaller than correlational studies suggest. Given that correlational studies are suggesting that at best 30 per cent of the variation in behaviour can be explained by intention there are obviously other factors worth exploring that may have a greater effect on behavioural change than intention. Webb and Sheeran (2006) argue that lack of control over the behaviour, circumstances that encourage habit formation and high social reactivity of the activity all reduce the impact of intention on behaviour.

Conclusion

Social cognition models have provided us with useful information about key factors involved in deliberate decision making about lifestyle behaviours. The fact that they generally explain less than half of the variation we see in health behaviours may be explained by the other roles that these lifestyle behaviours play in peoples lives; by the fact many lifestyle behaviours are habitual rather than deliberate and because change decisions will be influenced by both intuition and emotion as well as by cognitions.

Summary points

- Risk perception is a component of all social cognition theories of behavioural change.
- Perception of risk is not a good predictor of healthy lifestyle choices.
- Fear is not an effective motivator of lifestyle change.
- Self-efficacy is an effective predictor of positive lifestyle change.
- Stage theories of behavioural change recognise that lifestyle change is a process rather than an event.
- Past behaviour is a good predictor of future behaviour.
- Social cognition models can explain at best 50 per cent of the variation in behaviour.
- Social cognition models assume that behaviour is always the result of rational choice.
- Non-cognitive variables such as habit and enjoyment may have a role to play in behavioural change.

3 Eating

> Thou seest I have more flesh than another man, and therefore more frailty.
>
> Falstaff, in Shakespeare, *Henry IV, Part 1*

At the end of this chapter you will be able to:

- identify definitions of a healthy diet and problems with such definitions
- describe the extent of the obesity problem in the UK at present
- determine socio-demographic factors associated with obesity and poor diet
- pinpoint the consequences of poor diet and obesity for the individual and society as a whole
- describe and critically evaluate models of eating behaviour including genetic, socio-environmental and psychological models
- analyse the extent to which interventions aimed at increasing healthy eating are successful.

Definitions

Obesity and diet have a long history within medicine and health care. Tobias Venner in 1660 is reported as being the first physician to term the word 'obesity' and to suggest that it needs treatment (Haslam 2007). Subsequently, during the eighteenth century several authors suggested that avoiding obesity promoted good health, although the value of a good diet had been recognised much earlier. For example, Pythagoras suggests that 'No man, who values his health, ought to trespass on the bounds of moderation, either in labour, diet or concubinage'.

Hippocrates states that:

> Persons of a gross relaxed habit of body, the flabby, and red-haired, ought to use a drying diet ... Such as are fat, and desire to be lean,

> ould use exercise fasting; should drink small liquors a little warm should eat only once a day, and no more than will just satisfy their hunger.
>
> (cited in Haslam 2007: 32)

The connection between obesity and angina was emphasised in 1811 by Robert Thomas, who wrote:

> It is found to attack men much more frequently than women, particularly those who have short necks, who are inclinable to corpulency, and who at the same time lead an inactive or sedentary life . . . he should endeavor to counteract disposition to obesity, which has been considered a predisposing cause.
>
> (cited in Haslam 2007: 35)

More recently, the consequences of a poor diet have become the focus of media and political attention, with the detrimental affects of certain diets being highlighted. For example, the number of newspaper articles related to obesity increased from 62 in 1980 to over 6500 in 2004 (Saguy and Almeling 2005, cited in Campos et al. 2006a). It is estimated that obesity is responsible for more than 9000 premature deaths per year in England, and a similar proportion in Scotland, Wales and Northern Ireland (Canoy and Buchan 2007). Modelling suggests that moving towards the recommended diet could result in significant benefits in terms of both mortality and morbidity (see Table 3.1; Ofcom 2006).

Table 3.1 Premature mortality and morbidity improvements resulting from move towards recommended diets

	Premature mortality avoided	*Quality adjusted life years (QALYs) gained*
Increase fruit and vegetable intake by 136g/day	42,000	411,000
Reduce daily salt intake from average 9g to 6g	20,000	170,000
Cut saturated fat intake by 2.5% of energy	3,500	33,000
Cut added sugar intake by 1.75% of energy	3,500	49,000

The national guidelines suggest that a healthy diet is a balanced diet based on five major food groups: breads, other cereals and potatoes; fruit and vegetables; milk and dairy foods; meat, fish and alternatives; and foods containing fats and sugars (see Figure 3.1). The Department of Health

(1999b) defines good nutrition in the *Saving Lives: Our Healthier Nation* document as 'plenty of fruit and vegetables, cereals, and not too much fatty and salty food'. This definition is hardly specific, yet policy makers have continued with the concept of a 'balanced diet' gaining credence. The Food Standards Agency (FSA 2001) 'Balance of Good Health' has acted as the standard on which national guidelines are based. This has now been renamed the 'eatwell plate' (see Figure 3.1), based on the UK government's eight guidelines for a healthy diet:

1 Base your meals on starchy foods.
2 Eat lots of fruit and veg.
3 Eat more fish.
4 Cut down on saturated fat and sugar.
5 Try to eat less salt – no more than 6g a day.
6 Get active and try to be a healthy weight.
7 Drink plenty of water.
8 Don't skip breakfast.

The previous guidance (FSA 2001) was based on the five food groups (breads, cereals and potatoes; fruit and vegetables; milk and diary; meat, fish and alternatives; foods containing fat and sugar). It applies to most people including vegetarians, people who are a healthy weight for their height, as well as those who are overweight; however, it does not apply to

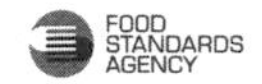

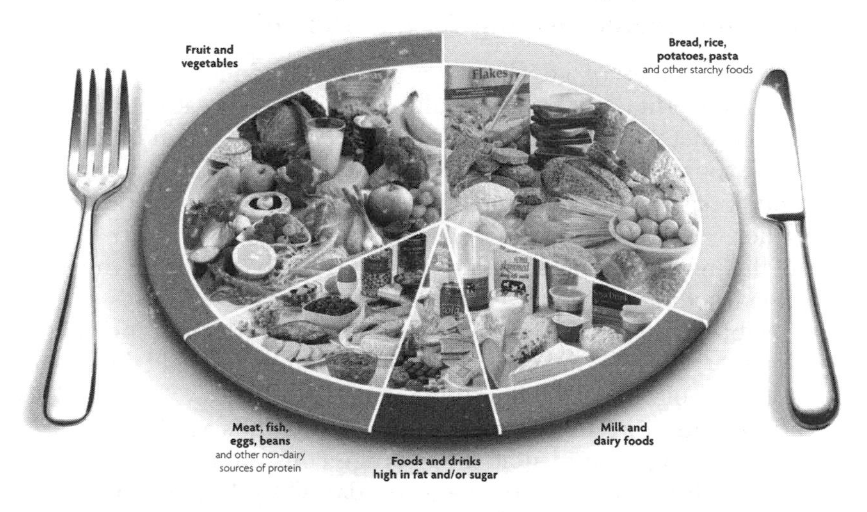

Figure 3.1 The eatwell plate (FSA 2008)

children under 2 years of age or those with special dietary requirements. The key message is that a balance of foods should be consumed to achieve a good healthy diet (see Figure 3.1). The message is to eat 'lots' of breads, cereals and potatoes, fruit and vegetables, 'moderate' amounts of milk, dairy and meat and 'sparing' amounts of fat and sugary drinks. Obviously, there is some uncertainty with this definition – 'lots', 'moderate' and 'sparing' are open to (mis)interpretation. Furthermore, the guidance does not include any information on portion sizes as this 'kind of information is potentially misleading' (FSA 2001: 6). This lack of certainty continues with the eatwell plate, although some change has occurred to try and clarify these uncertainties, for example, salt intake being limited to a suggested maximum of 6g and the definitions of portions being more clearly explained (140g of oily fish is a portion). Whether this clarification will have any impact on consumers is uncertain, and whether definitions based on gram weight are particularly useful is also unconfirmed.

Given this lack of certainty it is not surprising that many individuals are still confused and lack a basic understanding of the definition of a 'healthy diet'. Attempting to convey this information sensibly and coherently is not easy; it can be difficult to define and is subject to much revision and reinterpretation (Goode et al. 1995; Marshall et al. 2007). Where there is knowledge of what constitutes a healthy diet, and the need to limit unhealthy elements, for example, limiting fat, sodium and sugar intake, there is some indication that individuals did not have satisfactory nutritional knowledge of which foods are high in fat, salt and sugar (McCullough et al. 2004). This lack of nutritional knowledge can lead to unbalanced dietary patterns, with excesses of sugar and fat.

Government recommendations for a healthy diet

There are a number of governmental recommendations on diet and eating, although they can be essentially be reduced to eating a healthy and balanced diet. However, there are two specific recommendations: eat at least five portions of fruit and vegetables per day and reduce the consumption of salt to a maximum of 6g per day, and these will be considered further.

One of the major recommendations and the one that has been the focus of much marketing and advertising is that at least five portions of fruit and vegetables are consumed each day (WHO 2004a). A portion is approximately 80g (e.g. one medium apple, or three heaped tablespoons of peas). Do people actually follow this advice? In 2002, the National Diet and Nutrition Survey (Henderson et al. 2002) of adults aged between 19 and 64 years of age found that the average consumption of fruit and vegetables was less than three portions per day. Only 13 per cent of men and 15 per cent of women consumed the recommended five or more portions a day (Henderson et al. 2002). Social class differences are also apparent: those in the working class consumed 50 per cent less than those in professional groups. A particular area of concern is children's diet – research suggests that nearly 20 per cent of those aged between 4 and 18 years eat no fruit at all during a typical week (Strategy Unit 2008).Despite considerable effort, increased marketing commitment and expenditure towards increasing the consumption of fruit and vegetables, there has been little success (Strategy Unit 2008).

There are differences in 'healthy' consumption between the countries of the UK. To take one example, the consumption of fruit and vegetables between England, Wales and Scotland is presented in Table 3.2. The differences in the proportion of men and women eating more than five portions a day between the countries is considerable, with those in Wales reporting an almost twofold level of consumption compared to the English and Scottish survey respondents (obviously this could be a consequence of the survey methodology).

Table 3.2 Fruit and vegetable consumption in men and women from England, Wales and Scotland

Source of data	*Women's average daily portions of fruit and vegetables*	*Men's average daily portions of fruit and vegetables*	*Women eating five or more portions of fruit or vegetables a day (%)*	*Men eating five or more portions of fruit or vegetables a day (%)*
Health Survey England 2003	3.5	3.2	26	22
Scottish Health Survey 2003	3.2	3.0	22	20
Welsh Health Survey 2003	No data available	No data available	41	37

Evidence of the problem

Obesity is an excess of body fat leading to ill health (Canoy and Buchan 2007) and is commonly measured using the Body Mass Index (BMI). BMI originates from Quetelet's average man (Quetelet 1869) and is calculated using the equation weight (kg)/height (m^2). Among adults, the following categories have been used:

Not overweight/obese	BMI 25 or less
Overweight	BMI 25–30
Obese	BMI 30+

Although it is rather crude and imprecise, it is a useful measure of adiposity (WHO 2000) and correlates well with the risk of obesity-related diseases (Manson et al. 1995; Haslam and James 2005). However, BMI does not distinguish between fat mass and lean (non-fat) mass. For example, athletes and well-trained body builders have a very low percentage of body fat, but their BMI may be in the overweight range. Furthermore, the relationship between BMI and body fatness differs according to age and ethnicity: the relationship between BMI and body fatness is different in the elderly and non-Caucasian populations compared with younger Caucasian populations (Jackson et al. 2002; Chang et al. 2003; Snijder et al. 2006). A final problem with the BMI is that the distribution of fat over the body is not recorded.

In many studies, BMI is calculated using self-report height and weight (Adams et al. 2006; Chiolero et al. 2007). However, a systematic review has demonstrated that this self-report BMI may be lower than a measured BMI, i.e. some obese individuals are being misclassified as being non-obese based on self-reported BMI (Connor-Gorber et al. 2007). Importantly, this self-report misclassification is not random: moderately obese individuals are more likely to side with non-obese than severely obese, the latter having a BMI which is further away from the obese/non-obese cut-off value. Thus, it is likely that any association between obesity and health conditions is likely to be overestimated (Chiolero et al. 2007). As a result of such observations, Chiolero et al. (2007: 374) suggest that we be 'cautious with the interpretation of association observed between obesity defined using self-reported BMI and health conditions'.

In addition to overall BMI, the distribution of fat over the body has been linked to health outcomes. Studies have indicated that abdominal fat distribution is associated with increased disease risk, independent of overall obesity (Rimm et al. 1995; Snijder et al. 2006). Consequently, other measures of adiposity have been devised: waist circumference, waist-to-hip ratio, or the sagittal abdominal diameter (Lean et al. 1995; Onat et al. 2004).

BMI is used differently in children, as defining overweight and obesity is complicated by the fact that weight varies with height as children grow. It is calculated the same way as for adults but then compared to typical values for other children of the same age and biological sex. Thus the classification of a child as overweight or obese will depend on the reference population and the points of the distribution selected to define overweight or obesity (Butland et al. 2007).

Using the UK National BMI percentile classification system for children aged 2 to 15 years, overweight and obesity are categorised as follows:

Not overweight	85th centile or below
Overweight	Over 85th to 95th centile
Obese	95th centile or over

Measuring overweight and obesity in children is challenging as there is no universally accepted definition of childhood obesity. Consequently the International Obesity Task Force (IOTF) has developed an international classification system using data collected among children from six countries (Cole et al. 2000). The IOTF identifies the childhood percentile in the dataset corresponding to a BMI of 25 or 30 at age 18 and assumes that this percentile is the definition of overweight and obese tracking backwards to birth. The IOTF classification system is not designed for individual clinical diagnosis but is a useful epidemiological and surveillance tool (Butland et al. 2007). It is less arbitrary than the UK National BMI percentile classification system and better for comparing data between countries as the dataset is more ethnically diverse; however there is ongoing debate regarding which classification system is more robust (Jotangia et al. 2005).

Zaninotto et al. (2006) report on the prevalence and number of adults who are overweight or obese in the UK at present (see Figure 3.2). When the overweight and obese categories are collapsed, the results indicate the majority of people in the UK at present are at least overweight. Using this data it is estimated that between 12 and 15 million men and between 11 and 14 million women in the UK are either overweight or obese. Worryingly, it is also estimated that the number of women who are either obese or overweight will increase by 7 per cent by 2010 and the number of men by 10 per cent.

Obesity is a growing problem among children and young people as well: some 16 per cent of 2–15 year olds are obese. For children, it is estimated that there will be a 6 per cent increase in obesity by 2010, from

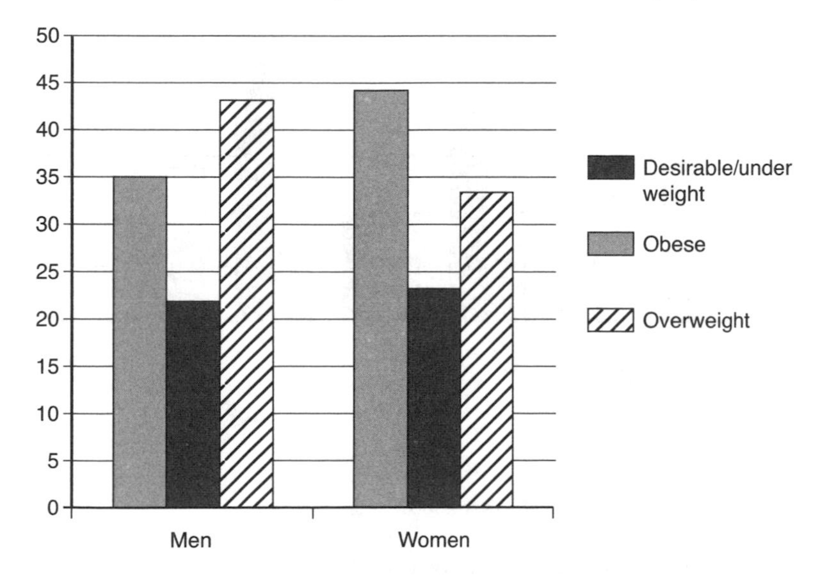

Figure 3.2 Prevalence of obesity and overweight in UK population

750,000 currently to over 800,000 (Zaninotto et al. 2006). Obesity has trebled in 20 years but there are sections of society that are differentially affected. People in the lowest social classes are particularly susceptible to becoming obese, the social class divide being particularly marked in women. Obesity rates also differ according to age, with obesity rates being highest among those in their fifties and sixties (McPherson et al. 2007). There are also differences according to ethnicity, with some ethnic minority groups more likely to suffer from obesity than others (McPherson et al. 2007). For men, the prevalence of obesity is greatest among the Bangladeshi population, with a large increase expected in Pakistanis (Figure 3.3). For women, it was predicted that obesity was expected to dramatically increase among the Black African and Pakistani populations, although the rates were predicted to decline for Black Caribbean women (Figure 3.4). There was some evidence that ethnic minority diets also differed, with greater consumption of fruit and vegetables but a greater addition of salt to cooking (DoH 2004a).

There are differences in the level of obesity between the different UK countries. In Northern Ireland, some 64 per cent of men and 53 per cent of women are overweight or obese (NISRA 2006). Similarly, in Scotland 64 per cent of men and 57 per cent of women are so classified (Scottish Executive 2005). The Welsh Health Survey did not report by males and females but found that 54 per cent of the sample was at least overweight.

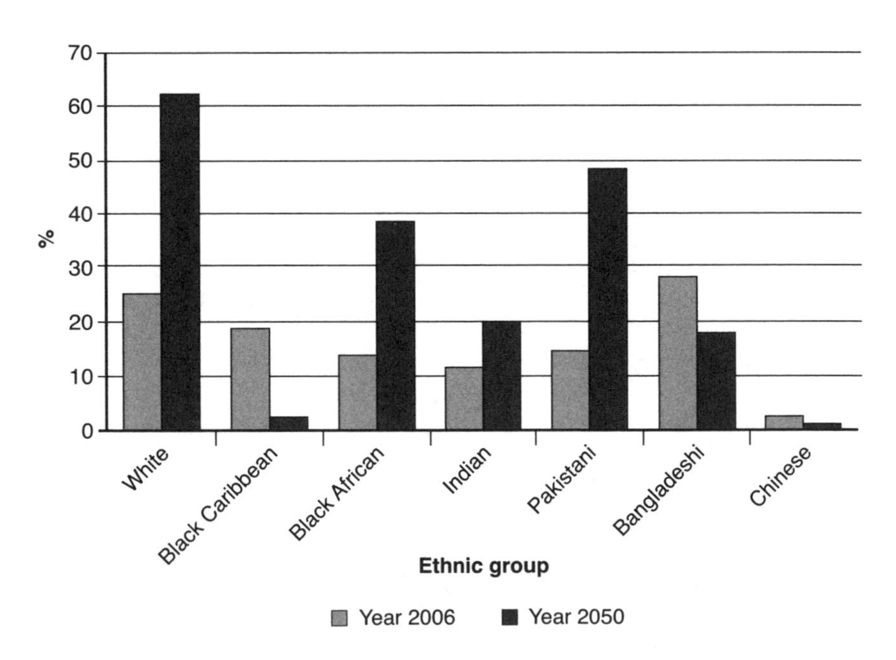

Figure 3.3 Actual and projected obesity levels for men (McPherson et al. 2007)

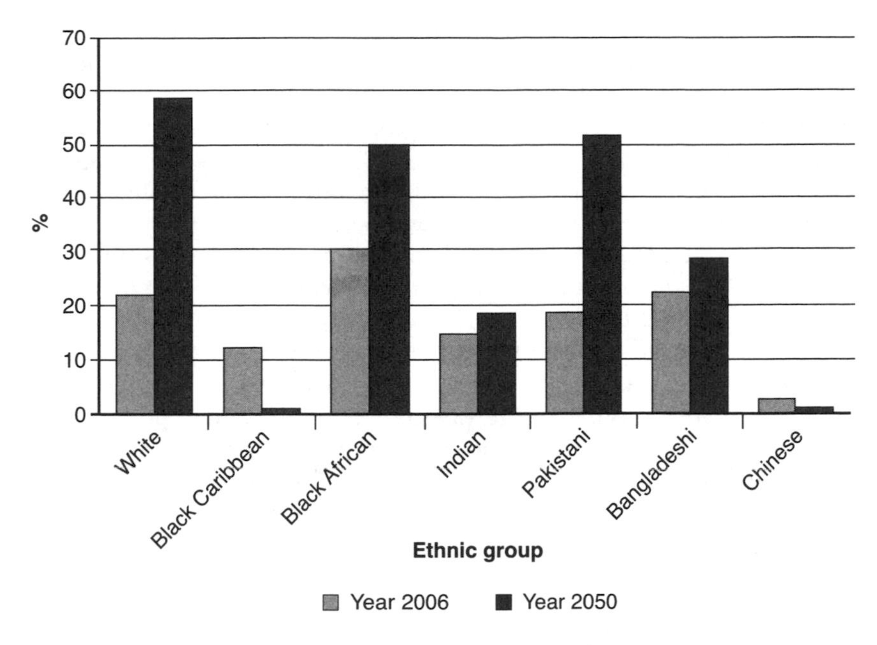

Figure 3.4 Actual and projected obesity levels for women (McPherson, et al. 2007)

In England, 65.2 per cent of men and 57 per cent of women were reported as being at least overweight. The results from the Health Survey for England show that the proportion of adults with a desirable BMI decreased between 1993 and 2005, from 41.0 per cent to 32.2 per cent among men and from 49.5 per cent to 40.7 per cent among women. There was no significant change in the proportion of adults who were overweight. The proportion who were categorised as obese (BMI 30+) increased from 13.2 per cent of men in 1993 to 23.1 per cent in 2005 and from 16.4 per cent to 24.8 per cent of women (Information Centre 2006).

However, Campos et al. (2006a) argue that there is no epidemiological evidence of an obesity crisis and calling for action on the 'obesity epidemic' is premature. They argue that the obesity epidemic is simply a product of tens of millions of people with BMIs formerly in the high 20s range gaining a modest amount of weight and thus moving into the BMI>30. Thus people are simply slipping over the borderline from one classification to another. Hence, this is a shift rightwards on the distribution curve with a proportion of people gaining 3–5kg more than a generation ago (Flegal et al. 1998). The average weight gain, Campos et al. (2006a) suggest, can be explained by '10 extra calories a day, or the equivalent of a Big Mac once every 2 months'. Which 'is hardly [an] orgy of fast food bingeing' (Campos et al. 2006a: 55).

The relationship between social class and health, and health behaviours has been recorded and recognised for well over 100 years (see Tables 3.3 and 3.4). Despite this the health gradient still remains and some have argued that it is increasing (Shaw et al. 2005). The influential Acheson report (1998) suggests that socio-economic differences account for 5000 deaths per year in men under the age of 65 years. In all age groups, people living on a low income have higher rates of diet-related diseases than other people. For example approximately 58 per cent more manual workers die prematurely compared to non-manual workers. Obviously this may be related to a number of different health-related dietary conditions (The National Diet and Nutrition Survey: DoH/FSA 2002). Obesity is more prevalent in those in social class V (i.e. working class) compared to those in social class I (i.e. upper class). Furthermore, central obesity (i.e. 'apple-shaped' or 'masculine' obesity when the main deposits of body fat are localised around the abdomen and the upper body) is more common in those from manual social classes than non-manual classes (see Table 3.3). Consequently, diabetes is more common in those in social class V compared to all other groups. Furthermore, premature death rate from coronary heart disease (CHD) is more than double in manual workers compared to non-manual workers for women, and more than half again for men. There is a similar discrepancy in breast and colon cancer survival rates: those in the lower socio-economic backgrounds have higher mortality rates from these conditions compared to those in other socio-economic backgrounds.

Table 3.3 Social class differences in risk factor prevalence, men

Risk (%)	*I*	*II*	*III(NM)*	*III(M)*	*IV*	*V*
Overweight or obese	58	63	60	64	59	57
Obesity	12	16	16	20	16	18
High waist to hip ratio	20	24	23	31	28	29
Untreated hypertension	28	31	30	33	28	33
Low physical activity	33	33	36	32	34	29
Consumption fewer than five portions of fruit and vegetables	64	71	79	80	78	83

Table 3.4 Social class differences in risk factor prevalence, women

Risk (%)	*I*	*II*	*III(NM)*	*III(M)*	*IV*	*V*
Overweight or obese	45	51	49	56	57	60
Obesity	14	18	18	24	25	28
High waist to hip ratio	18	18	18	22	24	27
Untreated hypertension	23	22	23	23	23	26
Low physical activity	37	40	41	42	43	40
Consumption fewer than five portions of fruit and vegetables	60	66	73	76	77	81

The National Diet and Nutrition Survey (DoH/FSA 2002) reported on a range of socio-demographic factors related to diet and obesity. For example, those in the low working-class group consumed more calories, considerably more fat, more salt and non-milk extrinsic sugars than those in the middle and upper classes. Furthermore those on low income eat a less varied diet compared to those in the upper classes. There are many reasons for these differences which will be explored later. However, it is worth recalling that these are not all psychological. The explanations also include some social factors, for instance the lack of access, availability along economies of scale and the potential fear of waste. This may also help to explain why those on lower incomes eat more processed foods which tend to be higher in saturated fats and salt (e.g. fast foods, white bread, processed vegetables and meat products). Similarly, people living on state benefits and reduced income eat less fruit and vegetables, less fish and less high-fibre foods: for example almost one-third had no fruit in the survey week (Henderson et al. 2002) and there is some evidence that there has been a decline in fruit and vegetable consumption in some of these lower social classes compared to those in the upper classes.

There are of course group differences with there being social class differences and differences across the country in terms of those eating the recommended intake of fruit and vegetables. It is even possible to explore the level of intake at a more local level. For example, the Welsh Health Survey highlighted that only 40 per cent reported eating five or more portions of fruit and vegetables, but this masks a range of between 34 per cent and 46 per cent (Figure 3.5).

It is no surprise that this poor diet in adults is also reflected in children. Consequently, children of semi-skilled and unskilled manual workers are

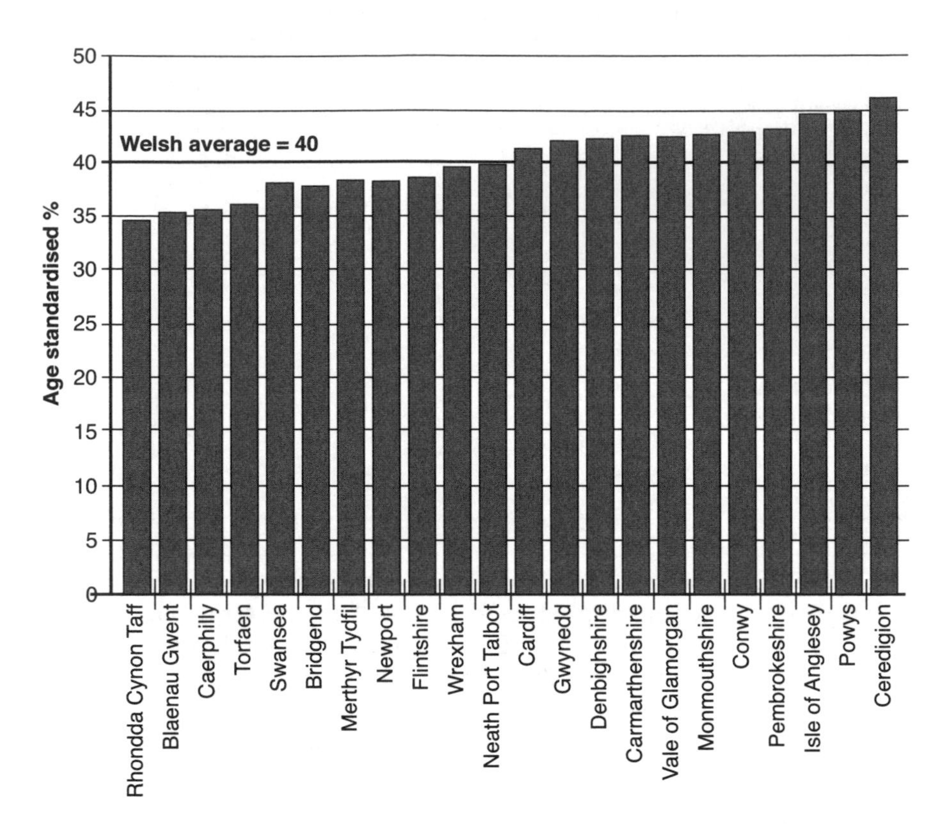

Figure 3.5 Adults who reported eating five or more portions of fruit and vegetables the previous day (National Assembly for Wales 2006)

more likely to eat fatty food, less fruit and vegetables, and more sweets than those children of professionals and managers. They have lower levels of vitamins such as folate, riboflavin, vitamin D and iron.

But why should there be this social class difference? More complex explanations will be presented later, but there may be something much simpler explaining the difference – cost. This simple explanation would assume that those in the lower social classes do not eat healthily because healthy foods cost more. However, even unpicking this simple explanation can lead into a more complex picture unfolding. For example, Frazão and Golan (2005) undertook a survey and found that a high dietary intake of sugars, total fats and sweets is cheaper than a high dietary intake of fruit, vegetables and meat. Both daily dietary cost and cost per unit energy were higher with a diet high in fruit and vegetable intake compared with a diet low in fruit and vegetable intake. Every extra 100g of fats and sweets eaten decreased diet costs by 0.05 to 0.4 euros, whereas every extra 100g of fruit and vegetables eaten increased diet costs by 0.18 to 0.29 euros.

Consequences of a poor diet

A poor diet can contribute to a range of illnesses, including both CHD and cancer (see Table 3.5). Poor diet also results in increased falls and fractures in older people (Vellas et al. 1990), low birth weight and increased childhood morbidity and mortality (Acheson 1998) and increased dental cavities in children (James et al. 1997). There is also evidence to support the link between poor diet and antisocial behaviour, not to mention growing concern over the economic implications of the population's weight gain.

Table 3.5 Diseases associated with obesity

Cardiovascular disease
Cancer
Diabetes
Stroke
Hypertension
Angina
Dental decay

The benefits of an improved diet have been highlighted in a number of public health documents and government policies. For example:

- Reducing cholesterol level by just 10 per cent would prevent some 25,000 deaths every year (Unal et al. 2004) which could be achieved by reducing saturated fat intake.
- The incidence of strokes could be decreased by increasing the consumption of fruit and vegetables.
- Hypertension could be reduced by reducing the salt intake and therefore have a positive impact on the incidence of cardiovascular diseases such as CHD/stroke (Davies et al. 2000).
- Approximately 40 per cent of endometrial cancer and 10 per cent of breast and colon cancers would be avoided by maintaining a healthy weight (i.e. BMI of 25 or less).
- Increased dietary fibre is associated with a decreased risk of colorectoral and pancreatic cancer.

Obesity may be a risk factor in a number of chronic diseases such as heart disease, stroke, some cancers and type 2 diabetes (Zaninotto et al. 2006). National Audit Office (2001) figures suggest that if there were one million fewer obese people in the UK, this would lead to around 15,000 fewer people with coronary heart disease, 34,000 fewer people developing type 2 diabetes, and 99,000 fewer people with high blood pressure. Greater awareness of the disease burden associated with obesity has led to concern over the economic implications of the population's weight gain. The

Health Select Committee (2006, as cited in McPherson et al. 2007) has estimated that the cost of obesity is £3.3–3.7 billion per year and that of obesity plus overweight is £6.6–7.4 billion. Based on Foresight extrapolations to 2050 the potential combined direct and indirect costs of obesity in the UK could rise to £52 billion per year (at 2008 prices) (McPherson et al. 2007).

The consequences of a poor diet are more than just obesity. For example, it has been suggested that around 30 per cent of all cancer deaths can be attributed to smoking cigarettes, but around 35 per cent can be attributable, in some part, to a poor diet (Doll and Peto 1981). A diet involving significant intake of high fat foods, high levels of salt and low levels of fibre appears to be particularly implicated (World Cancer Research Fund 1997). In addition to cancer, excessive fat intake has been implicated in disease and death from several serious illnesses including CHD. According to the Food Standards Agency (FSA) (2004), 73,000 cardiovascular deaths and 34,000 other deaths a year are related to the type and quantity of the food we eat. Obesity is an important issue in the poverty-poor diet-poor health cycle. Rayner and Scarborough (2005) estimated that food related ill-health is responsible for about 10 per cent of morbidity and mortality in the UK. The researchers concluded that the cost to the health service of dealing with poor dietary habits was significantly higher than the estimate for the annual cost of smoking, which is around £1.5 billion. They estimated that food accounts for costs of £6 billion a year (9 per cent of the NHS budget). It should be emphasised that this chapter will explore the obesity 'epidemic' and this side of the diet equation rather than the malnutrition side of a poor diet (although the latter has been suggested as costing the NHS some £7.3 billion a year, i.e. higher than the cost of obesity: Rayner and Scarborough 2005).

Obviously eating the right foods can prevent illness and promote health. For example, eating fruit and vegetables may offer protection against some forms of cancer (e.g. bowel). Block et al. (1992) suggested that on the basis of 132 of 170 studies, there is evidence to suggest that fruit and vegetables offer a significant protection against cancer and other studies have indicated that it is also of benefit for stroke and heart disease (Ness and Powles 1997). The precise mechanism by which fruit and vegetables improve health is unclear; however, a high fruit and vegetable intake may help to modify overall diet by increasing fibre and reducing fat and sugar intake. Fruit and vegetables also contain more than 100 beneficial compounds, many of which are antioxidants, which may reduce the risk of cancer and other chronic diseases by destroying free radicals in the body (European Heart Network 2002). It is estimated that eating five portions of fruit and vegetables per day would reduce mortality from CHD, stroke and cancer by 20 per cent (DoH 2000a). In fact, research suggests that increasing fruit and vegetable intake to five portions per day is the second most effective strategy in the prevention of cancer after smoking cessation (DoH 2000b). On the basis of this evidence current recommendations are to eat five or more portions of fruit and vegetables a day; however, less than 20 per cent of boys and 15 per cent of girls aged 13–15 were found to be doing so (Bajekal et al. 2003) and there is substantial evidence that adults are not following these recommendations either (Baker and Wardle 2003; Wardle and Steptoe 2003).

He et al. (2006) reported on a meta-analysis of studies exploring the link between fruit and vegetable intake and risk of stroke. The results indicated that an increased consumption of fruit and vegetables is associated with a reduced risk of stroke. Those having between three and five vegetable servings a day had an 11 per cent reduction in the risk of a stroke, and those with more than five servings per day had a reduction of 26 per cent, compared to those having less than three servings per day. The results indicated that 'both fruits and vegetables have a significant protective effect against stroke' (He at al. 2006: 324). In another study, Cade et al. (2007) examined the relationship between dietary fibre and the risk of breast cancer. Researchers found that fibre from cereals was inversely associated with the risk of breast cancer and that fibre from fruit had a borderline inverse relationship. A further model including dietary folate strengthened the significance of the inverse relationship between total fibre and pre-menopausal breast cancer. It was concluded that in pre-menopausal women, total fibre is protective against breast cancer, in particular, fibre from cereals and possibly fruit. Despite evidence highlighting the association between diet and health outcomes, in the United States life expectancy continues to increase and death rates from ischaemic heart disease continue to decline (National Center for Health Statistics 2004, cited in Flegal 2006). Since 1960 cardiovascular risk factors, with the exception of diabetes, have dropped at all BMI levels (Gregg et al. 2005) and research suggests a possible decrease in the relative risk of mortality associated with obesity (Flegal et al. 2005). There is thus some confusion over whether the relationship between mortality and morbidity and BMI is simplistically linear.

Flegal et al. (2007) attempted to clarify the association between BMI and all mortality causes. They examined data from the United States National Health and Nutrition Examination Survey (N = 2.3 million) dating back to 1971. It was found that being underweight was significantly associated with increased mortality from non-cancer, non-CVD causes, but not associated with cancer or CVD mortality. Being overweight was associated with significantly decreased mortality from non-cancer, non-CVD causes but not associated with cancer or CVD mortality. Obesity was associated with significantly increased CVD mortality but not associated with cancer mortality or with non-cancer, non-CVD mortality. Comparisons across surveys suggested a decrease in the association of obesity with CVD mortality over time. Thus Flegal et al. concluded that BMI-mortality associations vary by cause of death.

Why do people eat unhealthily?

As we have argued previously, eating is a lifestyle rather than simply a health behaviour. Diet has a number of consequences both health and non-health. It is interesting to note that Campos et al. (2006b) entitle their article 'Lifestyle not weight gain should be the primary target'. There have been a number of explanations for why people eat what they do and these have ranged from the genetic through to the social environmental, taking in media and cognitive factors along the way. Although it is impossible in one chapter to cover all of these different proposals, it is worth exploring some of these major explanations to review the background evidence before exploring in depth the major psychosocial theories that have been proposed to explain what people eat and why.

Genetic theories

Evidence from the robust twin and adoption studies have indicated that body weight is strongly influenced by genetic factors. Grillo and Pogue-Geile (1991) in an extensive review of the literature suggested that heritability accounted for approximately 70 per cent for weight and 60 per cent for BMI. These factors have been reduced somewhat by Bouchard and Pérusse (1993) who suggested there was a heritability of 40 per cent for BMI. More recently Herbert et al. (2006) suggest that there is a common genetic variant associated with adult and childhood obesity near the INSIG2 gene. The authors suggest that this gene was an 'important determinant of obesity'. However, these studies relate to obesity, rather than eating behaviour. Tholin et al. (2005) explored the genetic influence on eating behaviour and concluded that: 'On the basis of the results presented above, it is clear that eating behavior is strongly influenced by genes' (Tholin et al. 2005: 568). As most good psychology (and other) undergraduates will recognise however, a singular genetic hypothesis is simplistic and there is a need to appreciate the interaction between genetics and other, more socially derived factors.

The media

The media are often cited as one of the major reasons for the increase in diet problems in the developed world (Boyce 2007). Dietz and Gortmaker (1985) was one of the first studies to draw a link between media consumption (i.e. TV viewing) and the prevalence of obesity. Since this time, however, there have been a number of studies that have linked TV viewing and childhood obesity, with the common conclusion being that television viewing is an 'important contributing factor to childhood obesity' (Hancox and Poulton 2006: 171). There are a number of potential explanations for this link, but two predominate. On the one hand, it may be that watching TV encourages a sedentary lifestyle (Marshall et al. 2004); although there is limited exploration of whether media use displaces time spent doing physical activities. Alternatively, it may be that media advertising promotes unhealthy consumption and research has confirmed that this may be the case (Coon and Tucker 2002; Ofcom 2004).

Other explanations for the influence of media on eating behaviour include such descriptions as increased snacking with media use (Coon and Tucker 2002) and the body image presented by the media (Boyce 2007) compared to the use of media in public health campaigns (Miles et al. 2001).

Obesogenic environments

The speed with which obesity has become a global epidemic suggests that environmental or social influences have changed and are promoting weight gain in susceptible people (Hill et al. 2000). Terms such as toxic environment (Ebbeling et al. 2002) and obesogenic environment (e.g. Chopra et al. 2002) have been used to describe some of these influences. The term 'obesogenic environment' was coined by Swinburn et al. (1999), who argued that the physical, economic, social and cultural environments of developed worlds promote positive energy balance (i.e. calorie intake exceeding calorie output) and consequently weight gain and obesity. Industrialised societies have changed considerably since the 1950s. Food security ('The physical, social and economic access to sufficient, safe and nutritious food that meets the dietary needs and food preferences of a population, for an active and healthy life': UN 1998) has now been achieved and cheap transport is now available to the majority of the population. From this simple overview it can be seen how energy consumption has increased and energy expenditure decreased (Fox and Hillsdon 2007).

Examples of environmental influences that may encourage us to eat more than we need include the marketing of energy-dense drinks and snacks, for example through television advertising and vending machines in schools, and the documented increase in portion sizes (Swinburn and Egger 2002) where an average meal may provide up to 2000 kcal — almost the entire recommended daily intake for most adults (Ebbeling et al. 2002).

Time constraints on workers (and the increasing representation of women in the workforce) has led to an increase in demand for convenience food, pre-packaged foods with short preparation times, and in food consumption away from the home (McCrory et al. 1999; Schluter and Lee 1999). This has also led to a decrease in structured meals and an increase in snacking which are often (although not always) densely calorific along with the emergence of fast food restaurants which are associated with a high-fat diet.

On the other hand, the amount of sedentary time spent watching TV by children in the UK has doubled since the 1960s (Reilly and Dorosty 1999) and most European adults now spend more than three hours of each working day sitting (Martinez 2000). In order to expend energy, we need to buy specialist equipment either at home or in the gym, swimming pool or cycle path, but the costs of doing these things may form a barrier for some people (although, of course, it could be argued that exercise can be undertaken in an easy way by increasing our walking or running for example).

Psychosocial factors

There are a number of psychological explanations for individuals having a poor diet but before we explore these in further detail it is worth detailing some of the social barriers that exist.

Among the many influences on diet are availability, cost and time, which are external to the person. An example of such an external barrier to eating a healthy diet is costs: many studies have indicated that the *perceived* high costs of fruit and vegetables is a barrier for people on low income (e.g. John and Ziebland 2004). Socially deprived areas may lack local sources of reasonably priced, good-quality fruit and vegetables, causing a vicious circle of poor demand and supply. People on low income may have less access to cars and consequently out-of-town shopping centres and are thus unable to transport food in bulk (Caraher et al. 1998). Furthermore, there is a perception that fruit and vegetables are time-consuming to prepare and this is a frequently cited barrier (Anderson et al. 1998). Interventions to increase fruit and vegetable consumption among people on low income, or living in socially deprived neighbourhoods may need to include incentives and delivery schemes as well as motivational advice (Anderson et al. 2001).

Some key social factors associated with a poor diet include the following:

- *Low income and debt:* Healthier foods are generally more expensive than the less healthy alternatives. Fresh fruit and vegetables are less affordable.
- *Poor accessibility to affordable healthy foods:* Many local shops are closing and being replaced with larger, out-of-town stores. This is particularly an issue in deprived areas where such developments mean that there are increased costs within the local shops, poor quality foodstuffs and less choice remaining in the locality. The out-of-town public stores may have poor transport links and consequently not be as easily accessible as the local shops with poor quality and expensive food.
- *Factors involved in food production and the food chain:* The cheap nutrient content of easily available food stuffs such as TV-dinners may have high fat, sugar or salt content.

- *Poor literacy and numeracy skills:* These are barriers to maintaining a healthy diet, household budget, management and employment.
- *Food labelling:* The recently introduced food labelling agreement means that more information is available to the consumer. However, there is still some disagreement about the nature of the information provided and the value derived by the consumer from the information.
- *Food marketing:* The adverts to children usually focus on food that is high in fat or sugar. Consequently, the government is introducing new restrictions on what can be advertised and marketed to young children. However, there is still doubt about the finer details of this approach and given its recent introduction the success is yet to be assessed.

Improving diet and nutrition has been the subject of increasing UK policy focus in recent years. For example, *Choosing a Better Diet: A Food and Health Action Plan* (DoH 2005) outlines government's aims and objectives to improve diet and consequent health. It focuses on providing better information and aims to reduce the prevalence of diet-related disease, obesity and improve the nutritional balance of the average diet. It is also of interest to note that the government report is entitled *Choosing a Better Diet* and that Wardle (2007: 73) suggests, among others, that energy intake and expenditure are a 'consequence of behaviours (e.g. choosing foods . . .)'. But as we have seen there are considerable social factors that are associated with poor diet – the obesogenic environment highlights some of these – and consequently a simple *choice* model is not sufficient.

The essence of lifestyle and unhealthy and healthy behaviours is relatively simple. In the case of eating and diet, most people know that certain 'rich' foods (HFSS – high in fat, salt and sugar – foods) are bad for them, and that exercise is good for them (Bell and Esse 2002; Maio et al. 2007), yet many continue to eat too much and exercise too little. Eating 'rich' foods that provide excessive calories and salt content (i.e. HFSS foods) can result in positive sensations and rewards. HFSS foods are ever more present and there is a greater choice of foodstuffs on offer. Ironically, however, freedom of choice makes it more difficult to resist temptation and eat healthily. Other research also indicates that stress (Kruglanski and Webster 1996; Muraven and Baumeister 2000) and habit formation (Wood et al. 2002) also impede the ability to resist temptation.

The family is an important component of healthy eating. Children's dislike of fruit and vegetables was raised by many of the parents in studies (John and Ziebland, 2004). Hence, interventions cannot be described and enacted in a vacuum and approaches have to include the whole household. Women are more likely to shop and prepare the main meal and need to juggle the needs and tastes of their children and partners. Marshall (1995) highlighted that families tend to choose a narrow and repetitive range of fruit and vegetables that were not objected to by the rest of the family. Indeed, any intervention aimed at improving diet needs to take the social context – whether this is the family, peers or the wider context – into account.

Models of eating behaviour

Three core theoretical psychological perspectives have addressed the reasons why people have unhealthy diets. The developmental approach suggests that food preferences are learned in childhood and can be understood in terms of exposure, social learning and associative learning. The cognitive approach explores the extent to which cognitions predict and explain behaviour. The psychophysiological approach focuses on the biological aspects of eating and emphasises the importance of hunger and satiety. These approaches will be explored in more detail below.

Developmental approach

This approach suggests that diet is related to the development in early childhood. Based on research examining the facial expressions of newborn babies, there appears to be an innate preference for sweet and salty flavours and for the avoidance of bitter and sour tastes (Rosenstein and Oster 1988). Such preferences are thought to reflect an evolutionary background where sweetness predicts a source of energy and bitterness predicts toxicity. Because children eat what they like and leave the rest (Anliker et al. 1991) food preferences are important determinants of food intake in young children. The choices children make are particularly important when considering the overall nutritional quality of their diets, yet many show fear and avoidance of novel foods. The tendency to reject novel foods has been termed neophobia. Research has begun to reveal how early experience and learning can reduce the neophobic response to new foods, thereby enhancing dietary variety. For example, Birch and Marlin (1982) found that when 2 year olds were given varying numbers of opportunities to taste new fruits or cheeses, their preferences increased with frequency of exposure. Researchers found that between five and ten exposures to a new food were necessary before preference for that food increased.

In another study, Gerrish and Mennella (2001) investigated the acceptance of a novel taste (pureed carrot) by infants who had previously experienced a range of tastes that included many vegetables but not carrot. Exposure to fruit, carrots alone or a variety of vegetables resulted in an increased acceptance of pureed carrot. Furthermore, those who had been exposed to a variety of vegetables were also more likely to eat other novel foods. Researchers concluded that familiarity with a variety of flavours increased the acceptance of novel foods. The implication was that parents should expose their children to a wide variety of tastes to encourage the acceptance of novel foods. Given the role of parents in bringing food into the home, they play a major role in determining the foods to which a child is exposed. Consequently, exposure is a major factor in encouraging consumption.

There are important developmental, gender and individual differences in the strength of the neophobic response. For example, Hursti and Sjöden (1997) report moderate relationships between parent's and children's neophobia, while Koivisto and Sjöden (1996) report that males show greater neophobia than females, among both children and adults. The authors also confirmed that during childhood, the neophobic response to new foods decreases with age thus providing further support for the exposure hypothesis. Although repeated opportunities to taste and eat new food has been found to reduce neophobia and enhance acceptance, merely smelling or looking at the food has no such effect (Birch et al. 1987). This finding is consistent with the learned safety hypothesis which suggests that neophobia is only reduced as we learn that the food is safe to eat and does not cause illness (Kalat and Rozin 1973). Further evidence suggests that watching others consume the food may provide a form of 'exposure by proxy' or modelling which could also reduce rejection (Birch 1980; Hobden and Pilner 1995).

For infants and children, eating is typically a social event and others can have a considerable impact on children's food preferences and food selections. Support for the efficacy of social learning comes from Birch (1980), who demonstrated that children's preferences for and consumption of disliked vegetables were enhanced when children observed peers selecting and eating foods that the observing child disliked. Further support comes from a series of studies evaluating the 'Food Dude Programme' (see p. 80), a multi-component intervention combining video-based peer modelling together with rewards for eating fruit and vegetables. Evaluation of the programme showed that exposure to the 'Food Dudes' significantly increased fruit and vegetable consumption (Lowe et al. 2001; Lowe et al. 2002).

Research has also focused on the role of parents and teachers. Olivera et al. (1992) found a correlation between mother and child intake for most nutrients in preschool children and Contento et al. (1993) found a relationship between mother's health motivation and the quality of children's diets. Parental behaviour and attitudes are therefore central to the process of social learning, however this association is not straightforward, as parents often differentiate between themselves and their children in terms of food-related motivations and food choice (e.g. Alderson and Ogden 1999). In another study, Jansen and Tenney (2001) examined the consumption of high or low energy yoghurt drinks, with and without a teacher who was also drinking the product. Researchers found a preference for the taste was greatest for those taking the higher energy drink at the same time as the teacher. It was concluded that a preference for energy rich food was most easily established in the presence of an important adult. Based on these findings it is easy to see how observing a parent eating energy dense food could potentially encourage a child to establish similar food preferences.

The effectiveness of the role model has been found to differ depending on the relationship between the child and the model. For example, Birch (1980) and Duncker (1938, cited in Birch 1999) report that older children are more effective role models than younger children; Harper and Sanders (1975) report that mothers are more effective than strangers; and for older preschool children, adult heroes are more effective than ordinary adults (Birch 1999). Obviously this has been revealed with other lifestyle behaviours such as smoking (see Chapter 6).

The role of social learning is also shown in the impact of food advertising. In a content analysis of food advertisements airing during television programmes heavily viewed by children, researchers found that convenience, snack, fast foods and sweets comprised 83 per cent of advertised foods. Food companies and advertising agencies have denied that the content of advertisements or the number of advertisements play a significant role in causing weight gain; however, Lobstein and Dibb (2005) found that such a direct link was probable. A significant relationship between the proportion of children overweight and the number of advertisements per hour on children's television was found, especially those advertisements that encourage the consumption of energy dense foods. Furthermore they found a weaker negative association between the proportion of children overweight and the number of advertisements encouraging a healthier diet. The researchers concluded that the quantity of advertising on children's television appears to be related to the prevalence of excess body weight among children, while the content of the advertising also appears to have a specific effect. In light of this, 'junk food' advertising was banned to under 16 year olds from January 2007 such that advertisements of HFSS foods were not allowed during the following programmes:

- all pre-school children's programmes
- all programmes on mainstream channels aimed at children
- all cable and satellite children's channels
- programmes aimed at young people, such as music shows
- general entertainment programmes which would appeal to a 'higher than average' number of under-16s.

These restrictions did not apply a complete pre-watershed ban but applied to all programmes running any time of the day that has an 'above-average' audience of under 16 year olds. 'Above average' is defined as any programme that has a 20 per cent higher proportion of under 16 year olds viewing it than the UK average. Ofcom claimed that the new regulations will reduce the number of junk food ads seen by under 16 year olds by 41 per cent and the key group of under 9 year olds by 51 per cent. Although the ban has reduced the amount of adverts seen by children of 'junk food', the impact on diet is harder to judge.

In contrast to social learning, associative learning refers to any learning process in which a new response becomes associated with a particular stimulus. In terms of eating behaviour research has focused on the pairing of food cues with certain aspects of the environment, for example food has been paired with a reward, used as the reward and paired with physiological consequences.

Various studies have explored the impact of controlling food intake by rewarding the consumption of healthy food. For example, Birch et al. (1980) gave children food in association with positive adult attention and found that preference for that food increased. Similarly, the Food Dude Programme includes a significant reward component comprising a range of Food Dude prizes (stickers, pens, lunchboxes etc.). Evaluation of the programme found that there were some positive effects of reward alone, but not as great as when modelling and rewards were combined (Lowe et al. 1998).

Promise of a reward is a time-honoured parental tactic for promoting consumption of healthy food. Nevertheless, it has been argued that treating food consumption in this way may actually decrease liking for that food. Lepper and Greene's (1978) overjustification theory argues that offering a reward for an action devalues it for the child. In support of this a number of studies have reported decreased liking for foods when children are rewarded for eating them (e.g. Birch et al. 1982; Birch et al. 1984; Newman and Taylor 1992). Birch (1999) concluded that:

> although these practices can induce children to eat more vegetables in the short run, evidence from our research suggests that in the long run parental control attempts may have negative effects on the quality of children's diets by reducing their preferences for those foods.
>
> (Birch 1999: 53)

Discrepancies in findings between studies may arise from differences in outcome measures, the context in which rewards are given, or indeed the types of rewards offered (Wardle et al. 2003). Horne et al. (2004) argue that in order for rewards to be effective, it is important that they are highly desirable and that they indicate to the child that they are for behaviour which is enjoyable and high status.

Other studies have investigated the impact of using food as a reward. For example, Birch et al. (1980) presented children with foods either as a reward, a snack or in a non-social situation and found that acceptance increased if the food was presented as a reward. It is easy to generalise this finding to real life situations. High fat and sweet items are used repeatedly in positive contexts, for example on special occasions. The consumption of already pleasurable items in this way is reinforced. If children are given foods as rewards for approved behaviour, preference for those foods is enhanced (Benton 2004).

There is a wealth of literature exploring the association between food cues and the physiological responses that follow consumption. These responses can be positive, as the repeated association of food sensory cues with pleasant post-ingestive signals can produce learned preferences. For example there is something satisfying about high energy dense food. When children consumed yoghurts with novel flavours that varied in their fat content and hence energy density, their preference increased for flavours paired with the high but not low energy dense yoghurt (Johnson and Birch 1991). Thus, flavour and high caloric density can create taste preference as we tend to like foods that result in satiety. On the other hand, the association of a food with a negative gastrointestinal response such as nausea may result in the acquisition of a food aversion (Myers and Sclafani 2006).

The developmental model emphasises the importance of learning and focuses on the development of food preferences in childhood. From this perspective eating behaviour is influenced by exposure, social learning and associative learning. Nevertheless, there are some problems with this approach. First, much of the research carried out from this perspective has been conducted in the laboratory and the ecological validity of such approaches is questionable. Second, food can represent aspects of the self, is central to social interaction and communication and is a symbol of cultural and religious identity, factors that are largely ignored by the developmental model (Lupton 1995). Third, although the model includes a role for cognitions (as some of the meanings of food are considered to motivate behaviour) these cognitions are not explicitly described (Ogden 2003a). Finally, the model suggests that because food preferences are learned they are modifiable which is not always an accurate reflection of the current state.

Cognitive approach

Cognitive models of eating behaviour explore the extent to which cognitions predict and explain behaviour. Most research from a cognitive perspective has drawn on social cognition models and several models have been developed: the health belief model (HBM: Becker and Rosenstock 1984), protection motivation theory (PMT: Rogers 1985), health action process approach (HAPA: Schwarzer 1992), theory of reasoned action (TRA: Fishbein and Ajzen 1975) and its descendant the theory of planned behaviour (TPB: Ajzen 1985). All five models share the assumption that attitudes and beliefs are major determinants of eating behaviour, however they vary in terms of the cognitions they include and whether they use behavioural intentions or actual behaviour as their outcome measure (see Chapter 2 for an overview).

Social cognition models have been used extensively in the prediction of eating behaviour, for this reason the rest of this section will focus on research utilising the TRA and the TPB. The TRA seeks to explain behaviour which is under the control of the individual. With volitional behaviours it is argued that behavioural intention is the best predictor of actual behaviour. In turn, intention is predicted by two components: the individual's attitude towards the behaviour and the perceived social pressure to perform the behaviour (i.e. subjective norms). The TPB, however, seeks to be applicable to non-volitional behaviours and includes a component of perceived behavioural control in addition to attitudes and subjective norms. When PBC matches actual behavioural control, PBC is theorised to have a direct influence on behaviour.

Some research using the TRA and TPB has focused on predicting behavioural intentions. Research suggests however, that behavioural intentions are not that successful in predicting actual behaviour. In the nutrition literature for example, many studies have attempted to measure the degree of association between attitudes and consumption of foods. Axelson et al. (1985) performed a meta-analysis of such studies and found evidence for a small although statistically significant correlation between attitudes and behaviour (r = 0.18). Thus a superficial survey of this area may lead one to conclude that attitudes are not related to behaviour to an important degree. Consequently studies have also used the TRA and TPB to explore the cognitive predictors of actual behaviour. For example, Kassem and Lee (2004) used the TPB to predict soft drink consumption in pupils aged 13–18 years and found that the strongest predictor was attitude followed by perceived behavioural control and subjective norm, all of which were significant predictors. Attitude has also been found to be the best predictor of consumption of non-milk extrinsic sugars (Astrom and Okullo 2004), percentage fat intake and healthy eating, defined as a diet low in fat, high in fibre and high in fruit and vegetable consumption (Conner et al. 2002). The incorporation of perceived behavioural control has also received some support. For example, Masalu and Astrom (2001) used the TPB to predict between meal consumption of sugared snacks and drinks and found that PBC was the strongest predictor of behavioural intention (0.35) over and above attitudes (0.25) and subjective norms (0.28). It was also found that PBC had a significant direct effect on behaviour (0.18), although this was not as great as behavioural intentions (0.25). Subjective norm has been found to be a consistently poor predictor of eating behaviour.

Although the TRA and TPB have proved relatively successful in predicting eating behaviour, recent calls have been made to extend the models to include additional factors. For example, Sparks et al. (1995)

demonstrated that moral or ethical concerns added significantly to the prediction of intention to consume genetically modified foods. Paisley and Sparks (1998) examined the predictors of fat intake and included a measure of perceived need and found a significant increase in the variance accounted for, even after other important determining factors were taken into account. Researchers have also explored the role of ambivalence in predicting behaviour. Sparks et al. (2001) examined attitudes towards consumption of chocolate and meat. In line with previous research the results showed that attitude was the strongest predictor of intentions, however the relationship between attitude and intention was weaker in those with higher levels of ambivalence. Thus researchers concluded that holding both positive and negative attitudes towards a particular food will make it less likely that an attitude will be translated into an intention to eat it.

Trafimow (2000) argued for the addition of habit. Traditionally habit has been measured by the number of times behaviour has been performed in the past (Trandis 1977). Evidence to date, indicates past behaviour has a direct effect on current behaviour, even when TPB cognitions are taken into account. For example, Conner et al. (1999) used the TPB to predict alcohol consumption and found that a measure of past behaviour contributed to predictions of intentions over and above the contribution of attitudes, subjective norms and PBC. It was also found that past behaviour contributed to predictions of alcohol consumption over and above the contributions from intentions and PBC. Nevertheless behavioural recurrence does not constitute direct evidence for habitual processes. Verplanken and Orbell (2003) argue that habit is a psychological construct rather than behavioural recurrence and involves lack of awareness, difficulty to control, mental efficiency and repetition. Although repetition is a necessary requirement for a habit to develop, subsequent research has supported the hypothesis that frequency of past behaviour and habit are separate constructs (e.g. Verplanken 2006). Based on this conceptualisation, Brug et al. (2006) found that the addition of habit strength significantly increased explained variance in fruit intake and fruit intake intentions.

These cognitive models of eating behaviour explore the extent to which cognitions predict and explain behaviour. Cognitive models not only are informative with regard to their ability to predict behaviour but also provide a helpful insight into ways of influencing this behaviour (Stroebe and Stroebe 1995). However, there are several problems with this approach. First, most research carried out within this perspective devises questionnaires based on existing models. This means that the cognitions being examined are rather limited. It may be possible that cognitions central to the understanding of eating behaviour are missed out. Likewise, the cognitions that are incorporated in the models ignore the wealth of meanings associated with food and food-related behaviour (Ogden

2003a). Second, the cognitive approach assumes that behaviour is the consequence of rational thought; it fails to account for automatic processes and the role of affect. Third, although some cognitive models incorporate the view of others in the form of subjective norms, they have been criticised for their focus on individual level variables and for the assumption that the same set of cognitions are relevant to all individuals (e.g. Resnicow et al. 1997). Fourth, Sutton (1998) argues that models of health beliefs are ineffective at predicting behavioural intentions and even less effective at predicting actual behaviour. He argues that studies using these models explain between 40 and 50 per cent of the variance in behavioural intentions and only 19–38 per cent of the variance in actual behaviour. Thus a large proportion of the variance is left unexplained. Finally, Ogden (2003b) scrutinised articles published between 1997 and 2001 that tested or applied one or more social cognition models and highlighted several conceptual limitations. First, cognitive models do not enable the generation of hypotheses because their constructs are unspecific and therefore unable to be tested. Second, they focus on analytic truths as opposed to synthetic ones and the conclusions resulting from their application are often true by definition rather than by observation. Third, although intended to measure an individual's cognitions, questionnaires based on social cognition models may change rather than access the way a person thinks. Such an approach may also change subsequent behaviour.

Psychophysiological approach

The psychophysiological approach focuses on the biological aspects of eating and emphasises the importance of hunger and satiety. It explores the relationship between an individual's physiology, cognitions and behaviour and is implicitly related to both the developmental and cognitive approaches described earlier.

Food has several sensory properties which influence food choice and eating behaviour, for instance appearance, odour and taste. For example, MacDougal (1987) demonstrated that the degree of illumination used to display foods, influenced food choice. Likewise, Griep et al. (1995) and Reaich (1997) report an association between declining odour perception, malnutrition and a reduced food intake. Numerous studies have demonstrated that high palatability increases food consumption (e.g. Yeomans 1996; Yeomans et al. 1997; Yeomans and Symes 1999). Nevertheless there are inconsistencies in the literature (e.g. Rogers and Blundell 1990; Warwick et al. 1993). Shepherd and Farleigh (1989) suggest that inconsistencies may be due to the use of different measures of both sensory attributes and intake.

Psychopharmacology provides a useful means to understand the neurochemical basis for hunger and satiety. For example, the inverse relationship between tobacco smoking and body weight has been noted for over a century (Kitchen 1889, cited in Perkins 1992). It is commonly observed that smokers weigh less than non-smokers (Albanes et al. 1987) and gain weight after stopping (Williamson et al. 1991). Amphetamines have also been shown to have a dramatic suppressant effect on food intake and have been offered to dieters both legally and illegally for many years. Foltin et al. (1988) gave volunteers two cigarettes containing active marijuana or a placebo and found that active marijuana increased total caloric intake by 40 per cent. Finally, studies exploring the relationship between alcohol and food intake have been contradictory. In a mini-review Gee (2006) found that among eight studies reviewed, only one showed a significant difference in appetite ratings between the alcohol and no alcohol pre-load. However, in three of the eight studies reviewed, significant differences were found in energy intake following a high dose alcohol pre-load as opposed to a no-alcohol pre-load. Gee (2006) concluded that the effect of alcohol on appetite appears to be unsubstantiated; however alcohol's effect on energy intake does appear significant.

As well as recreational drugs, anti-psychotics and antidepressants have also been shown to influence hunger and satiety. Kaur and Kulkarni (2002) examined the effects of typical (i.e. chlorpromazine and haloperidol) and atypical (i.e. clozapine and risperidone) anti-psychotics on feeding behaviour in mice. Researchers reported increased food intake and body weight gain following administration of both types of anti-psychotic. Clozapine-induced hyperphagia (abnormally increased appetite) was significantly reversed after treatment with several serotonergic agents, thus serotonin may prove useful to counteract anti-psychotic-induced obesity. In line with this, selective serotonin reuptake inhibitors (SSRIs), a class of antidepressant, significantly attenuate body weight gain in rodents and weight loss in obese humans can be elicited via treatment with the serotonin precursor 5-hydroxytryptophan (Halford et al. 2007).

The psychophysiological approach has also focused on the relationship between stress and eating behaviour. The notion of stress–eating associations has received widespread scientific support, nevertheless research is often contradictory. For example, stress has been linked to both an increase in eating (hyperphagia) and a decrease in eating (hypophagia) and debate continues over what factors mediate or moderate this relationship. Support for stress induced hypophagia comes largely from animal studies (e.g. Robbins and Fray 1980); still no clear consensus has emerged. In a review of the literature Greeno and Wing (1994) concluded that chronic stressors such as lighting and noise tend to facilitate hypophagia, while mild stressors such as tail pinching and low intensity shocks often result in hyperphagia. Real world studies involving human participants have been just as inconsistent. Michaud et al. (1990) found that students consume more energy on the day of an examination than on a subsequent no-stress non-examination day (hyperphagia). In contrast, in one of the few naturalistic studies utilising a longitudinal design, researchers found that the vast majority of participants (72 per cent) demonstrated a hypophagic response to stress whereas only 28 per cent demonstrated a hyperphagic response.

Thus at times stress increases food intake while at others it causes a decrease. Greeno and Wing (1994) proposed two hypotheses to explain this paradox; the general effect model, which predicts that stress changes food intake in all exposed organisms, and the individual difference model which predicts individual differences in the vulnerability to stress-induced eating. More recent research has focused on the individual difference model and examined factors such as gender and dietary restraint. For example, Michaud et al. (1990) argue that stress is related to increased food intake in girls but not boys, and Wardle et al. (2000) argue that stress is related to increased food intake in dieters only. In contrast, Oliver and Wardle (1999) reported increased snacking behaviour in 73 per cent of participants regardless of gender or dieting status. Similarly, Cartwright et al. (2003) found that neither weight nor gender moderated the relationship between stress and eating. They did find, however, that stress was associated with eating more fatty foods, less fruit and vegetables, more snacking and a reduced likelihood of daily breakfast consumption.

The psychophysiological approach focuses on the biological aspects of eating and emphasises the importance of hunger and satiety. It examines the role of chemical senses, pharmacological drugs, neurochemicals and stress on food choice and eating behaviour. There are several problems with this approach. First, much of the research carried out within this perspective has been conducted in the laboratory and extent to which these findings would generalise to a more naturalistic setting remains unclear. Similarly, many studies have used animals and the extent to which research can be extrapolated to human behaviour is also unclear. Second, the psychophysiological approach minimises the social context surrounding food choice and eating behaviour. Like the developmental and cognitive models it ignores the diverse set of meanings which surround food choice and eating behaviour. Finally, the psychophysiological approach assumes that an individual will eat when hungry and stop when satiated; however, many individuals override the desire to eat, due to a desire for thinness. Similarly many override the drive to stop eating, due to the desire for a treat (Ogden 2003a).

Interventions to improve diet

Given the extent of the obesity problem in the UK and the potential considerable health difficulties associated with this, it is not surprising that the UK government (along with the separate legislatures) has developed strategic plans to counteract the looming difficulties. For example, the Food and Health Action Plan and the Activity Coordination Team is a cross-government group (led by the DoH) to improve public health through better diet. Examples of such action include:

- *Breastfeeding:* encouraging more women to breastfeed and to continue for at least six months.
- *Reform of the Welfare Food Scheme:* ensuring children in poverty have access to a healthy diet and increasing support for breastfeeding.
- *FIVE-A-DAY programme:* including the National School Fruit Scheme.
- *Food in Schools Programme:* promoting a 'whole school approach' and encouraging greater access to healthier choices within schools.
- *Work with the food industry:* addressing the amount of fat, salt and added sugar in the diet (with the Food Standards Agency).
- *New GP contract:* requiring practices to offer relevant health promotion advice to patients.

One such initiative is the school fruit and vegetable scheme (SFVS), part of the five-a-day programme to increase fruit and vegetable consumption. The scheme entitles every child aged four to six attending local education authority maintained infant, primary and special schools to a free piece of fruit or a vegetable on each school day. Initial evaluation of the SFVS was disappointing (Schagen et al. 2005). Researchers found that fruit consumption increased by about half a portion a day, but there did not appear to be any wider impact on diet. Furthermore, increased consumption was not sustained when children were no longer eligible to take part in the scheme. Researchers argued that the SFVS may have had a longer term impact if children were exposed to the scheme for a greater period of time, as the Year 3 pupils tested had been in the scheme for only four months (Schagen et al. 2005).

Two years after the previous survey, the Department of Health commissioned the National Foundation for Educational Research (NFER) to explore the impact of the SFVS further. The Year 3 pupils at this time had been involved with the scheme for two years and four months. Researchers found that overall daily fruit and vegetable consumption had risen from 3.65 portions to 4.41 portions per day. As in 2004, fruit consumption declined as children grew older, and the SFVS had not counteracted this effect. However, for the Year 3 children, the general increase in fruit and vegetable consumption had compensated for the decrease which occurs with age, hence they were eating as much as they did in Year 1. Although there was a significant positive change in fruit consumption, the increase over time was mainly in terms of vegetables. Further investigation suggested that school dinners had contributed to this change, with by far the biggest increase being vegetable consumption in those who ate school dinners. Although fruit and vegetable consumption increased, there was not a significant decrease in consumption of snacks and desserts overall. There was however a small yet significant decrease in snack consumption for those having school dinners, thus providing evidence to suggest that recent campaigns to improve school dinners are beginning to have an impact (Blenkinsop et al. 2007). Recent review evidence (The Strategy Unit 2008) suggested that there had been limited success in improving the population's diet and there was still considerable work to be done to try and improve the consumption of fruit and vegetables up to the recommended five portions or more per week.

In 2005 a documentary series was broadcast in which TV chef Jamie Oliver attempted to improve the quality and nutritional value of school dinners at a typical British school – a goal which ultimately led to a broader campaign called 'Feed me better'. Subsequently, the secretary of state for Education and Skills announced a £235 million package to improve the quality of school meals. At the same time the School Food Trust (SFT) was announced, a public body sponsored by the Department for Education and Skills (DfES) to provide support and advice to schools and parents. Since September 2006 every pupil taking a school lunch is guaranteed, by law, a balanced, nutritious meal. One of the aims of the SFT is to make sure that children are eating them (SFT 2006). Consequently, they launched a high profile campaign called 'Eat better, do better' to encourage children to see more clearly the link between good food and positive outcomes. Under the banner 'Eat better, do better' the SFT developed a series of initiatives which gives professionals, parents and pupils the information they need to make the right nutritional choice. One of the key targets for the Trust agreed with DfES was an increase in the uptake of school meals by 4 per cent by March 2008. In March 2007 the trust commissioned the Association for Public Service Excellence (APSE) to carry out its second annual survey of school food providers. APSE found that meal uptake in primary schools was down 1 per cent from 2005/06 to 41 per cent, while uptake in secondary schools was down 5 per cent from 2005/06 to 38 per cent. Furthermore only 17 per cent of primary services and 1 per cent of secondary services felt that the SFT would meet the 4 per cent target increase by March 2008 (Nicholas et al. 2007).

Despite considerable efforts over a number of years, there is limited evidence to suggest that educational approaches to dietary change (that is providing basic information about what constitutes a 'healthy' diet) alter children's eating habits (Bajekal et al. 2003; DoH 2005). Clearly, even if children do know what they should be eating, this does not necessarily translate into their dietary behaviour. In light of such evidence, a group of psychologists from the University of Bangor developed the Food Dude Programme (see Figure 3.6) based on underlying psychological principles.

The Food Dude Programme is specifically designed for 4–11 year olds to encourage the consumption of fruit and vegetables. The theoretical position of the programme is primarily based on research into learning and cognitive processes in particular peer modelling and rewards (Horne et al. 2004). Children watch a series of fun video episodes featuring the

Food Dudes, a group of positive role model kids who gain superpowers when they eat fruit and vegetables. The children are then given the opportunity to taste fruit and vegetables themselves. If they succeed in consuming these foods, then a variety of Food Dude stickers and prizes are given out as rewards. There is also a home pack to support the programme, which includes a diary to record fruit and vegetable consumption, plus tips and advice on healthy eating. By encouraging children to taste fruit and vegetables repeatedly, the programme helps them to discover the intrinsically rewarding properties of the foods. In the process, they also come to think of themselves as fruit and vegetable eaters in a school culture that is now strongly supportive of healthy eating (Food Dude Healthy Eating Programme 2006).

Initial evaluation of the Food Dude Programme showed that it resulted in large statistically significant increases in fruit and vegetable consumption at snack time and lunch time for both boys and girls in infant and junior schools (Lowe et al. 2001; Lowe et al. 2002). Successive studies have demonstrated that these positive effects are not confined to the foods

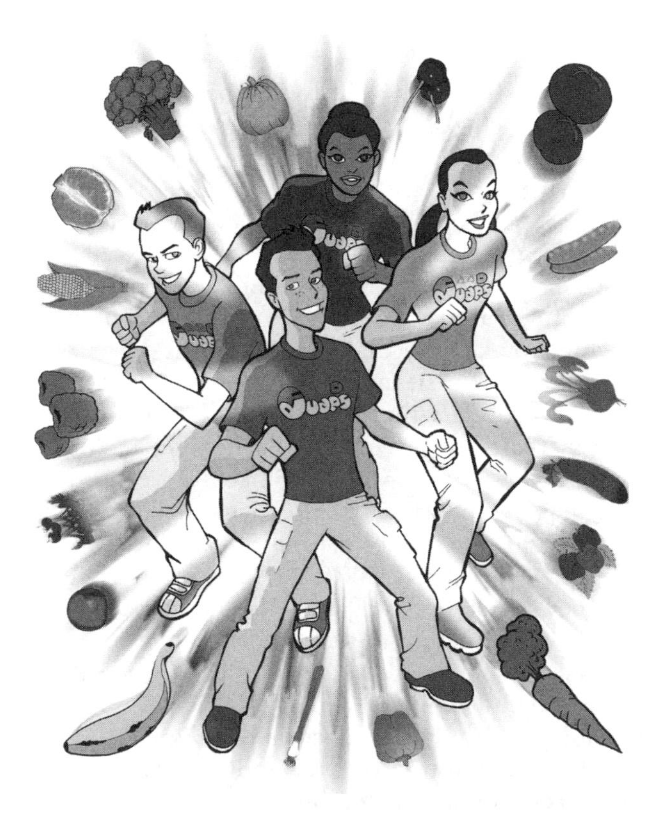

Figure 3.6 The Food Dude Healthy Eating Programme
(Reproduced with permission from Bangor University)

experienced during the programme, but spread to a wide range of other fruit and vegetables. The positive effects have been found to be general across contexts. For example, increased fruit and vegetable consumption at school was reflected by increased consumption at home. In one follow-up study, increases in fruit and vegetable consumption still persisted 15 months after the end of the intervention, highlighting the programme's long-term effectiveness (Lowe et al. 2007).

It has already been suggested that the price and availability of food may pose external barriers to eating a healthy diet. Therefore, ensuring that communities have good access to healthy affordable food is one of the UK government's strategies to improve public health and reduce health inequalities. Policy solutions for deprived communities without good access have focused on improving provision of food retail as part of wider recommendations for population dietary change. However, there is ambiguity over whether large-scale food retail interventions actually work. For example, in an uncontrolled before and after study conducted in Leeds, some small improvements in fruit and vegetables consumption were found, with the most positive impacts being seen in those who switched to the new supermarket compared with those who continued to use their existing provision (Wrigley et al. 2003). In contrast, utilising a controlled before and after design, one Glasgow study found no evidence for an intervention effect on fruit and vegetable consumption (Cummins et al. 2005). The quasi-experimental design utilised by the Glasgow study is important, as unadjusted changes within the intervention area were similar in magnitude to the Leeds study, suggesting that what was being observed was a product of general secular change as opposed to a direct effect of the intervention itself (Cummins and Macintyre 2006).

The food industry also plays a major role in helping individuals make healthier choices. Currently, both the FSA and the Department of Health are working with the food industry to encourage consumers to switch to healthier options. For example, the FSA have agreed new recommendations supporting traffic light front-of-pack labelling, which allows shoppers to see at a glance if a food product is high, medium or low in fat, saturated fat, sugar and salt. To underpin these recommendations, a series of consumer research projects were undertaken to explore peoples understanding of and preferences for a range of signposting concepts. Nonetheless, the FSA have agreed that it is important to assess the impact of the traffic light front of pack labelling system independently, the results of which will not be released until 2008 (FSA 2007).

At the level of the health practitioner, Kearney et al. (2005) report on a brief preventive intervention deployed in primary care consultations in a deprived area in North West England. At the centre of the scheme is a prescription for fruit and vegetables which GPs, nurses, health visitors and midwives issue to patients on an opportunistic basis. Each prescription contains four vouchers offering a £1 discount when £3 or more is spent on fruit and vegetables. As the health professionals issue the prescription they link it explicitly to key five-a-day messages. Evaluation of the intervention is not yet complete; however early feedback suggests that the intervention has a significant impact on patients in highlighting the connection between food and health. Furthermore clinicians express satisfaction with having a simple preventive intervention which takes only one or two minutes, and can be deployed effectively in routine primary care consultations. Primary care remains the public's preferred source of food and health information (Hiddink et al. 1997). It provides a natural setting for health promotion, which is usually long-term and characterised by trust. According to Bourn (2001) approximately two-thirds of the UK's population visit their GP at least annually, so primary care provides an unparalleled opportunity for health promotion and preventive interventions.

Hundreds of interventions to combat the obesity epidemic are currently being introduced worldwide, but there are significant gaps in the evidence base for such interventions and few been evaluated in a way that enables any definitive conclusions to be drawn about their effectiveness. Those that have shown an impact are limited to easily controlled settings and it remains unclear how promising small-scale initiatives would be scaled up for whole population impact (Butland et al. 2007). Counterweight is a primary care weight management programme for adults aged 18–75 years and is the only fully evaluated evidence-based primary care weight management programme in the UK. It is a low cost nurse-led programme which aims to help patients achieve a medically valuable weight loss of 5–10 per cent of initial body weight. The programme incorporates a structured pathway and guidance for the management of obesity and includes training for GPs and practice nurses. Patients are followed up at least quarterly for the first 12 months after the programme and reviewed annually thereafter. The programme is designed to empower the patient through increased patient participation, control and education, for example, through goal setting, relapse prevention management and tailored education materials. The programme centres on an interactive model of care, while drawing upon theory and evidence from learning theory, cognitive restructuring, self-efficacy, self-monitoring and stages of change (Counterweight Project Team 2005).

Evaluation of the Counterweight programme involving over 1500 patients showed that at 12 months, 33 per cent of patients achieved a clinically meaningful weight loss of 5 per cent or more. A total of 49 per cent of patients were classed as completers in that they attended the mandatory number of appointments in 3, 6 or 12 months. 'Completers' achieved more successful weight loss with 40 per cent achieving a weight loss of 5 per cent or more at 12 months. Thus results suggest that the programme provides an effective model for obesity management within general practice (Counterweight Project Team 2005).

When exploring the outcome of such interventions it has been demonstrated that self-efficacy is related to weight controlling behaviour (Dennis and Goldberg 1996; French et al. 1996). Self-efficacy regarding weight loss (Rodin et al. 1988), the ability to handle emotions and life situations (Jeffrey et al. 1984) and exercise have been related to later weight loss maintenance. Follow up data on weight maintainers have also shown that they have more confidence in the ability to manage the weight than the weight regainers (DePue et al. 1995).

The National Institute for Health and Clinical Excellence (NICE 2006a) has published recommendations on how to increase the effectiveness of interventions to improve diet and reduce energy intake. NICE recommends that interventions to improve diet should be multicomponent (i.e. including dietary modification, targeted advice, family involvement and goal setting), tailored to the individual, provide ongoing support, include behaviour change strategies and include awareness raising promotional activities as part of a longer term, multicomponent intervention rather than a one off activity.

Conclusion

Much research suggests that many people do not eat a sufficiently healthy diet. Several explanations have been put forward for why people eat what they do; these have ranged from the genetic, through to the social-environmental and the psychosocial. Countless interventions have been introduced to tackle British people's poor diet; however, the effectiveness of such interventions remains poor. Success is likely to be achieved only if there is a paradigm shift in thinking, not only by the individual, but also by society as a whole. Thus tackling the nation's poor diet is ultimately an issue about lifestyle.

Summary points

- Diet can not only affect health through an individual's weight but also play a role in the development of diseases such as CHD, cancer and diabetes.
- It is estimated that food-related ill health is responsible for about 10 per cent of morbidity and mortality in the UK.
- Healthy eating can be understood in terms of five major food groups and is important for promoting health and treating ill health.
- People living on a low income, in receipt of state benefits and those in social class V have higher rates of diet-related diseases, are more prone to obesity and eat a less varied diet than those in other social groups.
- Evidence from twin and adoption studies have indicated that body weight is strongly influenced by genetic factors.

- Eating behaviour has been shown to be influenced by the media, the environment and social barriers such as availability, cost and time.
- Three core psychological perspectives have addressed the issue of why people eat what they do: the developmental approach, the cognitive approach and the psychophysiological approach.
- The developmental approach emphasises the importance of learning and focuses on the development of food preferences in childhood. From this perspective eating behaviour is influenced by exposure, social learning and associative learning.
- The cognitive model explores the extent to which cognitions predict and explain behaviour.
- The psychophysiological approach focuses on the biological aspects of eating and emphasises the importance of hunger and satiety. In particular it examines the role of the chemical senses, pharmacological drugs, neurochemicals and stress on food choice and eating behaviour.
- Hundreds of interventions to improve diet and combat the obesity epidemic have been introduced worldwide; however, there are significant gaps in the evidence base and few have been evaluated in such a way as to enable any definitive conclusion to be drawn about their effectiveness.

4 Physical activity

> Lack of activity destroys the good condition of every human being, while movement and methodical physical exercise save it and preserve it.
>
> Plato

At the end of this chapter you will:

- understand the definitions of physical activity, exercise and sport
- review the current levels of physical activity in the UK and the individual home countries
- appreciate the relationship between physical activity and health
- explore the explanations of why some people engage in physical activity and some do not
- understand the importance of the obesogenic environment
- review the interventions (both at an individual and public health level) aimed at increasing physical activity.

Definitions of physical activity, exercise and sport

Physical activity, exercise and sport are all terms used comfortably in the lay arena that can be more problematic in academic and professional settings. Whereas the use of the term exercise implies a health-focused activity, the term sport has no such implications. Clearly agreed definitions of these terms are relevant for the promotion of lifestyle change. Physical activity can be defined as:

> Any bodily movement produced by skeletal muscles that results in energy expenditure and is usually measured in kilocalories (kcal) per unit of time.
>
> (Caspersen et al. 1985, cited in Buckworth and Dishman 2002: 28)

This definition of physical activity is undisputed and while broad is at least objective. However, under the umbrella of physical activity the subcategories of exercise and sport are less clearly delineated and involve a degree of subjectivity in definition. Exercise and sport are both terms recognised by most audiences but subtle differences in the way they are understood can be problematic and this can be of particular concern when interpreting research.

For activity to be defined as exercise Caspersen et al. (1985) require the activity to be purposeful. Consequently, they define exercise as:

> Planned, structured, repetitive bodily movements that someone engages in for the purpose of improving or maintaining one or more components of physical fitness or health.
>
> (Caspersen et al. 1985, cited in Buckworth and Dishman 2002: 28)

In adopting this definition, all physical activity that occurs indirectly, for instance through work, travel or play is not exercise.

However, Bouchard et al. (1990) prefer a wider definition of exercise that requires no intention: 'leisure-time physical activity'. This definition encompasses voluntary physical activity regardless of purpose, excluding only activity that is not voluntary and occurs as a result of other obligations, such as work, travel or caring responsibilities.

Both Caspersen et al.'s (1985) purposeful definition of exercise and the broader Bouchard et al. (1990) definition of exercise comfortably include recreational exercise that is health-focused such as aerobic classes, jogging or swimming. The Caspersen et al. (1985) definition can include all sport as long as you assume that everyone plays sport to improve fitness or health, which obviously may not be the case. Bouchard et al.'s (1990) definition avoids any issue of intention and so can include all amateur sporting activity but excludes all professional sportsmen and women. Consequently, the relationship between exercise and sport will depend first on which of the definition of exercise you adopt and second on how you define sport.

Sport is a term that is often defined in academic texts quite narrowly but adopted quite broadly in general use. Biddle and Mutrie (1991: 8) define sport as: 'Rule-governed, structured and competitive and involves gross motor movement characterised by physical strategy, prowess and chance'.

For Biddle and Mutrie (1991) sport is required to be both a formal, competitive game and to involve physical effort whereas in practice many activities that do not meet these criteria are understood to be 'sport'. For instance yoga is non-competitive but falls under the remit of the Sports Council. Darts involves little gross motor movement but is usually described as sport (Radlo et al. 2002). These vagaries in the way the term 'sport' is understood to make the relationship between exercise, which is the concern of health professionals, and sport problematic. Yoga is exercise as defined by the definitions earlier whereas darts is not. Nevertheless, darts is probably more usually described as a sport than yoga. Consequently, a linear relationship between these three levels of activity where sport is a subset of exercise and exercise subset of physical activity, although appealing for its simplicity, cannot describe the relationship effectively. A better model of the relationship is offered in Figure 4.1. Both exercise and sport are subsets of physical activity and the overlap between the two will depend on your definitions.

Initially government attempts to encourage more physical activity and so improve health focused on encouraging more people to take up sport as a leisuretime activity: 'Sport for all' (www.olympic.org, accessed July 2007). As recently as 1999 there was still a focus on encouraging sport:

> To help support the enthusiasm for physical activity and for better health, we will publish a *sports strategy* later this year which will promote greater scope for participation in sport and physical activity for all. It will build on many existing initiatives.
>
> (DoH 1999b: 25)

However, this enthusiasm did not last and during the period since the Department of Health (1999b) published *Saving Lives: Our Healthy Nation* the use of the term sport has become less common in policy documents. The decreasing emphasis on sport is presumably based on the rationale that the competitive element of sport was deterring participation and non-competitive organised exercise would be more attractive to the majority of adults. This approach also has not been as successful as public health professionals would like (DoH 2003; Scottish Executive 2005; National Public Health Service for Wales 2005; National Institute of Health and Clinical Excellence 2006). Consequently, the emphasis of public health initiatives in the twenty-first century has focused on encouraging individual, non-organised physical activity such as walking, cycling, gardening or housework. Sport and formal exercise have been losing

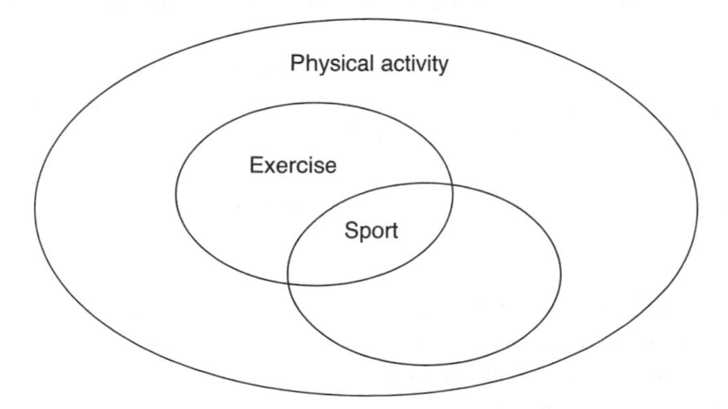

Figure 4.1 The relationship between physical activity, exercise and sport

credibility as potential sources of increased physical activity in the population. The current emphasis on physical activity and clear attempts to de-align physical activity from sport are evident in all public health documentation and policy (DoH 2003, 2004a; Scottish Executive 2005; Welsh Assembly Government 2003; National Institute of Health and Clinical Excellence 2006).

Government recommendations for physical activity

In 1999, the Department of Health document *Saving Lives: Our healthier Nation* recommended that adults took: '30 minutes of moderate exercise 5 times a week' (DoH 1999b). One problem with this recommendation is the use of the word 'moderate'. What is moderate for one person may be either intense or easy for the next. It is plausible that definitions of moderate may vary widely not only in the general population but also among health professionals. The Welsh Assembly Government's document *Healthy and Active Lifestyles in Wales: A framework for action* (Welsh Assembly Government 2003) does provide a definition of moderate:

> Moderate intensity activities include brisk walking, swimming, cycling, dancing, using stairs, sweeping and comparable intensity gardening or housework tasks.
>
> (Welsh Assembly Government 2003: 4)

The American position on appropriate levels of physical activity is similar to that in the UK. In 1999 the US Surgeon General stated that:

> Significant health benefits can be obtained by including a moderate amount of physical activity (e.g. 30 minutes of brisk walking or raking leaves, 15 minutes of running or 45 minutes of playing volleyball) on most, if not all, days of the week.
>
> (US Department of Health and Human Services 1999: 10)

The Surgeon General alludes to the relationship between intensity and duration and health benefits by suggesting that lower intensity exercise needs to be carried out for a longer duration to achieve the same health benefits as higher intensity exercise. Furthermore, the Surgeon General goes on to recognise the increasing benefits from increasing the duration or intensity of exercise:

> Additional health benefits can be gained through greater amounts of physical activity. People who can maintain a regular regimen of activity that is of longer duration or of more vigorous activity are likely to derive greater benefit.
>
> (US Department of Health and Human Services 1999: 10)

Both in the UK and in the United States, the guidelines introduce a suggestion that the appropriate level of exercise for good health is not definitive. Certainly, for weight loss there are arguments that higher levels of activity are necessary (Schoeller et al. 1997). There have been strong calls in Britain for the advice to change from moderate to vigorous, perhaps in recognition that a practitioner understanding of the term 'moderate' may be more vigorous than a lay understanding of the term 'moderate' (BBC News 2007). This call stems from a change in the American guidelines to make vigorous physical activity an integral aspect of the recommended physical activity levels (American College of Sports Medicine 2007). Furthermore, the American recommendations make explicit that physical activity in excess of the minimum recommendations will provide even greater health benefits (American College of Sports Medicine 2007). However, benefits would accrue from the majority of the population meeting the current government targets for physical activity. Church et al. (2007) found that 50 per cent, 100 per cent and 150 per cent of the recommended 150 minutes of physical activity a week all accrued increases in physical fitness and the relationship appeared to be linear. Consequently, Lee (2007: 2138) concluded: 'Even a little is good, more may be better'. Furthermore, there is considerable evidence, discussed in depth in subsequent sections of this chapter, that setting achievable goals is good practice in encouraging behavioural change (Ajzen 1998). Given the current levels of physical activity in Great Britain and other Western countries, increasing the recommended targets may be counter-productive if they are likely to be unachievable.

Evidence of the problem

Measuring physical activity

It is beyond the scope of this book to review and evaluate the full range of methods available to measure physical activity. For this purpose there are a number of exercise psychology and exercise physiology texts (Buckworth and Dishman 2002; American College of Sports Medicine 2005). Nevertheless, it would be inappropriate to evaluate levels of physical activity without acknowledging that different methodologies for measurement exist.

There are more than 30 different methods for measuring physical activity (Buckworth and Dishman 2002) and the selection of method hinges on appropriateness for the target population and the level of sensitivity and specificity necessary to answer the research question. A large-scale survey of population habits requires a less precise instrument than an individual activity assessment on which recommendations for an individuals' future behaviour will be based.

Methods can be categorised by what they measure: physiological response during physical activity, energy expenditure during activity, physiological adaptation to activity or direct/indirect observation of physical activity. The first three methods are objective assessments of activity whereas observation is a more subjective assessment. These methods can be evaluated by their ability to provide information on the type, duration, intensity and frequency of physical activity.

Epidemiological studies that provide measures of the physical activity of populations have typically utilised indirect observation methods, most usually questionnaires. Questionnaires range from self-report single-item questions to interviewer-administered questionnaires on lifetime physical activity. The more complex questionnaires will measure type, frequency, duration and intensity of activity providing many possible levels of analysis. The best studies will utilise a questionnaire that has been validated by an objective measure of physiological response to physical activity (such as heart rate monitoring) or an objective measure of energy expenditure (such as doubly labelled water) (Krista and Caspersen 1997). Questionnaires are cost-effective and practical whereas objective measures of energy expenditure are more precise but not practical for large-scale studies.

Current activity levels

Physical activity was measured in different ways in the English, Welsh, Scottish and Northern Irish Surveys (DoH, Social Services and Public Safety 2001; DoH 2003; Scottish Executive 2005; Welsh Assembly Government 2007) making detailed comparisons impossible. All the surveys asked participants about whether they met the governments' targets for weekly physical activity, enabling one comparison between all four surveys to be made (Table 4.1).

Table 4.1 Percentages of men and women living in the UK achieving the government guidelines for weekly physical activity

Source of data	*People achieving government guidelines (%)*	*Men achieving government activity guidelines (%)*	*Women achieving government activity guidelines (%)*
Health Survey England 2003	30.5	37	24
Scottish Health Survey 2003	38.5	44	33
Welsh Health Survey 2005–06	31	38	25
Northern Ireland Health and Social Wellbeing Survey 2001	28.5	30	27

Nearly a decade after the Department of Health (1999b) published its recommended physical activity levels and after ten years of policy and interventions attempting to encourage the population to meet these recommendations, still less than one-third of the populations of England, Wales and Northern Ireland are meeting these criteria (Table 4.1). Scotland has the best figures and even here considerably less than half the population are active. These figures are more alarming when broken down by age and it emerges that older people are even less likely to participate in physical activity (Table 4.2). The impact of at least a decade of interventions to increase physical activity, at first sight, does not appear very impressive. Any reversal of the downward trend in physical activity levels, however modest, would be encouraging.

The Health Survey for England (Primatesta 2004) looked at trends in physical activity between surveys carried out in 1997, 1998 and 2003. It did not find an overall trend for increasing activity although it found some increases in the proportion of older people meeting the recommended activity levels. Other surveys of activity report similar findings. The Department of Health, Physical Activity, Health Improvement and Prevention (2004) reports that since the late 1970s there has been a small increase in the proportion of people engaging in leisure activity but a reduction in routine physical activity, such as that achieved through necessary activities of work, travel or running a home. For example, the physically active aspects of housework have reduced, but most noticeably fewer people travel by foot or bicycle. The Office for National Statistics (2003) reported that distances walked annually dropped by 63 miles between 1975 and 2003. Similarly, distances cycled dropped by 16 miles in the same period. The proportion of people who travel by walking or cycling has declined by 26 per cent (Department of Health, Physical Activity, Health Improvement and Prevention 2004). Consequently, it has been argued that active transport is a key factor in the achievement of healthy levels of physical activity (Jones et al. 2007).

All four national surveys demonstrate the same sex difference in activity levels. Physical activity is the only lifestyle behaviour where men are more likely to achieve government guidelines than women (Table 4.1). Sport is a traditional male activity which may contribute to this finding. Indeed the Scottish Health Survey (Scottish Executive 2005) asked about types of physical activity and found that the most common physical activity in men was sport/exercise whereas in women it was heavy housework.

As both men and women age their activity levels decline. The Health Survey for England (DoH 2003) reports a decline in activity in men, from 53 per cent achieving government guidelines for activity in the 16–24 age group to only 8 per cent of men aged 75 and over. While considerably fewer young British women were active than young British men (Table 4.2) female activity levels remain stable over the lifespan at around 30 per cent, starting to decline only in those over 65, thereafter the decline is

Table 4.2 Percentages of men and women living in the UK achieving the government guidelines for physical activity broken down by age

Source of data	*% of ♂ 16–24*	*% of ♂ 25–34*	*% of ♂ 35–44*	*% of ♂ 45–54*	*% of ♂ 55–64*	*% of ♂ 65–74*	*% of ♂ 75+*	*% of ♀ 16–24*	*% of ♀ 25–34*	*% of ♀ 35–44*	*% of ♀ 45–54*	*% of ♀ 55–64*	*% of ♀ 65–74*	*% of ♀ 75+*
Health Survey England 2003	53	44	41	38	32	17	8	30	29	30	31	23	13	3
Scottish Health Survey 2003	59	57	45	40	35	23	13	36	40	39	35	28	16	6
Welsh Health Survey 2005–06	53	43	45	40	30	25	16	32	26	29	28	25	19	11
Northern Ireland Health and Social Wellbeing Survey 2001	38	34	36	34	23	20	15	27	32	35	31	24	17	7

marked, with only 3 per cent of women aged over 75 achieving the government guidelines. The fact that activity levels decline with age more markedly in men than in women goes some way to supporting the notion that men are achieving higher physical activity levels because they play more sport. Sporting participation decreases with age more markedly than any other physical activity (Scottish Executive 2005).

People in Scotland are generally more active than in the rest of the United Kingdom (Table 4.1). Although the same pattern of declining activity exists, the decline is less rapid. The Scottish Health Survey (Scottish Executive 2005) made a comparison with the 1998 survey reporting that activity levels have increased from 1998 to 2003 and these increases were particularly marked for men and women aged 55–74. The important question that emerges from making this comparison between activity levels in Scottish, English, Welsh and Northern Irish populations is why the Scottish are more active, particularly in later life.

The relationship between activity and social class as measured by the National Statistics Socio-Economic Classification (NS-SEC) (Table 4.3) is complex. In all three countries that made an NS-SEC comparison those who describe themselves as small employers or own account workers are the most likely to be participating in physical activity at the level recommended by the government. However, in Scotland the difference between this group and those who describe themselves as professional, managerial or intermediate is small and activity is lowest in those in routine occupations. In England and Wales those who describe themselves as professional, managerial or intermediate are considerably less active than people in the small employer/own account class and less active than those who describe their occupations as lower supervisory, technical, routine or semi-routine. Only the Welsh survey reports the activity levels of the long-term unemployed and those who have never worked and their activity is lower than all people in work apart from those in professional and managerial occupations. The relationship between NS-SEC and physical activity can be described by an inverted U-shaped curve, with those at either end of the NS-SEC scale being the least likely to be active. The slope of the curve is far less steep in people living in Scotland, where activity levels are far more consistent among the classes. The findings presented here are not entirely consistent with the conclusions by Hillsdon et al. (2005), who conclude from the population surveys they reviewed that people in lower social classes are more likely to be inactive. These data from the four National Health Surveys present a more complex non-linear picture.

While the national surveys did not present data on physical activity and ethnic minorities, the Health of Minority Ethnic Groups survey (Erens et al. 2001) measured participation in physical activity among the main minority groups in England. Compared to the general population, South Asian and Chinese men and women were much less likely to participate in physical activity of any kind. Bangladeshi men and women were the

Table 4.3 Percentages of adults living in England, Scotland and Wales achieving UK government guidelines for physical activity broken down by the NS-SEC of household reference person

Source of data	*Managerial and professional (%)*	*Intermediate (%)*	*Small employers and own account workers (%)*	*Lower supervisory and technical (%)*	*Semi-routine and routine (%)*	*Long-term unemployed or have never worked (%)*
Health Survey England 2003	28	30	39	36	33.5	Not available
Scottish Health Survey 2003	37	40	41	37.5	33.5	Not available
Welsh Health Survey 2005–06	27.5	26	38	34	32.5	28

Note: Data from Northern Ireland used the SEG rather than the NS-SEC so is not included

most inactive and were almost twice as likely as the general population to be classified as sedentary.

From all these various surveys we get a picture of activity in the UK of only a minority of the population achieving the government recommendations of physical activity. Physical activity is not consistent through the population. Women are less likely to be active than men. Activity declines dramatically during the lifespan in men, it declines more slowly in women so that activity levels in the two sexes become more similar as they age. The relationship between socio-economic class and physical activity is not linear and those at the top or bottom of the NS-SEC socio-economic classification are among the least active. People from ethnic minorities tend to be less active than the indigenous population.

Health consequences of low physical activity

Physical activity reduces the risk of premature mortality for everyone, regardless of their age, sex or ethnicity (Pate et al. 1995; US Department of Health and Human Services 1999; Warburton et al. 2006). The World Health Organisation has reported that physical inactivity is one of the ten leading causes of death, responsible for 1.9 million deaths worldwide each year. In England, the Department of Health, Physical Activity, Health Improvement and Prevention (2004) has estimated that adults who are physically active have a 20–30 per cent reduced risk of premature death. Warburton et al. (2006) have suggested that a 50 per cent reduction in risk from death is possible for the physically fit. The effect of physical activity on health manifests itself by its influence on a wide range of diseases. In particular, people who are physically active can achieve up to a 50 per cent reduced risk of developing the major lifestyle diseases: coronary heart disease, stroke, diabetes and cancers (Department of Health, Physical Activity, Health Improvement and Prevention 2004). All of these diseases are chronic diseases. While people diagnosed with chronic conditions face a shortened life expectancy, most will live for some years post-diagnosis, even if not for as long as they might have done if they had remained disease free. Not surprisingly, the World Health Organisation has calculated that physical inactivity leads to a considerable increase in disease-specific disability. Consequently, not only do inactive people face shorter lives, but also they face poor quality of life in the years preceding death.

While the relationship of physical activity to each disease is important in its own right, what makes physical activity so important is the strength of its effect over such a wide range of conditions. While physical activity can have a treatment function it is its preventative role that is so impressive and causes the Chief Medical Officer to conclude: 'physical activity is one of the main contemporary public health issues' (Department of Health, Physical Activity, Health Improvement and Prevention 2004).

Most people associate physical fitness with high levels of physical activity and inactivity with being unfit. Certainly it is irrefutable that physically active adults have higher levels of physical fitness (Pate et al. 1995). However, it is important to recognise that physical activity and physical fitness although related have independent effects on health (US Department of Health and Human Services 1999; Department of Health, Physical Activity, Health Improvement and Prevention 2004; Warburton et al. 2006). Associations with health are generally stronger for measured cardiorespiratory fitness than for reported physical activity (US Department of Health and Human Services 1999; Warburton et al. 2006) but a self-reported physical activity is still convincingly associated with reduced mortality (US Department of Health and Human Services 1999; Warburton et al. 2006). In short, cardiorespiratory fitness will benefit health but levels of physical activity that may not be of an intensity to alter physical fitness parameters may still have health benefits. In particular, for Type 2 diabetes an acute bout of physical activity will encourage the skeletal muscles to take up glucose, an immediate response to activity independent of any long-term benefits of physical activity. Similarly, the beneficial effects of physical activity for breast cancer, and colon cancer are both postulated to be mediated through metabolic mechanisms. For breast cancer, physical activity is proposed to reduce the risk by modifying circulating gonadal hormones concentrations (Pierce et al. 2007). For colon cancer the proposed mechanism is prostraglandin levels (US Department of Health and Human Services 1999).

Bodyweight and obesity

Levels of obesity in the UK are rising. The Chief Medical Officer describes it as a new and serious threat to health with nearly one-quarter of the population being clinically obese (see Chapter 3). This is a threefold increase between 1980 and 2002 (Department of Health, Physical Activity, Health Improvement and Prevention 2004). Obesity is often associated with physical inactivity. Indeed the Chief Medical Officer stated in 2004 that:

> Obesity is the main visible sign of inactivity, yet obesity is just one of possibly 20 chronic diseases and disorders for which low activity levels are a known contributory factor.
>
> (Department of Health, Physical Activity, Health Improvement and Prevention 2004: 20)

Physical activity is directly related to body weight. If your energy intake is equal to your energy output, your weight will remain constant. If your energy intake exceeds your energy output then you will gain weight. Physical activity increases energy expenditure and so decreases the likelihood that an individual will gain weight. However, it is possible that the Chief Medical Officer is overstating the case for the relationship between physical activity and body weight when he states: 'Obesity is the main visible sign of inactivity'. In making this statement he rather implies that activity can reduce the incidence of obesity. However, it is easier to influence the energy intake–output balance through diet than through activity (Dicken-Kano and Bell 2006). Physical activity, at the level suggested by the government, by itself can result in modest weight loss of around 0.5–1kg a month (Pate et al. 1995). Higher levels of physical activity can have more dramatic effects on body weight with exercise of 700 kilocalories a day producing at least as much fat loss as the equivalent dietary restriction (Sigal et al. 2006). However, this is more than double the government guidelines for physical activity and it is unlikely that many people could achieve this. Nevertheless, many health professionals and academics have called for new guidelines for weight loss physical activity to be established (Department of Health, Physical Activity, Health Improvement and Prevention 2004). The Chief Medical Officer recognises this in his 2004 report saying:

> 45–60 minutes of moderate activity per day may be needed to prevent the development of obesity … People who have been obese and have

managed to lose weight may need to do 60–90 minutes activity a day in order to avoid regaining weight.

(Department of Health, Physical Activity, Health Improvement and Prevention 2004: 5)

The evidence suggests that for physical activity to have a significant effect on bodyweight and in particular on weight loss then 30 minutes of moderate activity for five days a week is unlikely to be a high enough level of activity. However, if individuals who are moderately active are also likely to consume fewer calories, a combination of these two contributing factors to the energy balance equation together can be enough to maintain the energy balance equilibrium.

Why are people physically inactive?

The government guidelines for physical activity are not daunting and indeed are not as challenging as some health professionals would like, yet the majority of the population fail to achieve them (American College of Sports Medicine 2007). The complex picture of sex, age, socio-economic and ethnic differences in physical activity levels means the answer to the question of why people fail to engage in appropriate levels of physical activity will be complex. Indeed there may be a range of different answers for various cultural and demographic groups. However, an answer must be attempted in order to better inform public health interventions in the future, to enable the maximal uptake of healthy levels of activity that is possible within populations and to support individuals who would like to be physically active. Part of the solution to the problem of low levels of physical activity may be to turn the question on its head and consider why some people do achieve the physical activity guidelines. Investigations about why people do participate in physical activity are less common but may provide useful insights.

Socio-economic factors

Recent data from the Health Surveys of England, Scotland and Wales (Table 4.3) suggest that the relationship between physical activity and social class is not simple and not linearly related to access to resources. Levels of physical activity have been declining in the population and the cultural and environmental landscape may be implicated but, unlike the picture for diet and smoking, the implications of our changing environmental and cultural landscape are detrimental to people from many different occupational classes, not solely those in the lower occupational classes.

It is encouraging to see increasing recognition from policy makers of the importance of supportive social environments; illustrated by the emergence of the term obesogenic to describe environments that are adverse to physical activity and encouraging to excess calorific intake (Foster et al. 2006; Jones et al. 2007). Defining what constitutes an obesogenic environment is problematic but certainly includes cultural, social and physical characteristics (see Chapter 3). Furthermore, most people function in multiple settings adding to the challenge of understanding how an obesogenic environment impacts on its citizens (Jones et al. 2007). Many UK studies of environmental influences on physical activity have focused on a very specific and small aspect of the environment. A review of interventions that used the environment to encourage physical activity included 25 studies, 19 of which were studies aimed at encouraging the use of the stairs (Foster et al. 2006). While encouraging the use of the stairs is undoubtedly a worthwhile venture it is unlikely to increase the physical activity of any single individual by more than 10 minutes a day. The focus on encouraging stair use, often by decisional prompts, may reflect the difficulties with making significant changes to the environment. For instance, changing the environment to facilitate walking or cycling to work would probably require major changes. It might require the building of cycle paths, the provision of showers, lockers and bicycle sheds. It is hardly surprising that many 'environmental' interventions are focused on the simplistic directional change for stair use.

Jones et al. (2007) conclude in their review of research into environmental factors and levels of physical activity that the influence of the environment is probably small and the mechanisms are unclear. They argue that environmental factors and social demographic factors vary together making it difficult to evaluate whether the physical environment is influencing physical activity or whether it is actually an associated social factor such as ethnicity or poverty that is mediating the effect. They further conclude that the way individuals perceive their environment appears to have a stronger relationship with their physical activity levels than the objective environment. Jones et al. (2007) raise concerns that improving the environment by building more cycle paths, safe places to walk and so on may have its main effects on those who are already active rather than the sedentary. Better understanding of the mechanisms that mediate the link the environment to physical activity are required. The need for improved theorising is supported by NICE (2006b), which reports that physical activity interventions that are underpinned by psychological theory are more effective. Consequently, it seems that the effect of the environment on physical activity levels is influenced by other social demographic factors and mediated by psychological processes.

Psychological factors

Many different individual factors have been postulated to underpin physical activity behaviours. A perception of risk variously described as perceived personal threat in the HBM (Rosenstock 1974), threat appraisal in the PMT (Norman et al. 2005), and as beliefs in the TPB (Conner and Sparks 2005) has been found to correlate with exercise behaviours but effect sizes are consistently small suggesting that a perception of risk from lack of physical activity can account for only a small amount of the variation in behaviour (Harrison et al. 2002). Indeed, there are studies that report no relationship between a perception of risk and physical activity (Blue 2007). Interestingly, Blue (2007) finds the lack of relationship between perceived risk and physical activity in her study hard to accept and argues that her particular measure of risk perception may be at fault.

Another key factor in the HBM is a belief in the effectiveness of the behaviour, a variable which is also found in SCT described as an outcome expectation. The evidence to support the importance of this variable is not conclusive and once again any effect sizes are small (Rovniak et al. 2002) indicating that it plays only a small part in explaining any variation in physical activity levels in the population. So it would appear that perceptions and beliefs about the health risks and benefits of activity and non-activity play only a small part in explaining variations in physical activity behaviours. Some authors have argued that they may be necessary but are not sufficient to promote physical activity change. However, studies such as Blue (2007) that found no relationship between risk perception and activity levels raise the question as to whether a perception of risk is necessary at all.

Barriers to performing the physical activity have been found to be related to exercise behaviours but perceived behavioural control over potential barriers has been found to be a better predictor of physical activity than the objective barriers themselves. Hagger et al. (2002) found that including perceived behavioural control increased the amount of variation the original TRA model could explain from 37 per cent to 44 per cent. Consequently, the TPB, an adaptation of the TRA which includes perceived behavioural control (see Chapter 2) is now accepted as a more effective predictor of behaviour in the context of physical activity (Hagger et al. 2002).

Measures of social norm which are a key aspect of the theory of reasoned action and the theory of planned behaviour consistently predict little if any of the variation in physical activity indicating that social influences on intentions to exercise and exercise behaviour are less important than individual attributes (Godin and Kok 1996; Hagger et al. 2002). Some authors have argued that social norms are important but being more diffuse than individual attributes are harder to successfully operationalise and measure (Godin and Kok 1996). The better success of the more specific variable 'social support' in explaining variations in physical activity behaviour adds weight to this argument (Rovniak et al. 2002). Despite the failure to demonstrate that social norms are a major factor in predicting variations in physical activity Jones et al. (2007: 38) in their extensive review of obesogenic environments for the influential Foresight project still conclude that 'capturing the concept of social norm and modifying that norm' is one of the major public health challenges.

Probably, the most important psychological factor to emerge from social cognition research into physical activity behaviour is the concept of self-efficacy (Plotnikoff and Higginbotham 1998; Marshall and Biddle 2001; Hagger et al. 2002; Rovniak et al. 2002; Cox et al. 2003). Self-efficacy is distinguished from the conceptually similar control-focused variable 'perceived behavioural control' because it focuses on internal aspects of control such as perceived ability and self-agency whereas perceived behavioural control is externally focused. University students who reported higher levels of exercise self-efficacy were more likely to be physically active (Rovniak et al. 2002). McAuley 1992 and Armstrong et al. 1993 have reported that self-efficacy predicts both the adoption and maintenance of physical activity. Cox et al. (2003) found that self-efficacy for overcoming barriers was predictive of the adoption of physical activity and that increasing self-efficacy was critical to supporting positive changes in physical activity. Rovniak et al. (2002) argue that positive impact of self-efficacy on physical activity behaviour is mediated by the use of self-regulatory strategies. People with high self-efficacy are more likely to utilise self-regulatory strategies which in turn exerted a large total effect on physical activity in their study. Self-regulatory strategies include: goal setting, self-monitoring, planning and problem solving. Self-efficacy has been argued to be enhanced by: personal accomplishment or mastery, vicarious experience or verbal persuasion. Self-efficacy is not unrealistic optimism as it is based on experience so in consequence realistic goals and plans that an individual can achieve are essential to increase self-efficacy (Luszczynska and Schwarzer 2005). Self-efficacy is the central component of SCT (Rovniak et al. 2002) but has been included as an additional factor to increase the predictive power of many other social cognition models (Becker and Rosenstock 1987; Hagger et al. 2002). Self-efficacy can be argued to be the single most important factor in explaining physical activity behaviour and particularly in explaining change behaviour. People with high self-efficacy are more likely to be able to set achievable goals and overcome obstacles which in turn makes it more likely for them persist in their physical activity.

The transtheoretical model describes health behaviour adoption and maintenance as a process that occurs through a series of behaviourally and motivationally defined stages. In recognising that the practice of behaviours and in particular lifestyle behaviours is an ongoing process, this model was ground-breaking. Marshall and Biddle (2001) in their meta-analysis of the TTM and exercise behaviour felt that finding differences in variables such as self-efficacy between different stages was supportive of the TTM. However, Mutrie et al. (2002) found that although a written intervention to increase walking to work was effective, the processes of change did not explain movement through the stages of change. As has been argued in Chapter 2, you can argue that these are pseudo stages imposed on what is essentially a continuum. Other problems with evaluating the TTM are the failure to consistently operationalise the stages and the small number of long-term studies of changing physical activity. One longer-term study that evaluated the relevance of the TTM stages of change over an 18-month period was inconclusive about the relevance of stages of change. The majority of participants progressed from contemplation to action to maintenance in a linear fashion which could be argued to provide support for the TTM, but equally would support a continuum theory. Of particular interest was the failure of readiness to change to predict change, those assessed as less ready were just as likely to adopt exercise. The only variable from those postulated by the TTM to influence stage movement that consistently increased as exercise was established was self-efficacy (Marshall and Biddle 2001; Cox et al. 2003). Currently, the relevance of discrete stages to designing effective evaluations is still in question. However, the key concept of a process of behavioural change is without doubt of value to the investigation of physical activity.

The powerful influence of past behaviour over future behaviour (Hagger et al. 2002; Conner and Norman 2005) adds support to the argument for conceptualising physical activity as an ongoing process. Consistent patterns of past behaviours are often referred to as habits. In terms of the TTM when people are in the maintenance stage of behavioural change their behaviour is established and as past behaviour is an excellent predictor of future behaviour the continuation of their newly established habit should be assured. However, the dearth of longitudinal studies means it is not clear how long a behaviour must persist in order to be described as habitual. Habits in so much as they are acknowledged at all within the social cognitive framework are postulated to influence attitudes, social norms and perceived behavioural control through the positive feedback they provide to inform the cognitive decision to exercise. However, although the decision to start an exercise programme can be predicted from social cognitive variables, persistence is less predictable (Aarts et al. 1997). It may be more useful to conceptualise habits as established patterns of behaviour that may once have been initiated by rational choice but which are now under the control of specific situational cues that trigger the behaviour without cognitive effort. Aarts et al. (1997: 366) specifically define habitual exercise behaviour as 'mentally represented structures in which a certain situation is strongly associated with the goal to exercise that is chronically pursed in that situation'. Reasoned action as represented in social cognition models and habit can be considered as two extremes of a conscious decision-making continuum. In between may lie a number of heuristic decision-making strategies that involve varying degrees of cognition. Past physical activity is an important predictor of future physical activity (Hagger et al. 2002; Conner and Norman 2005) which suggests that developing physical activity habits are key to promoting long term positive changes in physical activity. While social cognition models may tell us something about the decision to take up exercise behaviour research now needs to focus on the formation of exercise habits. Aarts et al. (1997) suggest that a positive experience of physical activity is an essential aspect of habit formation, which leads us to the role of affect and enjoyment in physical activity. One caveat to the conclusion that establishing habits is the solution to promotion of physical activity is the concern that encouraging habit formation could encourage addictive behaviour which may have an overall deleterious effect on the individual. The other side of the coin to establishing physical activity habits is overcoming established sedentary habits (Puska 2001).

Traditional approaches to health behaviours have been negatively focused, looking predominantly at why people don't exercise. Furthermore, with the domination of social cognition theories, it can be argued that the emotional component has been marginalised. Consequently, enjoyment as a moderator of physical activity choices is seldom investigated. Nevertheless, studies that do consider affect report that long-term exercise is associated with increased positive affect during and following physical activity (Arent et al. 2000). When affect is considered in the context of social cognition theory it is evaluated in terms of its influence on components of the cognitive-decision making process. For instance it has been argued that the self-efficacy is increased with positive mood state. Furthermore, positive affect can feedback into attitudinal schema and increase positive attitudes (Aarts et al. 1997). Kiviniemi et al. (2007) have looked at affective associations and their relationship with cognitive beliefs. They conclude that affect can serve as a cognitive shortcut to behavioural choice, the decision about whether to exercise can be about whether an individual expects to enjoy the experience rather than a rational cost-benefits analysis. In this scenario social cognition models may be expected to predict the uptake of activity but enjoyment might be expected to predict adherence. The relationship between affect and cognition can be conceptualised using a dual-processing framework where both a rational choice decision-making process and a heuristic alternative, such as affect or some other sort of cognition-minimising shortcut are postulated to be available to the individual when faced with a choice. Finucane et al. (2003) neatly refer to the balance between affective and analytical thinking as 'the dance of affect and reason' and have argued that the emphasis in the dance will be mediated by a wide range of factors including both environmental conditions and individual characteristics. However, it is argued that as affective responses are immediate and cognitive decision-making strategies are slower that often the affective response dominates (Loewenstein et al. 2001).

Extensive evaluation of social cognition models' ability to predict uptake of physical activity leads to the conclusion that a perception of the risks of non-activity and the benefits of activity for health has at best a small impact of overall variation in physical activity behaviour. The concept of social norm as measured by social cognitive research consistently fails to predict exercise behaviour, although the more specific concept of social support is more successful which may suggest the diverse concept of social norms is worthy of more attention and better conceptualisation and measurement. The key factor to emerge from work on physical activity behaviour within the social cognitive framework is that external and internal measures of control, perceived behavioural control and self-efficacy are the best predictors of exercise behaviour and in well designed and operationalised studies have been found to predict more than 50 per cent of the variation in exercise behaviour (Rovniak et al. 2005).

The conclusion of the section on current levels of activity was that a decade or more of health promotion and policy interventions to increase physical activity levels in the population have been unsuccessful because only a minority of the population reach the government's arguably inadequate physical activity guidelines and more worryingly the trend in physical activity participation is still downwards, except in Scotland where a rise in physical activity levels was recorded between 1998 and 2003 (Scottish Executive 2005). It is therefore important to identify which interventions, if any, can be considered successful, which have not and plan future interventions on the basis of evidence of previous success.

Interventions to increase physical activity

Interventions to increase physical activity have been many and varied in many different settings with many different sections of society (Kahn et al. 2002; Hillsdon et al. 2005). Kahn et al. (2002) usefully differentiate between different interventions by categorising them as information based, behavioural or environmental/policy level interventions. Information-based interventions aim to change knowledge and attitudes about the benefits and opportunities for physical activity within a community. Behavioural interventions aim either to assist people in the development of behavioural management skills that enable them to adopt and maintain behavioural change and/or to create social environments that facilitate and enhance behavioural change. Finally, environmental/policy interventions aim to change the structure of physical and organisational environments to provide safe, attractive and convenient places for physical activity. While many interventions will straddle these definitions they do at least provide a starting point for evaluation.

Informational interventions can be as various as point of decision prompts at the bottom of a building where a choice of the lift or the stairs is available, to mass-media campaigns. In social cognitive terms an information intervention may attempt to change people's understanding of their susceptibility to health related problems associated with inactivity or the severity of such problems. Alternatively or as well as, an information campaign may highlight the benefits of exercise for the health of an individual. Most physical activity campaigns will take such a health-orientated focus although reference to social benefits or enjoyment is not uncommon. Research tells us that perceptions of risks and benefits explain at best small amounts of variation in physical activity (Harrison et al. 2002) which leads to the hypothesis that information campaigns designed to alter such perceptions are unlikely to promote large changes in activity. Kahn et al. (2002) in their review of informational campaigns found no evidence that informational only media-based campaigns were effective, in line with the theoretically derived conclusion that attempts to inform people of the benefits and costs of activity and inactivity are unlikely to facilitate substantial changes in behaviour. Similarly, Ogilvie et al. (2004) found no evidence that informational campaigns to increase active transport were successful. However, media-based informational provision was a consistent aspect of multicomponent interventions which were often successful at increasing physical activity (Kahn et al. 2002; W.J. Brown et al. 2006). Such multicomponent campaigns usually include self-help groups and other forms of social support (Kahn et al. 2002). Decisional prompts in buildings with a number of floors have been found to be effective in increasing the decision to take the stairs rather than the lift (Foster et al. 2006), although whether these are truly informational interventions is arguable as they don't necessarily provide information but rather identify a healthy choice for an individual over which they have immediate control and minimal perceived or real barriers. Hillsdon et al. (2005) in their evidence briefing to the Health Development Agency reported that brief advice from a health professional supported by written materials was likely to produce modest short-term (12 weeks or less) increases in physical activity. Information given on an individual basis can be seen as directly relevant to the individual, who cannot ignore their own susceptibility as easily as they can from media-based campaigns.

Behavioural interventions are more likely to be at a small group or individual level of intervention. Kahn et al. (2002) found that individually adapted behavioural change programmes were effective in increasing physical activity levels. Ogilvie et al. (2004) found that targeted behavioural change programmes were the most effective way to promote walking and cycling. Mutrie et al. (2002) found that a self-help intervention 'Walk in to Work Out' delivered via written materials successfully increased walking but not cycling at 6 months post intervention. Hillsdon et al. (2005) also found much support for interventions based in behavioural change. First, they concluded that interventions based on theories of behavioural change, that taught behavioural skills and were tailored to individual needs were associated with more long-term changes than interventions with no such theoretical base. Second, they concluded that regular contact with an exercise specialist resulted in sustained changes in physical activity. An exercise specialist seen regularly will provide social support and set appropriate goals that foster and develop self-efficacy (Rovniak et al. 2002). The majority of social cognition theories used to underpin physical activity interventions, be they the health belief model, the theory of planned behaviour or the TTM include either self-efficacy, perceived behavioural control or both. Consequently, the majority of behavioural change based interventions will include advice and help on goal-setting, overcoming obstacles and developing social support which facilitate uptake and maintenance of physical activity by increasing self-efficacy (Cox et al. 2003; Rovniak et al. 2002). Indeed Mutrie et al. (2002) postulate that the reason their intervention to increase active commuting was successful for walking but not cycling was because they were unable to provide solutions to major obstacles to cycling such as lack of segregation from motor traffic, or safe, covered places to leave a bicycle. Whereas, solutions to obstacles to walking such as getting wet were effectively resolved by the intervention materials that included information on purchasing effective waterproofs.

Wendy Brown et al. (2006) concluded that a range of different types of interventions can demonstrate small short-term improvements in physical activity in volunteer samples. A key finding from intervention studies is that theoretically based interventions are more likely to be effective and effective in the long term (Kahn et al. 2002; Hillsdon et al. 2005; NICE 2006b). Such interventions that focus on teaching behavioural change strategies and recognise the importance of developing self-efficacy and perceived behavioural control are more likely to result in sustained behavioural change. Improving self-efficacy involves careful self-regulatory goal-setting that challenges but does not overwhelm the individual so that self-efficacy is damaged. Such tailored interventions are costly in terms of expert time and require a specialist who has both the physiological and psychological skills base on which to base their recommendations for appropriate physical activity and the support required to sustain it.

Many public health interventions to increase physical activity in the community are not individualised, do not recognise the role of psychological processes in effective behavioural change and are carried out by professionals with no psychological training (NICE 2006b). For example, the National Institute of Health and Clinical Excellence (2006b) reports that although there are an estimated 600 exercise referral schemes in the UK, there is no evidence that such schemes successfully increase physical activity levels in the long term. Two trials suggested that exercise referral schemes were effective in the short term (6–12 weeks) but four studies reported no increase in physical activity over the longer term (12 weeks to 1 year). A more theoretical approach to exercise referral with appropriate psychological training of exercise providers may improve the outcomes from this wide-spread and major intervention. NICE (2006b) recommends that exercise referral schemes are properly evaluated.

Pedometers have become commonplace and the target of 10,000 steps a day is well known (Bennett et al. 2006; Slack 2006). Pedometers have been given away with cereal packets and promoted as an innovative and effective method of promoting physical activity. However, the National Institute for Health and Clinical Excellence (2006) concludes that there is no evidence that the use of pedometers increases physical activity levels either in the long or short term, although the longest follow-up reported was 24 weeks. Once again this is an intervention that is not based in psychological theory and that indeed could well be detrimental to the uptake of physical activity if the generalised goal of 10,000 steps a day is too many for an individual and this undermines their self-efficacy, perhaps preventing them achieving a more modest amount of walking. The moderately successful 10,000 steps Rockhampton Project (W.J. Brown et al. 2006) did demonstrate modest increases in physical activity in their community but only in women. However, the Rockhampton Project was a multi-strategy physical activity intervention based on a social-ecological framework which emphases interventions at multiple levels. Although 10,000 steps Rockhampton was a central coordinating theme, a clear secondary theme of the intervention was 'every steps counts' and was equally promoted during the campaign. The multi-level intervention involved social marketing, brief interventions by health professionals and positive changes to the environment.

NICE (2006b) and Hillsdon et al. (2005) found support for the short-term effectiveness of brief interventions in primary care. However, Hillsdon et al. (2005) and NICE (2006b) flag up the need for longer-term studies. While a 6 or 12 week increase in physical activity is promising, unless it is sustained there will be few health benefits from such a short period of increased activity. Exercise referral schemes were similarly promising in the short term but failed to deliver the long-term changes in physical activity that are necessary for improved health outcomes. NICE (2006b) indicates that follow-up sessions with the health professional would appear to increase the likelihood of sustained change.

So we can conclude that social cognitive research suggests that self-efficacy is key in predicting physical activity behaviour and interventions that focus on behavioural change and promoting self-efficacy are the most likely to achieve long-term increases in physical activity in their participants (Kahn et al. 2002; Cox et al. 2003; Hillsdon 2005). However, the most successful social cognition models seldom predict more than 50 per cent of the variation in physical activity found in any population (Rovniak et al. 2002). It seems that non-cognitive influences such as automatic habitual responses and/or affective responses to situations may be important in understanding how and why people choose or choose not to exercise. Enjoyment would appear to be key in the establishment of physical activity habits (Aarts et al. 1997). In order to influence individuals through an affective route, lessons may be learnt from persuasive literature where the salience of non-cognitive cues is already acknowledged. Effective promotional messages based on peripheral rather than cognitive cues are well established in many contexts such as advertising. The concept of social marketing, which will be developed in the final chapter, may well be of relevance.

Public health policy is focusing on the obesogenic environment and integrated health and transport strategies to promote active transport (Ogilvie et al. 2004; Foster et al. 2006; Jones et al. 2007). However, the evidence appears to be that the perception of the environment is more important than the environment per se (Jones et al. 2007). Consequently, environmental adaptations will need to be supported by behavioural interventions to support adaptation to the environment and positive changes in physical activity, or we run the risk of supporting only the physical activity behaviours of the currently active (Jones et al. 2007).

We need theories of behavioural change that do not simply view social factors as an adjunct but that incorporate socio-demographic, environmental and cultural factors as key factors in their theorising. Social-ecological models are a potential framework with which to investigate the multiple levels of influence on physical activity. Owen et al. (2000) have devised a behavioural settings model which attempts to model how the environment interacts with psychological and social factors in influencing activity behaviour. Owen et al. (2000) introduce the concept of behavioural settings which they define as:

> Those social and physical situations in which behaviours take place, by promoting and sometimes demanding certain actions and by discouraging or prohibiting others.
>
> (Owen et al. 2000: 155)

The value of such new theories is yet to be determined but they may well contribute to a better understanding of lifestyle behavioural choices.

Conceptualising physical activity as a lifestyle behaviour rather than a health behaviour acknowledges that physical activity is often not performed for its health benefits but for other purposes. A good example of how this may influence theoretical thinking is in terms of women's and men's health behaviours. Young men take more exercise primarily because they play more sport, probably for non-health reasons, consequently a health behaviour model would not be very predictive of their behaviour and interventions to increase participation based on health models would not be effective. Young women take less exercise and are not attracted to playing sport. Interventions to increase women playing sport or to increase the opportunities to watch female sport through the media have not been effective. Promoting exercise as a way to improve physical attributes may well be a successful, culturally embedded way of encouraging adolescent women to participate in exercise. Theories of body image may well be useful to develop robust theoretical models of young women's exercise behaviour.

When men and women reach middle-age the role of physical activity as a health behaviour may start to take precedence and health behaviour models may be more useful in predicting and intervening in physical activity. NICE (2006b) reported that brief physician interventions to increase physical activity are more effective with older adults supporting the argument that for older people lifestyle choices are more health-focused. A lifecourse perspective may well be crucial for effective promotion of physical activity (Hendry and Kloep 2002). Physical activity may have different connotations for different socio-demographic groups and its relevance and meaning may change over the lifespan. As a young adult it may serve a social function, an opportunity to compete and succeed or a method to improve the physique. For middle-aged adults it may have a primarily preventative function. For older people it may well have a treatment, control or rehabilitative function.

So a picture emerges of a situation where we require a model of behavioural change that is specific to or reflective of a person's place in the socio-environmental and lifecourse landscape. Different theories of behavioural change may then be relevant to different groups depending on their place in the lifecourse and their environmental resources. The attempt to develop a single theory of behavioural change may be futile. However, we may already have available a series of useful theories of behaviour and behavioural change that can be utilised by health professionals. The TTM was an acknowledgement of the fact that interventions may be appropriate at different stages in the process towards the regular adoption of physical activity. However, the relevance of the stages as conceptualised by the TTM have been challenged and it seems likely that identifying a person's resource capacity and their lifespan stage may be a more robust and practical way of distinguishing people for whom different interventions may be more effective (Hendry and Kloep 2002). Using a lifecourse perspective to conceptualise the process of participating in physical activity may be a effective way of identifying critical periods for the development of physical activity habits which along with self-efficacy are the most reliable predictors of future physical activity. Jones et al. (2007) have proposed a model of the potential determinants of physical activity which uses the environment and the lifecourse as the key axis between which the relevant factors interplay.

Conclusion

Levels of physical activity are low in the population and the establishment of positive physical activity habits is a key health promotional goal. Social cognition theory has identified self-efficacy and perceived behavioural control as key factors in the practice of healthy levels of physical activity, but at best such models can predict 50 per cent of the variation in physical activity. Research needs to move on and consider the role of non-cognitive factors in physical activity behaviour such as habitual practices and the enjoyment of activity. Furthermore, the recognition of the changing relevance of health to lifestyle choices as people progress through the life-course may enable health practitioners to select and utilise different behavioural change strategies to suit the time and place of the individual.

Summary points

- Physical activity can be defined objectively as: 'Any bodily movement produced by the skeletal muscles that results in energy expenditure and is usually measured in kilocalories (kcal) per unit of time' (Caspersen et al. 1985). However, definitions of exercise and sport are more subjective.
- Only a minority of the population achieve the government recommendations for physical activity.
- Women are less likely to be active than men. Activity declines dramatically during the lifespan in men; it declines more slowly in women so that activity levels in the two sexes become more similar as they age.
- The relationship between socio-economic class and physical activity is not linear and those at the top or bottom of the NS-NEC socio-economic classification are among the least active.
- People from ethnic minorities tend to be less active than the indigenous population.
- What makes physical activity so important for health outcomes is the strength of its effect over such a wide range of conditions.
- Perceptions of the risks of being sedentary and the benefits of physical activity can explain little or any of the variation in levels of physical activity.
- Self-efficacy is the best predictor of successful increases of physical activity.
- Past activity is a good predictor of subsequent physical activity. The establishment of good physical activity habits may be crucial in the promotion of physical activity.
- Enjoyment of activity may play an important role in the establishment of healthy physical activity habits.

- Perceptions of the environment may be more important than the objective environment for physical activity.
- A model of physical activity that is specific to or reflective of a person's place in the socio-environmental and lifecourse landscape is required.

5 Drinking

> O God, that men should put an enemy in their mouths to steal away their brains! that we should, with joy, pleasance, revel, and applause, transform ourselves into beasts!
>
> Cassio, in Shakespeare, *Othello*

At the end of this chapter you will:

- understand the definitions of sensible, hazardous, harmful and binge drinking
- be aware of the government guidelines for sensible drinking
- recognise the prevalence of harmful and binge drinking in Britain
- understand the relationship between health and alcohol consumption
- understand the demographic, socio-economic and environmental factors involved in excess alcohol consumption
- recognise the psychological factors involved in regular excess consumption of alcohol
- be able to evaluate current interventions to reduce excess alcohol consumption.

Definitions of alcohol and drinking

Alcohol

Alcohol is an easily identified chemical compound called ethyl alcohol, or more commonly ethanol. Its presence in drinks can be identified and quantified. In Britain the alcoholic content of drinks is clearly stated on the container as percentage volume. However, the quantity of ethyl alcohol can be measured as fluid ounces, millilitres, grams or units. One (UK) fluid ounce of alcohol is equivalent to 28.41 millilitres of alcohol. One millilitre of alcohol is equivalent to 0.79 grams of alcohol. One UK unit of alcohol is equivalent to 8–10 grams of pure alcohol (WHO 2000). A single pub measure of spirits (40 per cent alcohol), a small glass of wine

(12 per cent alcohol) or half a pint of standard strength beer (4 per cent alcohol) all contain 1 unit of alcohol (Plant and Plant 2006). However, many beers and wines are stronger than this and many servings larger. Reviews of alcohol consumption using different measures frequently standardise all their data back to grams of alcohol (Anderson et al. 1993; WHO 2000).

Alcohol is a substance that depresses the nervous system. It produces intoxication through its action on the brain and because of this can be considered a psychoactive drug, albeit a legal one. Intoxication leads to impairments in psychomotor control, reaction time and judgement making. Furthermore, intoxication leads to emotional changes and a decreased responsiveness to social expectations (Babor et al. 2003).

Drinking

Although we all drink many different types of liquids, 'drink' and 'drinking' are terms well understood to refer to the ingestion of alcohol. People can be easily categorised as smokers or non-smokers but categorising people as drinkers or non-drinkers (although just as straightforward) is not as useful. Smoking is simply damaging to health and it is advisable not to smoke (Plant and Plant 2006). The majority of the population do not smoke. However, 92 per cent of men and 86 per cent of women in Britain drink alcohol (DoH 2002a). Furthermore, the relationship between health and alcohol, although straightforwardly negative with excessive consumption, is considerably more complex at more moderate levels of consumption. Moderate consumption of alcohol has been associated with health benefits and reductions in mortality compared to non-drinking (Room et al. 2005). In the UK the promotion of sensible drinking, rather than total abstinence, is the crux of the majority of health-related anti-drinking campaigns (Department of Health, Social Services and Public Safety 2001; DoH 2003; Scottish Executive 2005; HM Government 2007; Welsh Assembly Government 2007).

We can define drinking per se as the ingestion of alcohol. However, for practical purposes we need to distinguish between different types of drinking: sensible drinking, hazardous drinking, harmful drinking and, of particularly pertinence to Britain, binge drinking.

Sensible drinking has been conceptualised as:

> drinking in a way which is unlikely to cause yourself or others significant risk of harm.
>
> (HM Government 2007: 3)

Harmful drinking on the other hand can be considered as:

> drinking at levels that lead to significant harm to physical and mental health and at levels that may be causing substantial harm to others.

> Examples include liver damage or cirrhosis, dependence on alcohol and substantial stress or aggression in the family.
>
> (HM Government 2007: 3)

Binge drinking reflects the time-frame of drinking and is a recent addition to policy documents. It reflects the importance of the pattern in which alcohol is consumed for health and social outcomes:

> Binge drinking is essentially drinking too much alcohol over a short period of time, e.g. over the course of an evening and it is typically drinking that leads to drunkenness. It has immediate and short-term risks to the drinker and to those around them.
>
> (HM Government 2007: 3)

Originally the term binge was used by health professionals to describe a prolonged drinking spree lasting at least two or three days. However, the term has been more broadly applied to describe a single drinking session that leads to drunkenness (Plant and Plant 2006; HM Government 2007).

Alcohol dependence and volitional drinking

In the past there has been a tendency to assume that the only serious problems with drinking were part of or due to dependence. However, it is now clear that there are a host of problems related to drinking that are not associated with dependence per se, including an increased risk of developing a range of chronic diseases (Room et al. 2005; French and Zavala 2007). Babor et al. (2003) argue strongly that the major problem with drinking is intoxication and that preventing intoxication from alcohol would prevent much of the social, physical and psychological harm that arises from alcohol. Intoxication is possible without dependence. Similarly, increased risk for a range of lifestyle diseases may occur in people who drink volitionally and are not dependent on alcohol. The concept of alcohol dependence has been recognised as a syndrome by the American Psychiatric Association and the criteria for alcohol dependence are shown in Table 5.1.

It is clear that a diagnosis of dependent drinking is a subjective judgement that will be depend on to cultural and societal expectations of drinking and drinking behaviour (Babor et al. 2003; Plant and Plant 2006). Furthermore, Babor et al. (2003) argue that although alcohol dependency is conceptualised as a clinical construct, it is actually a continuum disorder with milder degrees of habit or dependence present in the population. It is important to note that although consumption is not mentioned as an aspect of diagnosing dependency the higher the levels of consumption the higher the risk of clinical dependency (Babor et al. 2003).

Table 5.1 ICD-10 diagnostic criteria for alcohol dependence

- Evidence of tolerance to the effects of alcohol, such that there is a need for markedly increased amounts to achieve intoxication or desired effect, or that there is a markedly diminished effect with continued use of the same amount of alcohol.
- A physiological withdrawal state when alcohol use is reduce or ceased, or use of a closely related substance with the intention of relieving or avoiding withdrawal symptoms.
- Persisting with alcohol use despite clear evidence of harmful consequences as evidenced by continued use when the person was actually aware of, or could be expected to have been aware of, the nature and extent of harm.
- Preoccupation with alcohol use, as manifested by important alternative pleasures or interests being given up or reduced because of alcohol use; or a great deal of time being spent in activities necessary to obtain alcohol, consume it, or recover from its effects.
- Impaired capacity to control drinking behaviour in terms of its onset; termination or level of use, as evidence by alcohol being often taken in larger amounts or over a longer period than intended, or any unsuccessful effort or persistent desire to cut down or control alcohol use.
- A strong desire or compulsion to use alcohol.

(Adapted from World Health Organisation 1992a)

People become dependent on alcohol because of psychological and neurophysiological reinforcement. The positive outcomes from drinking – feeling euphoric, relaxed and so on – reinforce drinking behaviour. Alcohol interacts with neurotransmitter systems which can lead to sensitization and counter-adaptation which reinforce drinking behaviour. Alcohol's psychoactive properties are central to the development of dependency. Heavy drinking and dependency, in all likelihood, simultaneously reinforce one another. However, individuals will differ in their neurophysiological and psychological responses to alcohol and, consequently, in their risk of developing a clinical dependency. The majority of people who drink alcohol have not been diagnosed as dependent drinkers. Orton (2001) reported that 7.5 per cent of men and 2.1 per cent of women in Britain in the 1990s could be classified as dependent on alcohol.

The remit of this book is to consider lifestyle behaviours over which individuals have a level of control. Consequently, this chapter is focused on volitional rather than dependent drinking. Dependent drinking is a recognised mental health disorder with an associated repertoire of potential interventions that are in the main not appropriate to use with volitional drinkers wishing to reduce their alcohol consumption to sensible levels. However, as a caveat to that, it is clear that a diagnosis of alcohol dependency is subjective and, furthermore, that with a continuum disorder many people with no clinical diagnosis of dependency many nevertheless have a subclinical dependency (Babor et al. 2003).

Government recommendations for drinking

Sensible drinking

In 2007 in the policy document *Safe. Sensible. Social.* the UK government recommended that:

- Adult women should not regularly drink more than 2–3 units of alcohol a day.
- Adult men should not regularly drink more than 3–4 units of alcohol a day.
- Pregnant women or women trying to conceive should avoid drinking alcohol. If they do choose to drink, to protect the baby they should not drink more than 1–2 units of alcohol once or twice a week.

(HM Government 2007: 3)

Previous government recommendations have been framed in a weekly time-frame (Murgraff et al. 2007) and the recommendations that women drink no more than 14 units and men no more than 21 units of alcohol a week are probably the most well known drinking guidelines (Anderson et al. 1993; Scottish Executive 2005). Daily limits have been presented previously but usually alongside the weekly recommendations (Scottish Executive 2005). These current government recommendations, although similar to previous advice in terms of recommended quantities of alcohol, are presented solely in terms of daily drinking and are more flexible about quantity. Not all countries set the same drinking limits, although many governments are moving away from weekly to daily guidelines (www.alcohol.gov.au). The move towards using a daily limit of alcohol in government policy and health promotion reflects better understanding of the importance of patterns of drinking in health outcomes.

Harmful and hazardous drinking

The government defines harmful drinking for women as drinking more than 6 units a day or over 35 units a week. Harmful drinking for men is defined as more than 8 units a day or over 50 units a week (HM Government 2007). Intakes between the upper sensible limits of 14 and 21 units for women and men respectively and harmful drinking levels are considered hazardous (Anderson et al. 1993).

Binge drinking

The government acknowledges that wide variations in definitions of binge drinking exist by cautiously stating:

> Trends in binge drinking are usually identified in surveys by measuring those drinking over 6 units a day for women or 8 units a day for men. In practice, many binge drinkers are drinking substantially more than this level or drink this amount rapidly, which leads to the harm linked to drunkenness.
>
> (HM Government 2007: 3)

The Scottish Health Survey (Scottish Executive 2005) and the Welsh Health Survey (2005–06) use this definition of binge drinking in their national surveys. The Health Survey for England (DoH 2003) uses the definition 'more than twice the daily limits' which is the same thing if you use the upper daily limits from the *Safe. Sensible. Social.* policy document (HM Government 2007).

There is much debate about whether binge drinking should be defined as consumption above a fixed number of units (as we have described) or consumption that results in a particular blood alcohol content or consumption that leads to drunkenness. Furthermore, some authors argue that it should include an intentional component as many people understand 'binge drinking' as deliberately setting out to get drunk (Plant and Plant 2006). The most accepted definition of more than 6 or 8 units in one evening for women and men respectively has also been questioned. In the context of eating and drinking over an evening, 6 to 8 units may not induce the type of drunkenness implicitly understood to result from binge drinking (Plant and Plant 2006). On the other hand, more than 6 or 8 units (depending on your sex) is probably appropriate to reflect the level of alcohol necessary in one episode of drinking to increase your risk of cardiovascular events (Room et al. 2005). Some authors decry any objective measure of binge drinking, describing binge drinkers as people who have felt very drunk once or more in the past 12 months (Mathews and Richardson 2005). Despite the difficulties with defining binge drinking, concerns about this drinking pattern have increased (Room et al. 2005; Plant and Plant 2006; HM Government 2007) and binge drinking is now measured in the UK National Health Surveys in England, Scotland and Wales (DoH 2003; Scottish Executive 2005; Welsh Assembly Government 2003). Plant and Plant (2006) in their seminal text *Binge Britain* conclude that although the term 'binge' is now in general usage, the term 'heavy episodic drinking' may be a more accurate reflection of what is meant.

Evidence of the problem

It is beyond the scope of this book to review and evaluate the full range of methods available to measure drinking activity. However, it would be inappropriate to evaluate levels of drinking without acknowledging that different methodologies exist, particularly considering the variation in reported levels of population drinking identified later in this chapter.

Population levels of drinking can be estimated from per capita consumption. Per capita consumption is estimated from the following formula:

> Alcohol production + Alcohol Imports – Alcohol Exports / Population aged > 15
>
> (WHO 2000)

Clearly, per capita consumption is a very crude measure of alcohol consumption and is subject to errors due to: tourist consumption; stockpiling; waste and spillage, smuggling and duty-free sales among other things. Nevertheless, annual changes in per capita consumption can play an important role in informing public health policy. Per capita consumption also enables international comparisons in alcohol consumption (WHO 2000).

Collecting data from individuals can provide much more detail about drinking. Methods can be physiological: breathalyser tests, urine and blood samples or direct and indirect observational methods. Physiological measures are an objective measure of alcohol levels. Some indication of level of intoxication can be extrapolated from the amount of alcohol in the bloodstream but individual tolerances to alcohol will influence the levels of drunkenness displayed.

Surveys are probably the most common way to collect data about drinking in populations and involve indirect observation of drinking habits. Surveys can indicate who is drinking and describe both patterns of drinking and volume of consumption. They enable comparisons between subgroups within a population (WHO 2000). Indirect observation of drinking usually involves self-reporting of drinking. People can be asked about their drinking either by interview or questionnaire. Sometimes drinking is estimated from medical notes (Anderson et al. 1993). Non-response bias is a particular problem in drinking surveys. Alcohol consumption surveys usually yield response rates of between 60 per cent and 80 per cent (WHO 2000). If the non-responders are systematically different to responders in terms of consumption then estimates of drinking from these surveys cannot be considered representative. Issues of response bias are a common concern and one that afflicts many of the lifestyle surveys reported throughout this text. There are three main methods of asking people to assess their alcohol intake (see Table 5.2).

Often some combination of these three main methods may be utilised in one survey. Opinion is mixed about the reliability of these methods with some authors reporting that quantity-frequency (QF) measures underestimate drinking due to inaccurate recall and others that 'Last seven days' may miss irregular drinkers and underestimate drinking in that way.

An important issue for measurement of drinking is the validity and reliability of the instrument in question and unfortunately many widely used

Table 5.2 Methods of calculating alcohol consumption

Quantity-Frequency (QF)	Asks about usual consumption of alcohol and frequency of drinking
Graduated Quantity-Frequency (GQF)	Asks how often people drink specified amounts of alcohol in one day, usually starting with large amounts and graduating to small amounts
Last seven days	Asks people to indicate how much they drank on each of the previous seven days

(Adapted from World Health Organisation 2000)

measures of alcohol consumption have not been tested for such psychometric properties. Questionnaires are a subjective measure of drinking and ideally such tools should be validated by an objective physiological measure, although this is not as straightforward as it is for say physical activity. The validity of a physical activity questionnaire can be tested by measures of physical fitness that are relatively stable, certainly over the period needed for validation. However, physiological measures of drinking reflect drinking at only one point in time and do not provide a useful comparison for the validation of questionnaires that assess drinking habits. Therefore, work on the validity and reliability of alcohol consumption questionnaire is required. A wide range of different questions are utilised by various population surveys and standardisation of these approaches would provide the opportunity for more cross study comparisons.

Probably the most convincing evidence that self-report measures of drinking in any one study do, at the very least, place people in an appropriate place on the drinking continuum compared to their peers is the relationship between self-reported drinking and proven increased risk for a number of alcohol related conditions (Room et al. 2005).

Current drinking levels

Measurement of drinking behaviour varied in the English, Welsh, Scottish and Northern Irish health surveys (DoH 2003; Welsh Assembly Government 2007; Scottish Executive 2003: Department of Health, Social Services and Public Safety 2001 respectively). All surveys asked a wide range of questions about drinking habits utilising both 'quantity/frequency' and 'last seven days' methodologies. However, within these methodologies both the questions asked and descriptive statistics utilised differed. The Welsh Health Survey consistently reported overall percentages of consumption, including those who indicated that they hadn't drunk in the previous seven days. However, in the English and Scottish surveys data was presented as percentage consumption among those who reported drinking in the last week; only sometimes are the overall figures also provided. A significant minority of people, approaching 50 per cent in women in Wales, reported not drinking in the previous week (Table 5.3). Unsurprisingly the percentages drinking over the recommended daily units and the percentages binge drinking are far higher when those who didn't drink in the previous week are excluded (Table 5.3).

Table 5.3 Percentage of men and women reporting not drinking in the previous week

	Men reporting not drinking in the previous week (%)	*Women reporting not drinking in the previous week (%)*
Health Survey England 2003	28	37
Scottish Health Survey 2003	28	42
Welsh Health Survey 2005–06	30	47

Due to different questions asked by the four surveys, there are few comparisons available for all four. The best areas for comparison are the percentage exceeding daily recommended levels of units on at least one day during the previous week and the percentage binge drinking (exceeding twice the daily limits of more than 6 units or 8 units in a single drinking session for women and men respectively) on at least one day in the previous week. This data is available in three of the national surveys (English, Welsh and Scottish). The only point of comparison available for the Northern Ireland survey is the percentage exceeding weekly guidelines as this was measured in the Scottish survey as well.

The levels of drinking reported in national surveys (see Table 5.4) are higher than the figures presented in *Safe. Sensible. Social.* (HM Government 2007) which reported that overall 35 per cent of men and 20 per cent of women exceed the daily benchmarks on at least one day in the previous week. The *Safe. Sensible. Social.* figures were based on the 2005 General Household Survey (HM Government 2007). In the English Survey the overall percentages exceeding the daily limit on at least one day a week (Table 5.4) were more than 10 per cent higher than reported in *Safe. Sensible. Social.* (HM Government 2007). Self-report is known to be inaccurate, and people are generally understood to be optimistic about lifestyle behaviours, underestimating drinking and overestimating fruit and vegetable consumption (Plant and Plant 2006). However, Plant and Plant (2006) do acknowledge that some surveys, particularly of young people, may overestimate consumption. The variation in estimates of drinking levels between these various government documents gives cause for concern and highlights the importance of undertaking robust reliability and validity studies on drinking questionnaires. It is interesting that

Plant and Plant (2006) and Room (2004) are damning about government policy towards drinking in Britain. They point out that the Alcohol Harm Reduction Strategy for England (Prime Minister's Strategy Unit 2004) highlights control policies that are considered ineffective by most scientists (Room 2004; Plant and Plant 2006). Room (2004) and Plant and Plant (2006) suggest that government policy has been driven by a wish to cooperate with the beverage alcohol industry. Consequently, this may be why they prefer to cite the lower figures produced by the General Household Survey (ONS 2006a) than utilise the more worrying figures they themselves publish elsewhere.

Gender differences in alcohol consumption

Men drink more alcohol than women and they are more likely to exceed their daily and/or weekly guidelines, even though those guidelines are higher than those recommended for women (Table 5.4). This gender difference in alcohol consumption is consistently reported in the national surveys and elsewhere (HM Government 2007; ONS 2007) and furthermore is similar to the gendered drinking patterns of previous decades (e.g. Blaxter 1990).

Initially, the relationship between gender and drinking seems straightforward. Men drink more than women. However, when you include age in the analysis, some changing gender patterns emerge. In younger people aged 16 to 24 the gender difference in alcohol consumption is only 7 per cent in all three surveys (Table 5.5). In the 1984/85 health and lifestyle survey, young women drank far less than young men. In the more recent national surveys the gender gap in drinking is more pronounced in the older age groups (Table 5.5). The Health Survey for England has been collecting annual data since 1998 and consequently has more previous comparison points than the other surveys. It reports that binge drinking among men has remained stable, increasing by only 1 per cent between 1998 and 2003. However, there has been a 2 per cent increase in female binge drinkers from 11 per cent in 1998 to 13 per cent in 2003. Given the initial percentages for men and women, this is proportionally significant. As this is cross-sectional data it is difficult to tell whether younger women will continue to drink as much alcohol as their male counterparts as they age. However, it is an indication that drinking alcohol is a gender role activity that is changing and that it is more acceptable for young women to drink.

A number of authors and surveys have expressed concern about the increased levels of drinking in young women (HM Government 2007; News 2007). Plant and Plant (2006) suggest that the high levels of binge drinking reported by young British women is unusual and has not been reported in the majority of other Western countries. A number of explanations for the high levels of binge drinking in young British women have

Table 5.4 Drinking prevalence rates in men and women taken from the national surveys

Source of data	*Men reporting exceeding four units of alcohol on at least one day in the previous week (%)*	*Women reporting exceeding three units of alcohol on at least one day in the previous week (%)*	*Men reporting binge drinking in the previous week (%)*	*Women reporting binge drinking in the previous week (%)*	*Men reporting exceeding weekly limits (%)*	*Women reporting exceeding weekly limits (%)*
Health Survey England 2003	*62* 47	*49* 30	*36* 28	*22* 14	No data available	No data available
Scottish Health Survey 2003	*63* 47	*57* 36	*37* 28	*28* 18	27	13.5
Welsh Health Survey 2005–06	45	26	27	12	No data available	No data available
Northern Ireland Health and Social Wellbeing Survey 2001	No data available	No data available	No data available	No data available	25	14

Notes:
Figures in italics are based on people who reported drinking in the previous week.
Figures in roman are overall percentages

Table 5.5 Percentages of men and women in different age groups exceeding daily recommended limits on at least one day in a week

Source of data	*% of ♂ 16–24*	*% of ♂ 25–34*	*% of ♂ 35–44*	*% of ♂ 45–54*	*% of ♂ 55–64*	*% of ♂ 65–74*	*% of ♂ 75*	*% of ♀ 16–24*	*% of ♀ 25–34*	*% of ♀ 35–44*	*% of ♀ 45–54*	*% of ♀ 55–64*	*% of ♀ 65–74*	*% of ♀ 75*
Health Survey England 2003	*77*	*71*	*66*	*63*	*57*	*40*	*27*	*70*	*61*	*56*	*50*	*40*	*24*	*14*
Scottish Health Survey 2003	*81*	*69*	*64*	*64*	*59*	*47*	*32*	*76*	*70*	*63*	*56*	*46*	*35*	*17*
Welsh Health Survey 2005–06	47	57	53	51	45	28	12	40	35	34	32	20	11	4

Notes:
Figures in italics are based on people who reported drinking in the previous week
Figures in roman are overall percentages

been proposed although there is little evidence to support any of these hypotheses. It has been suggested that women in the UK have more social freedom than women in other countries and that alcohol advertising has been especially targeted at young women (Plant and Plant 2006). However, other potential factors such as the rising age of first pregnancy and increasing equality for women in society are also factors in other countries where young female drinking has not risen so remarkably. The policy document *Safe. Sensible. Social.* (HM Government 2007) suggests that agencies should be working to make drunkenness unacceptable but it would appear that drunkenness is becoming more socially acceptable for young women in the UK. Whatever the reasons for the surge of drinking in young women, health professionals are alarmed (News 2007) about the potential consequences in terms of later health problems and are anxious to evaluate whether this is an acute feature of young adult life in women who will then reduce their drinking in later life or whether this trend of increased drinking in young women will persist through the life course (HM Government 2007).

As men and women get older the amount they drink decreases, and this is more noticeable in women. This is cross-sectional data so we cannot be sure whether this is an effect of ageing or a cohort effect. Young women have been previously highlighted as drinking more than previous generations of young women (Blaxter 1990). However, it is not possible to say how this generation of young women will drink when they are older. In Blaxter's (1990) study older men and women both reported lower levels of drinking than their younger counterparts. If we extrapolate from this data we might expect the current generation of young women to reduce their drinking as they age but still drink more than women of previous generations.

Socio-economic differences in alcohol consumption

There are few clear socio-economic trends in alcohol consumption evident from the National Surveys. Only the English and Scottish surveys present socio-economic daily drinking patterns stratified by sex and no clear socio-economic patterns emerge for either sex (Tables 5.6 and 5.7). The Welsh survey only presents average daily consumption on a drinking day by socio-economic class and then only for adults, not stratified by sex; again no socio-economic patterns emerge (Table 5.8). There was no socio-economic pattern in female binge drinking in Scotland but binge drinking was more common for men living in households of lower socio-economic classification. Binge drinking was also more common in the most deprived areas of Scotland. Similarly, the English Survey reported that binge drinking was less common in people who reported having a managerial or professional job.

The Scottish survey also asked about weekly consumption and here reported a reversed socio-economic classification and alcohol consumption relationship from that reported for binge drinking. Scottish women living in managerial and professional households were more likely to exceed the weekly limit of 14 units than women living in households with lower socio-economic classifications. Weekly consumption showed a linear relationship with class, being lowest in women living in households classified as semi-routine or routine. However, there was no such clear pattern of weekly consumption and socio-economic classification of the household in Scottish men. In contrast, *Safe. Social. Sensible.* reports that drinking over sensible guidelines is more common in areas of high deprivation and

Table 5.6 Percentage of men in different socio-economic groups exceeding daily limit on at least one day in a week (age standardised)

Source of data	*Managerial and professional (%)*	*Inter-mediate (%)*	*Small employers and own account workers (%)*	*Lower supervisory and technical (%)*	*Semi-routine and routine (%)*	*Long-term unemployed or have never worked*
Health Survey England 2003	60	63	68	66	64	Not available
Scottish Health Survey 2003	58	65	63	70	67	Not available

Table 5.7 Percentage of women (among women who drink) in different socio-economic groups exceeding daily limit or binge drinking on at least one day in a week (age standardised)

Source of data	*Managerial and professional (%)*	*Inter-mediate (%)*	*Small employers and own account workers (%)*	*Lower supervisory and technical (%)*	*Semi-routine and routine (%)*	*Long-term unemployed or have never worked*
Health Survey England 2003	48	52	48	47	52	Not available
Scottish Health Survey 2003	51	56	52	55	58	Not available

Table 5.8 Overall percentage of adults in Wales in different socio-economic groups with an average consumption above the daily limits on days that they choose to drink

Source of data	*Managerial and professional (%)*	*Inter-mediate (%)*	*Small employers and own account workers (%)*	*Lower supervisory and technical (%)*	*Semi-routine and routine (%)*	*Long-term unemployed or have never worked (%)*
Welsh Health Survey 2005–06	36	39	36	43	41	29

that alcohol related deaths were three to five times higher in people living in areas of high deprivation (HM Government 2007). Jefferis et al. (2006) also reported social gradients in drinking. Their data is particularly interesting because it is prospective, longitudinal data rather than the cross-sectional snapshot of current drinking behaviour that is presented in the national surveys. Jefferis et al. (2006) found clear social class patterns in drinking but of a non-linear pattern. They report that the least educated men were both more likely to report that they were non-drinkers or that they were binge drinkers than more educated men. The picture for women was more complex with educated women being more likely to report binge drinking in their twenties than less well educated women but being less likely to report binge drinking in their thirties. These longitudinal data suggest differential socio-economic effects in men and women and differential socio-economic effects for different drinking patterns. These differential effects reported by Jefferis et al. (2006) are similar to those found in the cross-sectional data from the National Surveys.

Ethnicity and alcohol consumption

While none of the national surveys present data on ethnic differences in drinking patterns the Health Survey for England focused on ethnic minority health in their 1999 survey (Erens and Laiho 2001). In England in 1999, men and women from all minority groups, except the Irish, reported less alcohol consumption than that reported by the general population. People from ethnic minority groups were more likely to report that they were non-drinkers. 30 per cent of Chinese men, 33 per cent of Indian men and over 90 per cent of Pakistani and Bangladeshi men were non-drinkers. The percentage of non-drinkers was even higher among women from all ethnic minorities, with 99 per cent of Bangladeshi women being non-drinkers. In all ethnic minority groups, apart from the Irish, the levels of alcohol consumption were also lower than the general population. Erens and Laiho (2001) reflect that general social norms might result in some under-reporting of alcohol consumption, particularly among minority groups that prohibit alcohol such as Muslim communities. Many interviews were not conducted in private, the presence of other family members may have contributed to the problem of under-reporting. These data are currently ten years out of date and it is probable that the picture may be changing. When we consider the change in female drinking habits over a similar period these figures should be viewed with considerable caution. It is possible that older people from ethnic minorities are maintaining the habits that they practised in the 1990s but younger people may well have different attitudes and practices from their parents and grandparents.

From these data from the national surveys of lifestyle behaviours in the UK we get a picture of younger people drinking more than older people. A cursory glance at gender differences would suggest that men drink more than women but a closer look at the relationship between sex, age and drinking suggests that young women's drinking is becoming more similar to men's. Unlike smoking, no straightforward linear socio-economic patterns in drinking emerge. We see different socio-economic effects on patterns of drinking in men and women. Whereas men at the lower end of the socio-economic scale are more likely to 'binge' drink than their professional or managerial counterparts, in women there is either no socio-economic influence on drinking reported or professional and managerial women are found to drink more. The most interesting phenomenon in drinking patterns for health professionals are the habits of women, which appear to be undergoing a cultural revolution not apparent in men. The implications of increased levels of drinking in young women now, and of how they continue to drink as they progress through the lifecourse have the potential to significantly influence future health outcomes.

Consequences of excessive drinking

The relationship between drinking and health is complex. Alcohol undoubtedly has a predominantly negative effect on the health of populations. However, at the individual level it has been suggested that alcohol can have positive effects on health outcomes but only for certain restricted patterns of consumption (Room et al. 2005; French and Zavala 2007). Alcohol is different from the other lifestyle disorders presented here, except perhaps for drug abuse, in that it impacts directly on the health of individuals, through the physiological effects of ingesting alcohol and also indirectly through the behavioural changes that excess alcohol consumption can initiate.

Indirect health consequences of drinking

The indirect implications of drinking alcohol are not the major concern of this text. Nevertheless, a brief résumé of the indirect consequences of such behaviour is appropriate not least because these indirect and unusually short-term consequences of alcohol consumption may prove useful in the promotion of health drinking patterns which will have the long-term health consequences of more direct interest to health professionals.

People under the influence of alcohol are more likely to behave aggressively and this can lead to physical violence that can harm themselves and others (Room et al. 2005; Plant and Plant 2006; HM Government 2007). Offenders are believed to be under the influence of alcohol in 46 per cent of incidents of domestic violence and 44 per cent of acquaintance violence. HM Government (2007) reports that among young people who report binge drinking, only a quarter become involved in antisocial behaviours or disorder. However, Budd (2003) reported that 39 per cent of binge drinkers aged 18–24 had committed an offence in the previous year. The relationship between drinking and violence is not simple and varies in different countries. An extra litre per capita of ethanol consumption raises the homicide rate by twice as much in northern European countries as it does in southern European countries (Room et al. 2005) which may be due to different societal patterns of drinking. Drinking also has the potential to make people more vulnerable targets of other people's criminal behaviour; 15 per cent of rape victims recorded by the 2001 British Crime Survey were raped when they were under the influence of alcohol. Heavy drinking has also been linked to increased numbers of sexual partners (see Chapter 7) which increases the risk of sex-related infections.

People under the influence of alcohol are also more likely to have accidents. Motor vehicle accidents are the most common form of unintentional alcohol related injury (Room et al. 2005). The World Health Organisation (2002) estimates that 20 per cent of motor vehicle accidents worldwide are alcohol related. HM Government (2007) reported that in 2005 6 per cent of road casualties and 17 per cent of all road deaths occurred when someone was driving while over the legal limit for alcohol. From 1980 to 1999 the number of people killed or seriously injured annually in drink-driving incidents fell from 9,000 to fewer than 3,000 which is a significant reduction in alcohol related incidents. However, the number of people killed or seriously injured in drink-driving incidents since 1998 has stabilised and new strategies to reduce such unnecessary fatalities may be indicated.

Direct health consequences of drinking

Alcohol has been implicated in more than 60 medical conditions, predominantly with negative, but occasionally with positive, consequences (Room et al. 2005). It has been recognised that the relationship between alcohol consumption and health is not always linear. Patterns of drinking, especially irregular heavy drinking have been linked to an increase risk of cardiovascular disease (Room et al. 2005)

For coronary heart disease, stroke, diabetes, and also for the indirect consequences of alcohol consumption discussed above, irregular patterns of heavy drinking are associated with pharmacological and physiological effects that increase the risk of cardiovascular disease and increase the risk of injury to self and others. Episodic heavy drinking, even when the overall volume of alcohol intake is low, has been found to increase the risk for a number of cardiovascular conditions. This association is physiologically consistent with the increased clotting, lower threshold for ventricular fibrillation and elevation of low density lipoproteins that occur after heavy drinking (Room et al. 2005).

However, regular low to moderate alcohol consumption is associated with physiological mechanisms linked to favourable cardiac outcomes; these positive effects are believed to be mediated by the influence of alcohol on lipids and haemostatic factors. Another drinking pattern that appears positive for cardiovascular disease is drinking with meals (Room et al. 2005). French and Zavala (2007) reported that there is a J-shaped relationship between alcohol consumption and total mortality with moderate drinkers having the lowest mortality rates, heavy drinkers the highest and abstainers/light drinkers somewhere in between.

In other diseases a linear relationship between consumption and disease does exist. Breast cancer risk increases linearly with increased alcohol consumption: 10 grams of alcohol a day (an average UK unit) increases the relative risk of breast cancer by 9 per cent. A daily consumption of between 30 and 60 grams a day increases the relative risk by 41 per cent (Cancer Research UK 2002). It has been argued in Chapter 4 that the positive effects of exercise on breast cancer risk are mediated by the influence of physical activity on circulating oestrogen. Similarly, the relationship between alcohol and breast cancer is also thought to be mediated by effect of alcohol on circulating oestrogen.

Alcohol is also implicated in a range of psychiatric disorders that arise from its pharmacological effects. Depression, epilepsy and alcohol addiction are all serious health problems that can be caused by excessive alcohol consumption (Room et al. 2006; Plant and Plant 2006; HM Government 2007). Furthermore, alcohol consumption exacerbates existing conditions such as depression or anxiety.

Drinking is also associated with weight gain and with rising levels of obesity (Plant and Plant 2006). Oesterle et al. (2004) suggest that young women who drink to excess are at increased risk of weight gain. However, in contrast to this the Scottish Health Survey reported a relationship between drinking and obesity in men but not in women (Scottish Health Executive 2003).

The disorders most commonly understood to be related to alcohol consumption are liver diseases, although many people who have liver disorders are not heavy drinkers. Cirrhosis of the liver can be an alcohol-related disease, although only 39 per cent of cirrhosis cases are alcohol-related. In 2005 4,160 people in England and Wales died from alcoholic liver disease (HM Government 2007). This is a significant increase of 41 per cent since 1999 when 2,954 people died from alcoholic liver disease. Alcohol is also implicated in oral cancers of the mouth and throat (Room et al. 2005).

In England and Wales alcohol-related injury or illness accounts for 180,000 hospital admissions a year (HM Government 2007). Alcohol-related deaths in the UK have more than doubled between 1991 and 2006 from 6.9 per cent to 13.4 per cent per 100,000 (ONS 2008). A summary of the major disease and injury conditions related to alcohol and the percentage of incidents that are attributable to alcohol is presented in Table 5.9.

Table 5.9 Global mortality burden (deaths in thousands) attributable to alcohol by major disease categories – 2000 (adapted from Rehm et al 2003)

Disease conditions	*Men*	*Women*	*Total*	*% of all attributable deaths*
Conditions arising during the perinatal period	2	1	3	0.2
Malignant neoplasm	269	86	355	9.7
Neuropsychiatric conditions	91	19	111	6.2
Cardiovascular diseases	392	–124	268	14.9
Other non-communicable diseases (diabetes, liver cirrhosis)	193	49	242	13.4
Unintentional injuries	484	92	577	32.0
Intentional injuries	206	42	248	13.7
Alcohol-related mortality burden all causes	1,638	166	1,804	100
All deaths	29,232	26,629	55,861	3.2

One area of concern is the numbers of people living with chronic diseases who regularly drink above the sensible drinking guidelines. Many people with diseases such as diabetes, coronary heart disease and hypertension where alcohol is implicated in the aetiology and progression of the disease continue to drink beyond their diagnosis (see Table 5.10) (HM Government 2007).

Table 5.10 Percentage of people not drinking sensibly despite diagnosis (from HM Government 2007)

Condition	*Men (%)*	*Women (%)*
Hypertension	42	10
CHD	34	6
Stroke	33	7
Diabetes	35	8
Kidney disease	26	6
Depression	42	16

Why do people drink more alcohol than is sensible?

The UK has a long tradition of both sensible and harmful drinking. The consensus of surveys has traditionally been that the majority of adults consume alcoholic beverages at least occasionally and that most people drink moderate amounts that do not have harmful effects (Plant and Plant 2006). Plant and Plant (2006) suggest that most people drink alcohol because they enjoy the taste and the disinhibiting effects of such drinks and because consuming them is a sociable thing to do.

Paglia and Room (1999) suggest that young people start to drink as part of the developmental process of identity formation. It can be a symbolic behaviour that facilitates social bonding and peer status among peers. Alcohol can provide youth with a seemingly adult status (Paglia and Room 1999). Alcohol consumption at any age can be functional providing pleasure, alleviating boredom, satisfying the desire for sensation seeking or acting as a coping or escape mechanism.

Alcohol serves an important social function. It enhances social integration and facilitates the development of relationships (Kuther and Timoshin 2003). It is hardly surprising that people drink most at a period in their lives which is normally associated with the development of stable adult relationships (Paglia and Room 1999). Increased levels of drinking in newly divorced people may be in part due to the breakdown of stable relationships and the desire to establish new relationships (HM Government 2007). Social isolation is a key factor in poor health outcomes (Cacioppo and Hawkley 2003) so the positive social function of alcohol in enabling people to develop social relationships should not be overlooked.

Socio-economic factors

The relationship between socio-economic factors and drinking is not simple. There is some evidence that people from the most deprived walks of life are more likely to binge drink, develop non-functional addiction to alcohol and to die from conditions with a primarily alcohol-related aetiology (HM Government 2007). However, regular consumption at levels above the recommended limits is more likely in people from higher socio-economic groups, particularly women (Department of Health, Social Services and Public Safety 2001; DoH 2003; Scottish Executive 2005; Welsh Assembly Government 2007). Alcohol in UK culture can be considered to have no class boundaries.

Psychological factors

Many different psychological factors have been postulated to underpin volitional drinking behaviours. A perception of risk variously described as perceived personal threat in the HBM (Rosenstock 1974), threat appraisal in the PMT (Norman et al. 2005) and as beliefs in the TPB (Conner and Sparks 2005) is an integral aspect of most social cognitive modules of behaviour. However, similarly to other lifestyle behaviours there is little evidence that perceptions of risk can explain much if any of the variation in drinking behaviour (Minugh et al. 1998).

Marcoux and Shope (1997) reported that the theory of planned behaviour successfully predicted alcohol use in adolescents, explaining 26 per cent of the variation in alcohol use in their population of nearly 4000 adolescents. Intention to drink predicted 26 per cent of the variation in drinking behaviour. 76 per cent of the variation in intention to drink was explained by attitudes, social norms and perceived behavioural control. Murgraff et al. (2007) argue that the TPB is the most successful predictive model of health behaviour. Murgraff et al. (2007) may draw this conclusion because of the power of the TPB variables to predict 'intention to behave' rather than actual behaviour. Interestingly, Murgraff et al. (2007) conclude that intention is not a sufficient prerequisite for action and propose an intervention to reduce 'Friday Night' consumption among moderate drinkers that utilises implementation intentions. Implementation intentions and the related practice of goal setting all stem from the recognition of the important of self-efficacy and are practical approaches to increasing self-efficacy (Rovniak et al. 2002). Consequently, although Murgraff et al. (2007) cite the TPB as the theoretical basis of their study, it could be argued that social cognitive variables are also involved.

Kuther and Timoshin (2003) investigated the role of social cognitive variables in predicting alcohol use. They reported that social cognitive variables explained 76 per cent of the variation in self-reported alcohol use in more than 200 college students. This is a considerably higher percentage than Marcoux and Shope (1997) found the TPB could predict, supporting the argument made previously that SCT is a better predictive model for drinking than the TPB. In particular, outcome expectations about the likelihood and desirability of the positive and negative consequences of drinking as well as self-efficacy predicted self-reported drinking. Those who believed they could control their drinking drank less. Blume et al. (2003) reported that low self-efficacy was associated with greater levels of drinking. Williams et al. (2007) found that self-efficacy was a key factor in predicting improved drinking habits in individuals identified as drinking unhealthily in the primary care setting. Similarly, Murgraff et al. (2007) found that self-efficacy was implicated in a slight reduction in binge drinking in young women who had moderate weekly alcohol consumption.

In contrast to other lifestyle behaviours where social norms have been argued to play little or no part in the explanation for variations in behaviour, social norms are consistently reported to be useful in explaining variations in drinking behaviour (Delaney and Ames 1995; Ames and Grube 2000; Dijkstra et al. 2001; Yang et al. 2001; Kuther and Timoshin 2003; Ramos and Perkins 2006; Barrientos-Gutierrez et al. 2007). However, McMillan and Conner (2003) report that in studies evaluating the TPB social norms are consistently the weakest predictor of intention across a wide range of health behaviours including sensible drinking.

There is a rational explanation for this apparent contradiction. McMillan and Conner (2003) conclude that the way that social norms are traditionally conceptualised with the TPB does not account for the various ways in which social influence is exerted and is particularly inappropriate for drinking. Traditionally, social norms are conceptualised and measured within the TPB framework by asking about the social approval or disapproval of others and are described as injunctive social norms by McMillan and Conner (2003). However, studies that report strong relationships between social norms and drinking behaviour ask about descriptive social norms. That is to say they ask individuals how much they think their peers are drinking. Kuther and Timoshin (2003) looked at both descriptive peer norms and descriptive parental norms, and found both were associated with levels of drinking in students, although the relationship was stronger for peer norms. Similarly, in the workplace the descriptive drinking norms within that organisation and among colleagues were strongly associated with drinking behaviours both within and outside the working environment (Barrientos-Gutierrez et al. 2007).

The relationship between perceptions of peer drinking norms and individual drinking has led to the utilisation of social norms theory in alcohol interventions. Social norms theory postulates that behaviours can be influenced by potentially incorrect perceptions of how members in a social group think and act. An individual could overestimate the acceptability of drinking among his or her peers or may underestimate the practice of health behaviours (Ramos and Perkins 2006). Social norm theory is conceptually similar to the concept of unrealistic optimism that is well recognised in a number of health-related behaviours (Weinstein 1984). Interventions based on social norms theory attempt to challenge individual perceptions of normative drinking behaviours among their peers and have met with some success (Paglia and Room 1999; Ramos and

Perkins 2006). Kuther and Timoshin (2003) also report the importance of drinking for socialisation. They reported that students who reported higher levels of drinking were significantly more likely to report high levels of social support.

The transtheoretical model of behavioural change (TTM) was first developed to use with smoking but has been utilised with many other lifestyle behaviours, including drinking (Kurz 2003). As has been found in other lifestyle behaviours the concept of drinking reduction as a process is useful but the value of the actual stages as conceptualised in the original TTM are hard to evaluate.

Prochaska et al. (2004) have stated that the TTM is one of the most promising solutions to the problem of alcohol abuse on college campuses. Prochaska et al. (2004) reported that of 1,500 first and second year students about 70 per cent were in the pre-contemplative stage for stopping abusing alcohol. They go on to outline an ambitious whole campus approach to reduce drinking, which is broadly based on TTM theory. Prochaska et al. (2004) report that their multiple interventions, including decreasing the availability of alcohol, increasing the number of alcohol-free activities, creating a climate that discourages high-risk drinking, challenging inaccurate perceptions of peer-drinking norms (a social norm theory based strategy) along with a number of other strategies did reduce binge drinking, police complaints, and admissions for alcohol poisoning. The most dramatic effect was on student awareness of alcohol policies with 97 per cent of students on the campus in question, rather than 73 per cent nationally, being aware of drinking policies. While such a comprehensive and multilevel strategy is encouraging and some of the results are positive it is difficult to conclude that the TTM is the effective component of the multilevel programme as some interventions were TTM based, others utilised strategies that were derived from other theories and others had no clear theoretical premise. The key advantage here of utilising the TTM is providing a framework and focus for the intervention.

In contrast to Prochaska et al.'s (2004) entirely positive evaluation of the usefulness of the TTM for changing drinking behaviour, Ramos and Perkins (2006) found less support for the TTM in their evaluation of a programme to encourage sensible drinking. They report that more than half of their sample moved from being precontemplators to being in the action stage, although the time frame of their Alcohol Intervention Programme was only 3–4 weeks. This presents a challenge to the TTM which conceptualises stage change as far slower. Ramos and Perkins (2006) argue that the kind of conceptual change they witnessed is not possible and that there may be an element of social desirability coming into play with students anxious to demonstrate the kind of behaviour changes that they perceive were required. Nevertheless, Ramos and Perkins (2006) remain positive about the value of TTM for promoting changes in drinking behaviour.

However, Williams et al. (2007) found that measures of readiness to change did not predict either future heavy episodic drinking or future overall consumption in 312 primary care patients who drank unhealthily. They found that self-efficacy predicted lower consumption and less heavily episodic drinking and concluded that interventions that support self-efficacy such as motivational interviewing might have greater utility than stage-based interventions for promoting behavioural change in people who drink unhealthily.

In conclusion, there is some evidence that social cognition theories can predict sensible drinking in populations. In particular, social norms when conceptualised as descriptive social norms are important in understanding drinking behaviour. As with other lifestyle behaviours, risk perception appears to have little or no value in predicting drinking behaviour. Similarly to other lifestyle behaviours, the role of self-efficacy in promoting drinking behavioural change looks promising.

Interventions to reduce drinking

The Nuffield Council on Bioethics (2007) has argued that public health policies should be about enforcement and it proposes an 'intervention ladder' as a useful way of conceptualising public health interventions and their impact on an individual's choice (see Table 5.11 and discussion of interventions for smoking cessation).

In terms of drinking, current UK government policies are firmly focused on strategies from the final two rows of the table, although certain limited strategies from higher in the table such as taxation on alcohol and limited legal restrictions on drinking in some contexts are in place.

Plant and Plant (2006) raise concerns that the Alcohol Harm Strategy for England ignores the evidence of the ineffectiveness of alcohol education and the effectiveness of taxation as preventative drinking measures: a picture which is mirrored in the other national policy documents (Plant and Plant 2006). The strategy highlights policies of alcohol education and voluntary agreements with the alcohol industry which have no credence with professionals in the field. The strategy ignores advice from experts such as the Academy of Medical Sciences (2004) who argue that even modest increases in alcohol taxation could substantially decrease alcohol related mortality and under-aged drinking. The following discussion on interventions to reduce risky drinking will consider all the levels of intervention proposed by the Nuffield Council on Bioethics in turn (Table 5.11).

There are certain groups, more influential in the United States, who would support prohibition and the criminalisation of alcohol but even in the United States and certainly in Britain these are a minority voice and there is no likelihood of prohibition becoming policy in the UK. However, alcohol is illegal for certain age groups in various countries. In the United States, you cannot legally drink alcohol before you are 21, whereas in

Table 5.11 The intervention ladder

Level	*Description*	*Drinking example*
Eliminate choice	Introduce laws that entirely eliminate choice	Prohibition
Restrict choice	Introduce laws that restrict the options available to people	Remove alcohol from supermarkets
Guide through disincentives	Introduce financial or other disincentives to influence behaviour	Increase taxes of alcohol via taxation
Guide through incentives	Introduce financial or other incentives to influence people's behaviour	Fund alcohol free events
Guide choices	Changing the default policy	Recommend sensible levels of alcohol consumption
Enable choice	Help individuals to change their behaviour	Provide drinking cessation schemes

(Adapted from Nuffield Council on Bioethics 2007)

Britain you may drink alcohol in private from the age of 5 but may not purchase or drink alcohol in a public place until you are 18. Consequently, some interventions, particularly school-based interventions in the United States, have a goal of total abstinence. The rationale for such a stance is not only to limit damaging drinking in young people in the present but also to reduce the risk of problem drinking later as it is well established that the earlier a person starts to drink, smoke or use illegal drugs the higher the risk of later abuse (Hawkins et al. 1997; Foxcroft et al. 2003). In Britain, where the legal situation is different, there is more of a problem with binge drinking in young people. However, many countries with equally lax laws about the age of drinking do not report the same incidence of binge drinking that is reported in Britain (Plant and Plant 2006). Nevertheless, there is evidence that increasing the minimum drinking age would reduce drinking in young people (Klepp et al. (1996).

Taxation as a public health measure is a familiar practice in smoking. It is an effective intervention only if people drink less in response to rising price. It will be an effective health intervention only if people who are currently drinking hazardously or dangerously drink less. If moderate drinkers are more affected by a price change than heavy drinkers, as Manning et al. (1995) have suggested they may be, then using taxation to decrease the risk of alcohol-related disorders may not be effective. A contrasting argument is the 'alcohol prevention paradox' (Kreitman 1986) which suggests that reduction of harm at the population level is best achieved through the reduction of per capita consumption. There are considerably more moderate drinkers in the population so a modest reduction in drinking in this group is easier to achieve and generates more benefit than a reduction in the drinking of the smaller number of heavy drinkers.

There is evidence that people drink less if the price of alcohol increases (Room 2004) and that those of particular concern, heavy drinkers and young people, both respond to price increases by drinking less (Sutton and Godfrey 1995). However, the effectiveness of raising taxes is not clear cut, with consumption of popular drinks such as beer and wine being less responsive to price rises than other alcoholic beverages. Paglia and Room (1999) suggest that adolescents are particularly responsive to the price of alcohol and that increasing the price of alcohol would be effective in reducing heavy drinking and related harm among this cohort. Room (2004) and Plant and Plant (2006) have concluded that the power of the alcoholic beverage lobby is one reason why alcohol taxation as a public health measure has not been adopted.

Funding of alcohol-free events is perhaps the least well researched type of intervention. It has been utilised as part of whole campus, multifaceted interventions but its effectiveness is hard to evaluate as it is usually only one of a number of interventions simultaneously rolled out to change the drinking habits of a whole community (Prochaska et al. 2004).

Guiding and enabling choice strategies are often but not always combined as interventions. Consequently, they will be evaluated together. Interventions that guide or enable choice are many and varied and can be usefully categorised as early drinking interventions aimed at adolescents and young people or as interventions for established drinkers. Similarly to other lifestyle behaviours, a failure to properly evaluate the effectiveness of such intervention programmes is common (Foxcroft et al. 2003) and the majority of studies follow up their participants only in the short term. Definitions of long and short term differ between evaluations of lifestyle behaviours. In the exercise literature a short term follow-up would generally be defined as 12 weeks or less. Foxcroft et al. (2003) define short term as less than 1 year of follow-up, medium term between 1 and 3 years of follow-up, and anything over 3 years as long-term follow up. Nevertheless, the same message emerges, the majority of programmes follow up their programme participants only in the short term and for the purposes of promoting long-term healthy drinking we need to understand their effectiveness over the long term (Foxcroft et al. 2003).

Early interventions in drinking

Many interventions to encourage sensible drinking are aimed at adolescents and young people with the goal of preventing the establishment of unhealthy drinking habits. The rationale for a predominance of interventions for this age group includes the indisputable fact that young people are the heaviest drinkers in society (HM Government 2007; see previous discussion on pp. 120–123). Furthermore, there is a tacit assumption that 'bad leads to bad' although the evidence to support that this is always, or even usually, the case is not compelling. As Paglia and Room (1999) argue, bad beginnings do not always have bad ends and many people who experiment with excessive drinking in their youth are not excessive drinkers in their mid to late twenties. Nevertheless, it is indisputable that it is in adolescence that drinking begins, so encouraging sensible drinking in this cohort continues to be high on public health agendas.

Many early drinking interventions are educational in nature. In essence these are risk communication messages and the evidence from psychological research is that improving risk perceptions will have little impact on levels of drinking. Unsurprisingly then, there is little evidence that alcohol education and health promotion have any positive effect on drinking habits in Britain (Plant and Plant 2006) or the United States (Paglia and Room 1999). These campaigns are heard and understood because knowledge increases in targeted populations (Paglia and Room 1999; Plant and Plant 2006) so it is not that the message is failing to reach the designated audience, rather the message has no impact on behaviour. Worryingly, there is evidence that educational programmes to reduce drinking can have the opposite effect and increase drinking (Duryea and Okwumabua 1988; Hopkins et al. 1988). It is possible that young people who may be attracted to unconventionality or rebelliousness could be attracted by the described risks that are intended to prevent initiation of drinking.

There are a great many school and university based programmes focused on preventing the early onset of drinking and promoting sensible drinking. Community programmes to delay the onset of drinking or promote the early adoption of sensible drinking habits also exist (Foxcroft et al. 2003). Foxcroft et al. (2003) reviewed the effectiveness of programmes designed to prevent excessive drinking in young people. Worryingly, Foxcroft et al. (2003) found very little evidence that any of these programmes were effective. Among the studies with medium-term follow-up that met the methodological guidelines the majority, 19 studies, found no evidence of intervention effectiveness. Several of these studies had previously reported short-term effectiveness which demonstrates the importance of longer term follow-up. For instance, Werch et al. (1998) developed a robustly theoretically derived programme based on the multi-component motivational stages (McMOS) prevention model which postulates there are stages of habit initiation that parallel the stages of behavioural change described in the transtheoretical model (TTM). The study also incorporated factors derived from the health belief model, social cognition theory and behavioural self-control theory. Werch et al. (1998) reported success in altering short-term alcohol consumption but these effects were not sustained at one-year follow-up. This intervention looked promising and utilised a set of activities for families to work through together. What was not clear from this programme was which of the theoretical factors that underpinned the programme was successful in producing the short-term change. This is acknowledged by the authors who recognise that the 'active' ingredient of successful prevention programmes needs to be established.

There were fewer studies that reported long-term follow-up of over three years in Foxcroft's 2003 review. Of those that did, the Iowa Strengthening Families (ISF) Programme and the Preparing for Drug Free Years (PDFY) Programme (Spoth et al. 2001) were the most promising. Similarly to other successful interventions for drinking, this intervention was delivered through the school but based in the family. Both interventions were theoretically derived. The PDFY was based on the social development model and the social control model. The ISA was based on the biopsychosocial model, resiliency model and the social ecology model of adolescent substance use. Both programmes aimed to develop pro-social bonds within the family and coping skills of the adolescent. Spoth et al. (2001) reported that both interventions delayed initiation of drinking and reduced current use compared to the control group and these differences persisted for four years past baseline. Interventions like this are reassuring and suggest that it is possible to intervene positively in adolescent drinking. However, great care must be taken to identify the active ingredient in successful interventions, given the very many programmes that fail to deliver positive change. Foxcroft et al. (2003) raise a note of caution when interpreting these findings in a British context. The majority (84 per cent) of the studies included in their review took place in the United States; only two British studies met the methodological criteria to be included in the review. The different legal position and promotion of abstinence until 21 in the United States compared to sensible drinking in the UK may render extrapolation to the British context unsafe. Consequently both Foxcroft et al. (2003) and Mulvihill et al. (2005) in their evidence briefing for the Health Development Agency conclude: 'there is currently a lack of review-level evidence for the effectiveness of interventions in reducing alcohol misuse in young people' (Mulvihill et al. 2005: 36).

One study that is unusual and interesting because it reports negative findings was based on a social norms theory but within a social marketing context. Wechsler et al. (2003) investigated the effectiveness of social norms marketing interventions to reduce students' heavy drinking. Social norms marketing derives from social norms theory which was discussed earlier in the chapter. A typical social norms marketing message would be: 'Most students have 5 or fewer drinks when they party' (Wechsler et al. 2003: 485).

Social norms marketing is popular in the United States. Wechsler et al. (2003) compared US colleges where social norms drinking marketing programmes were active with those where no such programmes exist. They reported that there was no difference in the quantity, frequency or volume of alcohol consumption or in measures of drunkenness or heavy episodic drinking. However, in the colleges where social norms drinking marketing existed, increases in alcohol use and percentage of students drinking only 20 or more drinks a month were reported. It would appear the social norms drinking marketing does not reduce heavy drinking and can increase lower level drinking. Wechsler et al. (2003) conclude that while social marketing strategies are a palatable solution to the problem of heavy drinking, they are at best ineffective and at worst counter-productive and tougher measures aimed at limiting access to alcohol and controlling the marketing practices of the beverage industry are more likely to be effective in reducing drinking.

There are two concerns from these studies on early drinking interventions. First, there are a wealth of studies that report no reduction in any measure of drinking. Second, research has failed to consistently test and tease out what is effective. It is important to recognise that the successful interventions are consistently theoretically derived although the key influential factors on their success are not well articulated. We need to identify what factors are working. It is plausible that the skills-based interventions are increasing refusal self-efficacy. Other factors that strengthen relationships are clearly potential mediators but work is required to establish what is effective and to avoid future interventions that are ineffective.

Interventions to change established drinking

Many interventions to challenge established drinking are aimed at addictive drinkers. Nevertheless, interventions to challenge less serious drinking problems do exist. As predicted by psychological research education, health promotion messages that inform people about the risks of drinking are as ineffective in established drinkers are they are in early drinkers (Paglia and Room 1999; Babor et al. 2003; Room 2004; Plant and Plant 2006). However, there is evidence that informational campaigns and in particular mass media campaigns and health warning labels do have a role to play in the promotion of sensible drinking. In multilevel campaigns where an informational message is supported by programmes to support sensible drinking decreases in drinking levels have been reported (Paglia and Room 1999).

Intervening in primary care is the most common way for non-informational based interventions to reach their audience of established drinkers (Mulvihill et al. 2005). In Britain, brief counselling interventions in primary care settings are the most common way that people who volitionally drink too much will receive support (Mulvihill et al. 2005). It is likely that many people who are drinking non-volitionally and who perhaps warrant more intense intervention are also treated in this way and so the effectiveness of these interventions for volitional drinkers may be underestimated if participants with a serious addictive disorder are included.

Brief interventions for alcohol use are well researched. They have many advantages. They are acceptable to individuals with less severe drinking problems for whom more intensive treatment would not be acceptable. They can be administered by a wide range of health professionals in many settings and are inexpensive (Moyer et al. 2002). Brief interventions, although varied, have been described by Moyer et al. (2002) as having the six features shown in Table 5.12. Such a format for brief interventions is also recognised by Williams et al. (2007), who state that brief alcohol counselling interventions generally include assessment, feedback, advice and goal setting.

Table 5.12 Key features of brief interventions

1	A goal of reduced or non-problem drinking rather than abstinence
2	Delivered by a health professional as opposed to an addiction specialist
3	Directed at volitional rather than dependent drinkers
4	Addressing individuals' level of motivation to change drinking habits
5	Being self (as opposed to professionally) directed and/or
6	Having the following ingredients: feedback of risk; encouraging responsibility for change; advice; menu of options; therapeutic empathy; enhancing self-efficacy

(Adapted from Moyer et al 2002)

Level of motivation derives from the stages of change component of the TTM which acknowledges the importance of the individual's motivational state. Self-efficacy is another key social cognitive variable which has been consistently found to predict behavioural change. Consequently, the theoretical underpinnings of such an approach are clear. Interestingly, Williams et al. (2007) found that readiness to change did not predict reduction of drinking in their cohort of people identified in primary care as drinking unhealthily whereas levels of self-efficacy did predict a reduction in drinking. Williams et al. (2007) argue that in the busy primary care setting, formal assessment of readiness to change may not be necessary.

Brief interventions, while following this basis framework, can vary and in particular the length of a brief intervention, although intuitively short can range from one 5-minute session to brief multi-contact interventions. Many studies have found that brief interventions can reduce drinking (Poikolainen 1999; Moyer et al. 2002; Mulvihill et al. 2005; Williams et al. 2007) However, Mulvihill et al. (2005) in their comprehensive review conclude that multi-contact brief interventions are more effective than single very brief sessions. Moyer et al. (2002) raise a note of caution that many studies report only short-term follow-up of a year or less. Given that Foxcroft et al. (2003) in their review of interventions aimed at young people found that most of the short-term effectiveness of interventions had disappeared at medium-term follow-up, the lack of long-term follow-up of brief interventions needs to be addressed. Some authors have found that brief interventions are only effective in women (Poikolainen 1999). However, others report equal effectiveness in both men and women (Moyer et al. 2002; Ballesteros et al. 2004).

There is a significant body of work on workplace drinking norms that suggest that changing workplace drinking norms to support sensible drinking could be key in changing drinking behaviours both in a work and non-work context (Barrientos-Gutierrez et al. 2007). The challenge will be to develop interventions that can successfully change group-based norms. Challenging descriptive social norms in interventions with young people has been utilised with some success (Paglia and Room 1999; Prochaska et al. 2004). Similar work-based interventions may well be a useful additional strategy for established drinkers.

Some general practitioners offer lifestyle-based advice that is not formally recognised as a brief drinking intervention. There was conflicting evidence about the effectiveness of such a strategy with some studies finding that advice from the doctor did reduce drinking whereas others found no reduction in drinking. Such discrepancies may arise from the differential styles of delivering advice. Cognitive behavioural therapy has also been found to reduce drinking in some studies (Mulvihill et al. 2005). There is also modest evidence that self-help materials can reduce drinking, particularly for people actively seeking help for their drinking (Mulvihill et al. 2005).

Conclusion

Many people drink more alcohol than is good for them. Drinking is most prevalent in the young where peer group drinking has been postulated to encourage and support excessive drinking. Similarly, workplace drinking cultures in adults have been found to play a significant role in supporting excessive drinking. It has been argued that reducing the availability and increasing the cost of alcohol are the best way to reduce excess drinking, although the government has continuously resisted calls to increase the cost or limit the sale of alcohol. Interventions that attempt to build self-efficacy for reducing alcohol consumption and that challenge perceived social norms for drinking are the best way to help people change their drinking habits within a culture that is generally complicit in excess drinking.

Summary points

- Alcohol contributes to the aetiology and progression of a wide range of lifestyle diseases.

- Many people drink more alcohol than is sensible for their health.
- Young people are the most likely to drink heavily and to binge drink.
- Young women are drinking more than they did in previous generations.
- Clinical dependency is the extreme end of a continuum between dependent and volitional drinking. Many people will have established drinking habits that are difficult to overcome without being strictly clinically dependent.
- The availability and low cost of alcohol has been implicated in the early establishment of drinking in young people.
- Perceived social norms within university and workplace environments have been postulated to support excessive and episodic heavy drinking.
- Brief interventions for alcohol use that have a goal of non-problem drinking rather than abstinence, can be delivered by non-addiction specialists and usually include assessment, feedback, advice and goal setting.
- Brief interventions for alcohol use have been found to reduce drinking in the short term although long-term effects on drinking have not been established.
- Interventions that develop self-efficacy for reducing drinking have been found to be effective.

6 Smoking

> To cease smoking is the easiest thing I ever did. I ought to know because I've done it a thousand times.
>
> Mark Twain

By the end of this chapter you will:

- understand the extent and demographics of tobacco smoking in the UK currently
- review the health and economic consequences of tobacco smoking
- review the explanations of why people start to smoke, and continue to smoke
- review the transtheoretical model of change and how this has been applied to smoking, and smoking cessation
- understand the approaches to smoking cessation at both an individual and population based level.

Definition of smoking

Defining tobacco smoking is, at its most simplistic, unproblematic: 'Tobacco products are products made entirely or partly of leaf tobacco as raw material, which are intended to be smoked, sucked, chewed or snuffed. All contain the highly addictive psychoactive ingredient, nicotine' (WHO 2007b). However, of course the term suggests two elements: 'smoking' and 'tobacco'. So do both have to be in existence? If tobacco alone is sufficient then, of course, either tobacco snuff or chewing tobacco could (or should) be included. If it is simply 'smoking' then herbal cigarettes would be safe, as would other non-tobacco products. To counter this, a variety of legislatures have ensured that both smoking and tobacco are included. For example, the State of Queensland, Australia, passed amendment of the Tobacco Products (Prevention of Supply to Children) Act 1998:

> it has been established that the deliberate inhalation of smoke from the combustion of any matter is injurious to health, whether or not the smoking compound contains addictive substances such as nicotine. Furthermore, the smoking of non-tobacco products, such as herbal cigarettes, leads to at least a similar degree of exposure to carbon monoxide and tar as conventional cigarettes.

Tobacco has been available in Europe since the sixteenth century and has been used in a variety of forms: snuff, chewing tobacco, cigars and pipes. It is only since the start of the twentieth century that cigarettes have predominated and now, worldwide, they are the most popular form of tobacco consumption. Successful marketing campaigns in the UK, Europe and elsewhere in the developed world and more recently in the developing world have led to the widespread adoption of cigarette smoking.

Cigarette smoking remains the single most avoidable cause of death and disability in the UK and the Western world and this is a consequence of the constituents in the cigarette (Fiore et al. 2000, 2008). Of the people alive in the world today, 500 million are predicted to die from the use of tobacco (Peto and Lopez 1990). Not just tobacco but also the additives, the filters and the wrappings all contribute to the harmful effects of cigarette smoking. Tobacco smoke contains over 4000 different gases and particles, including nicotine, tar and gases (e.g. carbon monoxide, ammonia, hydrogen cyanide, formaldehyde).

There is considerable variation in the prevalence of smoking worldwide. In sub-Saharan Africa less than 10 per cent of the population smoke, whereas in Japan this figure rises to above 50 per cent, and in Indonesia 69 per cent, with almost three-quarters of the Vietnamese population smoking (Edwards 2004).

Government recommendations for smoking

The UK government targets for smoking are to reduce adult smoking rates (from 26 per cent in 2002) to 21 per cent or less by 2010, with a reduction in prevalence among routine and manual groups (from 31 per cent in 2002) to 26 per cent or less. The Department of Health's tobacco programme is split into 'strands', each of which it is hoped will contribute to an overall reduction in smoking. These strands include the following.

Smoke-free legislation

From March 2006 in Scotland, April 2007 in Northern Ireland and Wales and from July 2007 in England virtually all enclosed public places and workplaces became smoke free, including all pubs, clubs, membership clubs, cafés and restaurants.

Reducing exposure to second-hand smoke

Second-hand smoke (also known as 'environmental tobacco smoke' (ETS) or 'passive smoking') is a mixture of sidestream smoke from the burning tip of a cigarette, and mainstream smoke exhaled by a smoker. Legislation such as that introducing smoke free public buildings and workplaces has reduced the exposure to ETS.

Tobacco media and education programmes

A key strand of the UK government's tobacco control programme is the provision of an ongoing media and education campaign. There are four overall strands to the campaign, as recommended by international best practice (Schar and Gutierrez 2001):

- *Motivation:* provides smokers with new and motivating reasons to quit
- *Support:* outlines the choice of NHS support available
- *Reducing exposure to second-hand smoke:* demonstrating that second-hand smoke is dangerous, not just unpleasant
- *Product and pack:* links the health messages back to the product, giving the smoker another reason to quit.

Reducing availability of tobacco products

Price increases have been a highly successful way of helping people become non-smokers: UK budget changes to tobacco duty have been directed towards increasing the real cost of cigarettes and thereby increase economic pressures on smokers. However, a careful line has to be drawn to ensure that the increase in prices is not too extensive so as to increase the extent of tobacco smuggling.

NHS Stop Smoking Services and NRTs

The UK government has set up a NHS Stop Smoking Service. Services are now available across the NHS in the UK, providing counselling and support to smokers wanting to quit, complementing the use of stop smoking aids, nicotine replacement therapy (NRT) and bupropion (Zyban).

Reducing tobacco advertising and promotion

The UK has a comprehensive ban – just like many other countries in Europe and beyond – on tobacco advertising and promotion.

Regulating tobacco products

This strand of the government's tobacco control programme concerns regulating the contents of tobacco products and the labelling of packaging.

Evidence of the problem

Despite the health effects of smoking being known since the 1960s, and the health impact being publicised, some 12 million individuals still smoke in the UK: 25 per cent of men and 23 per cent of women (ONS 2007). These figures have shown a substantial decrease since the early 1970s: for example in the 1970s the comparable figures were 51 per cent of men and 41 per cent of women smoking. Much of this decline occurred in the 1970s and 1980s, after which the rate of decline slowed. Although the number of people smoking has decreased considerably, this is mainly due to the established smoker giving up; the number of young people starting to smoke remains, broadly, the same (ASH 2008).

The prevalence of smoking is not the same in different groups: about one-third of those in the manual groups smoke compared to less than 20 per cent of the professional and managerial groups. Similarly, smoking is the highest in the 20–24 year age group (about 36 per cent) and the lowest in the over 65 years (about 15 per cent). This reflects both the fact that many former smokers will have quit and also that about a quarter of smokers die before reaching retirement age (ONS 2007). The lowest rate is among elderly people, possibly because non-smokers tend to live longer than smokers. It is also of interest to note that the rate of smoking has decreased more significantly in men compared to women.

Smoking prevalence is dropping throughout the UK. In the years since the Health and Lifestyle Survey based in England (Blaxter 1990), there has been a 9 per cent decrease in smoking rates in men living in England and a 8 per cent decrease in women living in England (see Table 6.1). Although the Scottish smoking rates are noticeably higher than those for England, Wales and Northern Ireland, their rate of decrease is similar because their smoking rates were higher initially. The Scottish Health Survey reports an 8 per cent decrease in smoking rates for men between 1995 and 2003 and a 5 per cent decrease for women during the same period (Scottish Executive 2005). Smoking rates in women are not dropping as quickly as they are in men in all four countries. Indeed in Northern Ireland, it is striking that while male smoking rates have dropped from 39 per cent to 26 per cent, female smoking rates have dropped by only 1 per cent; in essence the percentage of women smoking has not changed significantly at all and remains at a similar level to the 1983 figure of 29 per cent of women smoking (Department of Health, Social Services and Public Safety 2001). This huge difference in rates of stopping has resulted in

Table 6.1 Current smoking prevalence rates in men and women

Source of data	*Men reporting smoking (%)*	*Women reporting smoking (%)*
Health and Lifestyle Survey (Blaxter 1990)	36	32
Health Survey England 2003	27	24
Scottish Health Survey 2003	32	31
Welsh Health Survey 2003	27	26
Northern Ireland Health and Social Wellbeing Survey 2001	26	28

Northern Ireland being the only country in the UK where the percentage of women smoking is greater than the percentage of men. An explanation for such a marked difference from other UK countries is not offered by the Northern Ireland survey. However, different patterns of gender-related lifestyle behaviour in countries that are so geographical close is evidence of the complexities of socio-demographic influences over life-style behaviours. It could be argued that gender influences smoking behaviour and changing gender role expectations have led to these changes (e.g. Kirkland et al. 2004) but this cannot explain why gender mediates smoking behaviour so differently in Northern Ireland compared to the rest of the UK. Some other socio-demographic factor is likely to be interacting with gender here and it might be hypothesised that it is perhaps poverty, women may be more prone to using smoking as a way of coping with the stresses or be more likely to be in unskilled employment (e.g. Blaxter 1990).

Health consequences of smoking

Doll and Hill (1952) were the first to link smoking and cancer and this initial report has been followed by numerous studies highlighting the link between poor health and tobacco smoking. The statistics surrounding tobacco smoking are, indeed, shocking and regularly reproduced by the advocates of smoking bans and the health establishment. For example, in the UK it is suggested that annually some 120,000 people die as a result of their smoking habit (440,000 in the United States). Every year, tobacco smoking kills 5 million people worldwide (Perkins et al. 2008) or about one person every six seconds. Deaths caused by tobacco smoking in the UK are higher than the number of deaths caused by road traffic accidents (3,500), other accidents (8,500), poisoning and overdose (900), alcoholic liver disease (5,000), suicide (4,000) and HIV infection (250). Almost a half of all regular smokers will be killed by their habit. A man who smokes cuts short his life by 13.2 years and female smokers lose 14.5 years (ASH 2008).

In terms of morbidity, smoking has been linked to a whole host of diseases and chronic conditions including heart disease, throat cancer, stomach and bowel cancer, lung cancer, leukaemia, peripheral vascular disease, premature and low weight babies, bronchitis, emphysema, sinusitis, peptic ulcers dental hygiene problems and can worsen the effects of asthma, and infections (see Table 6.2 for overview).

Table 6.2 Illness associated with smoking

System	*Illness*
Cardiovascular	Aneurysm Angina (20 × risk) Beurger's disease (severe circulatory disease) Coronary artery disease Myocardial infarction (2–3 × risk) Peripheral vascular disease Stroke (2–4 × risk)
Musculoskeletal	Back pain Ligament injuries Muscle injuries Neck pain Osteoporosis Osteoarthritis Rheumatoid arthritis Tendon injuries Low bone density Hip fractures
Visual	Cataracts (2 × risk) Posterior subcapsular cataract (3 × risk) Optic neuropathy (16 × risk) Macular degeneration (2 × risk) Nystagmus Ocular histoplasmosis Tobacco amblyopia
Genito-urinary	Erectile dysfunction Impotence (2 × risk) Decreased fertility in women Pregnancy complications (e.g. premature rupture of membranes, placenta previa or placental abruption, miscarriage, still birth, low birth weight, reduced lung function in infants)
Digestive, metabolic	Gum disease Duodenal ulcer Colon polyps Crohn's disease Diabetes Stomach ulcer Tooth loss
Respiratory	COPD

Table 6.2 Illness associated with smoking (continued)

System	*Illness*
Cancers	Lung (90% associated with smoking)
	Mouth and throat (90% associated with smoking)
	Breast (60% increased risk)
	Pancreatic (2 × risk)
	Oesophageal cancer
	Stomach
	Liver
	Bladder (2–5 × risk)
	Kidney
	Cervical cancer
	Myeloid cancer
	Urinary tract cancer
Other conditions	Depression
	Psoriasis (2 × risk)
	Hearing loss
	Sudden Infant Death Syndrome (SIDS)
	Exacerbates:
	Asthma
	Chronic rhinitis
	Diabetic retinopathy
	Graves' disease
	Multiple sclerosis (MS)
	Optic neuritis
	Coughing, sneezing, shortness of breath
	Common colds, influenza, pneumonia

Stopping smoking reduces the risks of many of the conditions highlighted in Table 6.2 although there are time lags in the reduction in risk of developing these conditions. Those who quit smoking by the age of 40 years retain almost the same life expectancy as lifelong non-smokers (suggesting that it is the chronic effects of smoking that are important). Even those who quit by the age of 50 or 60 can gain several years of life expectancy compared to those who continue to smoke (Doll et al. 2004). Thus quitting smoking at any age brings with it health benefits.

Economic implications

Of course, the impact of smoking is not only health related: there are severe economic implications. Smoking kills people at the height of their productivity, and therefore deprives families of their breadwinners and countries of their healthy workforce. Smokers are also more likely than non-smokers to retire from work early due to ill health (Husemoen et al. 2004). Tobacco is estimated to result in a global loss of $200 billion (WHO 2004b). The economic impact imposes costs on individuals, the health care system of the country and society. At an individual level, somebody smoking 20 cigarettes a day will spend approximately £2,200 per year on their habit, with individuals on the lowest income spending proportionately more of their income on cigarettes than those with higher incomes.

In terms of the health care system, a large proportion of hospital admissions and GP appointments are related to illnesses associated with smoking (Milner and Bates 2002): one-third of a million hospital admissions are related to smoking. Parrott and Godfrey (2004) suggest that smoking costs the British economy £1.4–1.5 billion per year (or about 0.16 per cent of gross domestic product) including £127 million to treat lung cancer. Each year, more than 34 million working days are lost in England and Wales due to smoking-related illnesses.

Obviously, economic benefits also result from stopping smoking, saving an individual almost £2500 per year. By reducing ill health, smoking cessation also reduces healthcare costs. If the government's targets (DoH 2002b) were met, then there would be a reduction in 6,300 heart attacks and 5,000 strokes by 2010 and therefore save the NHS some half a billion pounds (Naidoo et al. 2000).

It was in the early 1950s that the classic study (Doll and Hill 1952) was carried out and the health effects of smoking are well known by almost the whole adult population (see Arnett 2000). Given that there is this level of understanding, why do people continue to start smoking, and when they do continue to do so? It is important to note that there is a difference in the explanations offered for why people start smoking and for why people continue to smoke: these will be treated independently.

Why do people smoke?

It would be assumed that given the extreme negative consequences associated with tobacco smoking, nobody in their right mind would start smoking – but they do. Indeed, around a quarter of the population in the Western world smoke, so why do people start smoking? It should be highlighted, of course, that many smokers do not see the risk associated with their behaviour. Weinstein et al. (2005) are among many that report that smokers underestimate their risk of lung cancer relative to other smokers and to non-smokers, and demonstrate a lack of understanding of smoking risks. Consequently, it raises the possibility of whether individuals are making their risk decision on a lack of accurate information. However, Peretti-Watel et al. (2007) suggest that it is a *risk denial* rather than a lack of information about the health consequences of tobacco smoking. Consequently, the health education message is not necessarily about informing the (potential) smoker of their risks but should be about changing the way they process the information in order to ensure that they produce beliefs and limit their capacity to generate self-exempting beliefs. Similarly, although using different terms, Dillard et al. (2006) suggest that smokers have an 'unrealistic optimism' associated with their smoking behaviours and the potential health risks. However, the conclusion was the same: the lack of quitting behaviour was associated with unrealistic optimism and there was (is) a need for health educators to address such false beliefs.

It is usually teenagers who experiment with smoking, with very few smokers starting after the age of 25 years (Piasecki 2006). There are a number of reasons why people start smoking, but these are mainly related to psychosocial motives (Jarvis 2004). Research has also indicated that teenagers underestimate the health risk of smoking (Slovic 2000) and they also believe that they will quit before they do themselves serious damage (Arnett 2000). Hence, they smoke in spite of knowing the health damage effects of smoking: they know of them, they just don't think it will impact upon them. Furthermore, health is defined in terms of fitness and beauty (Murray and Jarrett 1985) and smoking is not thought to harm these features.

Usually children or teenagers experiment with smoking and this leads to further smoking behaviour. One of the major reasons for experimenting with cigarettes is social pressure from peers or older siblings to experiment with tobacco. Early studies suggest that those who experiment with just four cigarettes become regular smokers (Salber et al. 1963). Obviously this suggests that the prevention of smoking should begin early in schools and target young people before they have experimented with smoking.

From a psychological perspective, a number of explanations have been proposed to account for people's smoking. For example, the behavioural perspective has been applied by researchers attempting to explain the initiation of cigarette smoking among adolescents (Akers 1977). In short this perspective suggests that the smoking behaviour is learned according to the key learning processes of classical conditioning, operant conditioning, observational learning and cognitive processes (see Table 6.3 for explanation of how individual elements can be applied to smoking).

The social learning perspective suggests that the major influence on adolescents' cigarette smoking is a behaviour learned by modelling and social reinforcement. The most consistent and powerful predictor is whether their friends smoke (Urberg et al. 1990). The other significant influence is family; adolescents are more likely to smoke cigarettes if their parents smoke (Bricker et al. 2005; Huver et al. 2006) or their siblings (e.g. Brandon and Brandon 2005). For example, Bauman et al. (1990) found that lifetime parental smoking was strongly correlated with adolescent smoking. However, as adolescents develop, parents generally become less influential as compared with peers (Valante et al. 2005) and often the media (e.g. Gutschoven and Van den Bulck 2005).

Why do people continue to smoke?

The explanations for why people continue to smoke are, unsurprisingly, multifaceted. Although these are overlapping and complementary three

Table 6.3 Behavioural explanation of smoking development

Concept	*Rules*	*Example*
Classical conditioning	Behaviours acquired through associative learning	Having a cup of coffee and a cigarette equals relaxation
Operant conditioning	Behaviour is likely to increase if it is positively reinforced by the presence of a positive event, or negatively reinforced by the absence or removal of a negative event	Smoking is positively reinforced by social acceptance
Observational learning	Behaviours are learned by observing others	Parents or friends smoking
Cognitive factors	Other factors such as coping mechanisms or self-image may contribute	Belief that smoking looks 'cool'

broad themes are evident: biological, social and psychological (which, evidently, covers all possible variables). These factors can be described as predisposing factors (see Figure 6.1) which are the foundations for awareness, information and motivational factors that all result in intent, and ultimately (although often weakly) behavioural state (Seegar et al. 2007). The model highlights that behavioural intent can be determined by three types of motivational factors: attitude towards a new behaviour (e.g. the pros and cons), social influences (e.g. norms, modelling and pressure) and self-efficacy explanations. These are all influenced by distal factors: awareness (knowledge, relevance and risk perception) and information (message, channel and source) and the predisposing factors.

These factors have been modified in a number of different ways and presented in a variety of models as previously outlined in Chapter 2. It is, of course, possible that these individual models are not sufficient to explain smoking behaviour given the physiological and social context in which the behaviour operates and it is important to ensure that the multi-faceted nature of smoking is recognised.

Social factors

The social context in which smoking develops and is maintained is key. The social factors implicated in the initiation of smoking behaviour (e.g. parents, siblings and peers) all have a part to play in the maintenance of this behaviour. Although the relative importance of these various groups has been debated, most research has agreed that they do have a role.

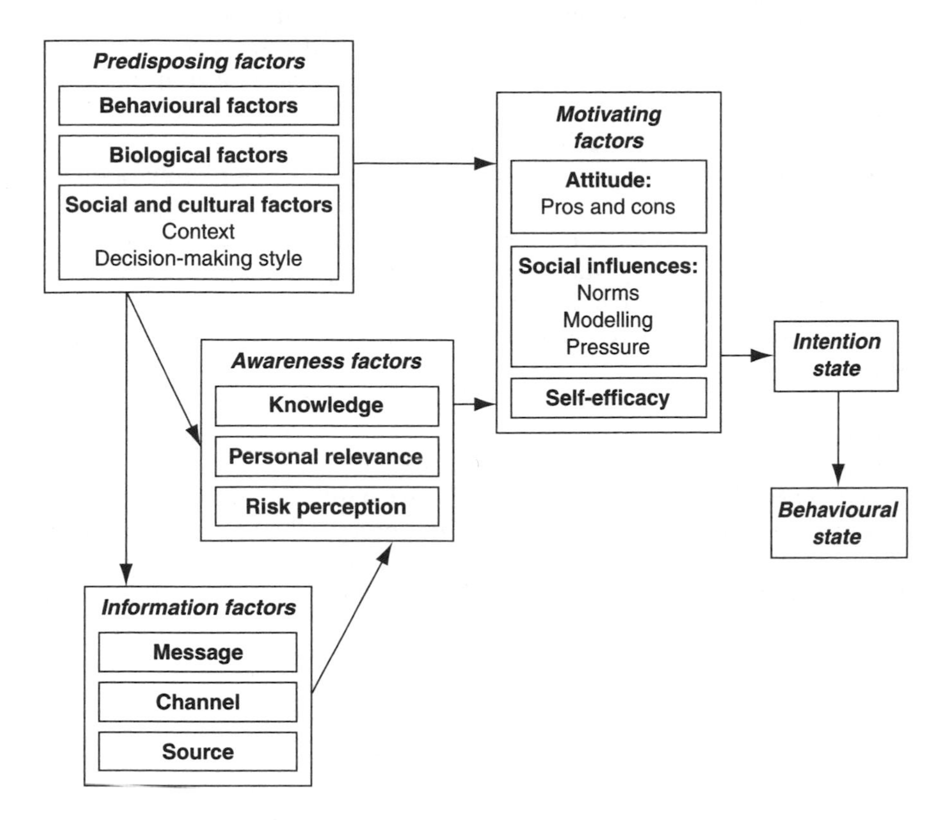

Figure 6.1 Integrated change model (Segar et al. 2006)

Smoking is a social activity for many but this can differ from individual to individual and from cigarette to cigarette (Perkins et al. 2008). Thus, for somebody at work, smoking a cigarette may provide an opportunity to escape from the drudgery of the workplace and to have a break. In contrast, down the pub, the sharing of a cigarette was a means of strengthening social bonds with friends. For low-income mothers, smoking was used as a means of having a break after a certain number of activities or tasks or as a means of coping when something went wrong (Graham 1987; Bottorff et al. 2000; Irwin et al. 2005).

Psychological factors

Several psychological variables have been implicated in the continuance of smoking. A number of models explored in Chapter 2 have been used as predictors of smoking. Models of health behaviour such as the health belief model, the protection motivation theory, the theory of reasoned action and the health action process approach have been used to examine the cognitive factors that contribute to smoking initiation. Obviously the distinction between these forms of models and the social explanations presented earlier is somewhat tenuous: there is a clear overlap between these factors and attempting to explain smoking (or any) lifestyle behaviour mono-theoretically is a flawed task.

However, another approach is based on the theory of planned behaviour (Ajzen 1991) which appears to be one of the most popular and successful model for studying health behaviour (Armitage and Conner 2001). The TPB has been successful in predicting smoking among adolescents (e.g. Higgins and Conner 2003; McMillan et al. 2005; Conner et al. 2006). These studies have provided good predictions of intentions and subsequent behaviours.

According to the TPB the proximal determinants of behaviour are the intentions to engage in the behaviour. Intentions reflect an individual's decision to exert effort to perform the behaviour and is assumed to be a function of a number of related factors (see Chapter 2). Smoking could be assumed to be different from some of the other behaviours discussed in this book. In particular, smokers might become addicted (whether psychologically or biologically) to cigarettes, but this should not suggest that they have lost control over their behaviour but that it is a difficult behaviour to change in the sense that their perception of control over the behaviour appears incomplete.

Biological explanations

The biological model suggests that smoking is a result of individuals becoming physically dependent on nicotine and the multitude of chemical substances found in cigarettes. The nicotine entering the lungs from a cigarette is transported through the blood supply to the brain, where it leads to an activation of the autonomic nervous system (ANS). Consequently, there is an increase in heart rate and blood pressure which leads to the body becoming more aroused and alert. Once the person has stopped smoking, the level of nicotine reduces as do the 'positive' effects of smoking. From this, a model of nicotine regulation can be proposed: smokers continue to smoke in order to avoid withdrawal symptoms (Schacter et al. 1977). However, there are some people who stop smoking for a number of years (and hence all of the nicotine has disappeared from their bodies) but then start smoking again. Furthermore, there are smokers who are known as 'chippers' who smoke a few cigarettes a day for a number of years but do not increase the amount they smoke (hence they do not show tolerance). Because of these issues it is recognised that the biological theories are not the complete picture; there must be other social and psychological factors involved.

Interventions to reduce smoking

Evidence suggests that the majority of smokers want to stop smoking (DoH 2003; Brunnhuber et al. 2007), so why is the non-smoking figure not lower? Each year in the UK about one-third of smokers are very keen to quit smoking, although the majority fail within days (Jarvis 2004). Just over a half of smokers do succeed in quitting smoking before they die, although for many it is too late (Stapleton 1997). However, what can health care professionals do to try to decrease smoking levels and improve the success of those attempting to quit?

There must be a complex approach to smoking cessation: it can be either methods aimed at preventing people starting smoking (which is preferable) or getting those who are smoking to quit. At the same time these approaches can be at either the population level or the individual level.

It has been suggested, of course, that getting people to stop smoking should be the cornerstone of every health care professional's advice to patients and clients who smoke. However, although it undoubtedly has benefits, quitting can be fraught with difficulties. People may get irritable, depressed, anxious or restless and will crave tobacco. In light of these factors a range of pharmacological treatments have been developed to help relieve them. For example, there are sprays, chewing gum, patches and inhalers, all of which can work to help people stop smoking (Cummings and Hyland 2005). However, there must also be a psychological element to cessation or there will be no cessation. For example, at its most basic there must be a motivation to give up smoking. Before the methods that have been used to promote smoking cessation are explored, it is worth considering how research into the effectiveness has been defined.

Definition of outcome criteria

What makes a successful quitter? Although on the one hand this should be a relatively simple answer it is of course responded to differently by different researchers and practitioners. For example, how long does cessation have to be before they are categorised as 'successful'? Some have argued for two weeks, others for three months and some for six months. The Cochrane collaboration has resolved some of these difficulties by establishing a common set of criteria, but these are still some variation in interpretation of these. In light of these difficulties, West et al. (2005) have suggested a common set of standards (the Russell Standard – RS) for research studies thereby allowing for a better comparison of outcomes:

- *Duration of absence:* either six months (RS6) or twelve months (RS12) follow-up periods. Shorter periods of follow-up and abstinence are not accurate, sufficient to predict long-term cessation or have a significant impact on health (with exceptions in certain cases, for example pregnancy and pre-surgery).

- *Abstinence:* a self-reported abstinence of smoking no more than five cigarettes from the start of the abstinence period.
- *Biochemical verification:* this is required at the final follow-up and expired carbon monoxide is the best method for detecting recent smoking activity.
- *Intention-to-treat:* all randomised subjects should be included in the calculation of abstinence rates (with the unavoidable loss to follow-up excluded).
- *Protocol violators:* participants who violate the protocol should be followed up in their original treatment group and classified according to their smoking status.
- *Blind follow-up:* follow-up data should be collected blind to treatment allocation.

Stopping people smoking

Cigarette smoking remains the single most avoidable cause of death and disability in the UK and the United States and as such, public policy has stressed the need to reduce tobacco smoking in the population. Encouraging smoking cessation is now recognised as an important part of public health. Anthonisen et al. (2005) report that those that stopped smoking as a result of a cessation programme had 46 per cent lower mortality rates than those who continued to smoke. Interestingly, other studies have suggested that interventions to improve smoking results in beneficial changes in other health behaviours (Tang et al. 1997), so getting people to stop smoking can have positive consequences not just on the health benefits derived from quitting tobacco.

Clinical smoking cessation includes (either alone or in combination) behavioural and pharmaceutical interventions and they range from brief advice and counselling to intensive support, administration of medications that contribute to reducing or overcoming dependence in individuals and in the population as a whole (Raw et al. 2002). In contrast, public health interventions can be defined as those interventions, probably with the same aim, that are conducted at a population level.

There are US guidelines for the treatment of tobacco dependence, referred to as *The Guidelines* (Fiore et al. 2000, updated in 2008), which indicate which treatment approaches have been found to be most effective. Of course, knowing *what* works is not sufficient to enable practitioners to help smokers succeed in breaking powerful tobacco dependence. Obviously what is required is *learning* how to put these approaches into practice and enabling an evaluation of the effectiveness of the evidence base.

Figure 6.2 displays a modified model based on that provided by *The Guidelines* (Fiore et al. 2008) that demonstrates the simple measures that should be taken by health care professionals in order to promote smoking cessation. This model emphasises that tobacco use status should be assessed and documented for each patient seen by a health care professional. Furthermore, even those who have never smoked or are abstinent for an extended period of time also require support. It also stresses the importance of NRTs in the initial 'treatment' of the smoker (see Figure 6.2). It is perhaps worth highlighting at this stage that these interventions are based on the transtheoretical model of change and as such demonstrate the greater theoretical basis of smoking cessation interventions compared to other lifestyle behaviours (e.g. physical activity, illicit drug taking).

Population level approaches to promoting smoking cessation

Efforts to increase the rates of smoking cessation are aimed at convincing smokers to attempt to quit and to encourage those who have tried to try again with, perhaps, more efficacious methods of cessation. Obviously the more smokers that the intervention reaches, the greater the chance of success. Hence, the approach that has been taken is one that are repeated interventions that impact on all smokers. For example, higher taxes on tobacco products, comprehensive advertising bans, pack warnings, anti-tobacco education campaigns and smoke-free policies (Frieden et al. 2005; Biener et al. 2006; Hammond et al. 2007).

At the outset, the population level approach to public health interventions has to be assumed to be the more efficacious than individual level approaches; it is cheaper and can get the message to a greater number of individuals than the clinical measures ever can. The most significant population level smoking intervention in recent years has been legislation to restrict smoking in public places. Since March 2006 in Scotland, April 2007 in Northern Ireland and Wales and July 2007 in England all public places and workplaces became smoke free. The introduction of this change was not particularly controversial: the proportion of the population supporting such a change was high. For example, 88 per cent supported restrictions in the workplace, 91 per cent supported restrictions in restaurants and 65 per cent in pubs (ONS 2006a). It is interesting to speculate on both the extent of the smoking ban and its implications. For example, smoking in cars is allowed as long as the vehicle is not used for work purposes (e.g. taxi drivers or couriers). Although many view their car as their own personal space the law can regard them as public spaces: the car's occupants are subject to legal requirements regarding seat belts, car standards, driving conduct and mobile phone use. Surely it could be argued that smoking in cars when others are present should be banned (several Australian states have introduced this)? Taking this one step further, the fear of the smoking ban was that it would increase smoking in the home and therefore secondary smoking by children and

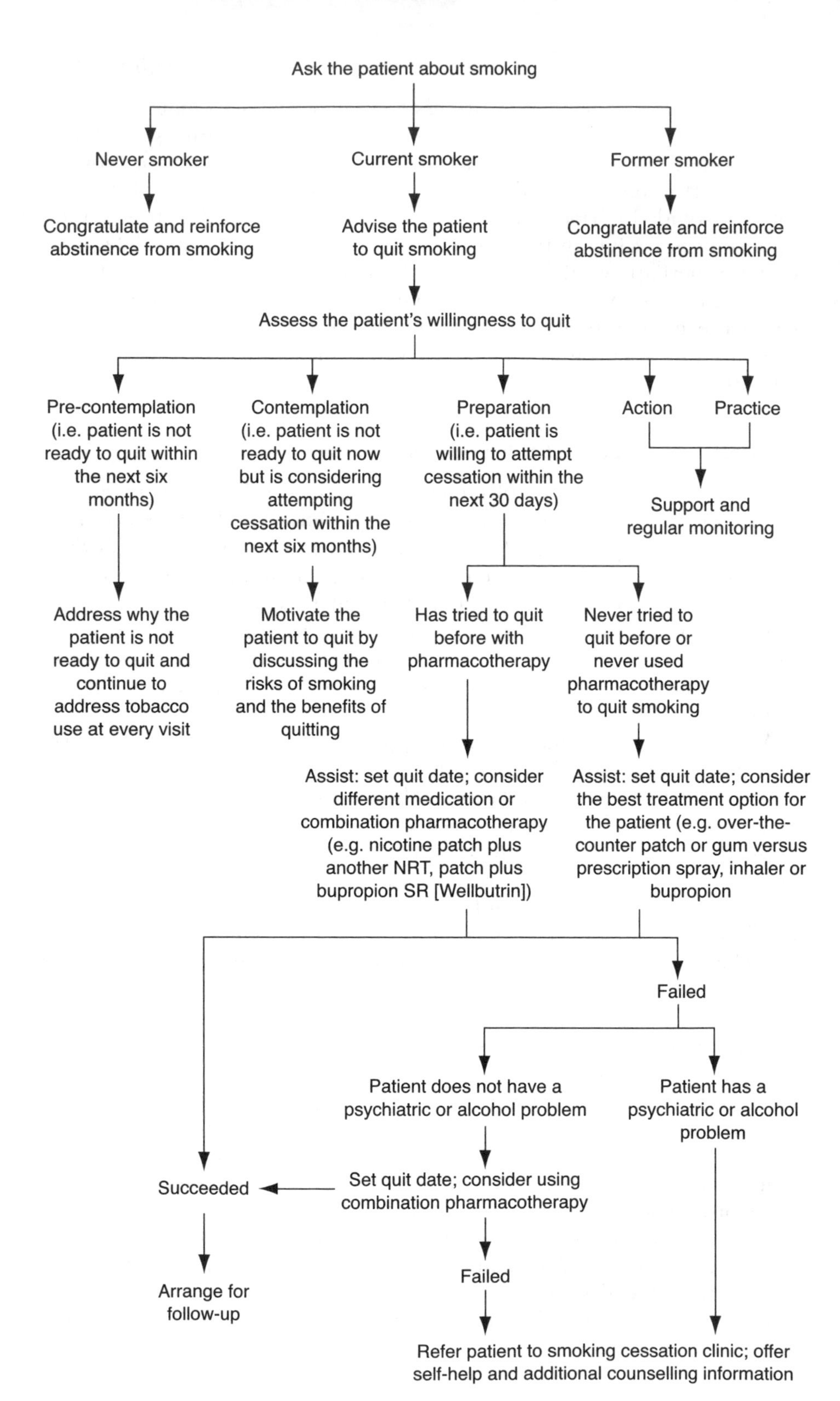

Figure 6.2 Smoking cessation

others. However, this does not seem to be the case, with early research reports suggesting that there was little increase in home smoking with the ban (Phillips et al. 2007). Homes are now the primary source of smoke exposure so will homes ever become legally smoke free places? Surely it would be an authoritarian state that banned smoking in people's homes?

An interesting perspective and debate was raised by the Nuffield Council on Bioethics (2007), which argued that public health policies should be about enforcement and proposed an 'intervention ladder' as a useful way of conceptualising public health interventions and their impact on an individual's choice (see Table 6.4).

Table 6.4 The intervention ladder

Level	*Description*	*Example*
Eliminate choice	Introduce laws that entirely eliminate choice	Compulsory isolation of those with an infectious disorder
Restrict choice	Introduce laws that restrict the options available to people	Remove unhealthy foods from shops
Guide through disincentives	Introduce financial or other disincentives to influence behaviour	Increase taxes on cigarettes
Guide through incentives	Introduce financial or other incentives to influence people's behaviour	Tax breaks for bicycle purchases
Guide choices	Changing the default policy	Change the standard side dish from chips to salad
Enable choice	Help individuals to change their behaviour	Free stop smoking programmes
Provide information	Inform and educate public	Encourage people to eat five a day
Do nothing	Or monitor situation	

In the case of smoking, how does this fit into the ladder? On the one hand, it can be seen that currently the UK government 'guides by disincentives' and 'restricts choice' to a certain extent. The ban on smoking in public places is significant as it is the first legistative attempt to alter lifestyle choices made by governments for many years. However, it could be argued that the government should totally eliminate choice and should ban smoking totally. On the one hand, smoking is a behaviour which is avoidable: society and civilisation would not suffer considerably if it was banned across the UK. Certainly, the Nuffield Council on Bioethics (2007) would argue that this would be important and that enforcement should be used, this curtailment of individual freedom being ethically justified. Their argument concerns proportionality: can the enforcement benefits outweigh the interference in people's lives? Smoking is a dangerous lifestyle behaviour that has its roots in social, physiological and psychological elements. Its dangers are obvious to most and it can kill not only the individual but also the innocent bystander. Is this sufficient to 'eliminate choice' (to use the phrasing of the Nuffield Council, equivalent to 'ban', 'coerce' or 'outlaw')? Obviously, libertarians would argue that smoking is a right of the individual and if individuals want to chose this behaviour then this is their right; consequently it is up to health promoters, health psychologists and health care professionals to promote smoking cessation and not to severely curtail our freedoms. An editorial in *The Times* (13 November 2007) argues that 'John Stuart Mill held that the only justification for state coercion was to prevent harm, or "evil", being done to others. It is a stretch to say that ... smoking at home meets this definition.'

Of course, public health interventions have impact on different socio-economic groups. This is a major issue since those in the lower socio-economic groups have higher rates of smoking than other groups, and this significantly contributes to the socio-economic inequalities (Jarvis and Wardle 1999).

The greatest decline in smoking rates has been seen in the higher income smokers and the current overall national cigarette smoking prevalence of the 26 per cent (see Figure 6.3) masks a differential decrease in the different socio-economic status (SES) groups, with high levels of smoking still found in the deprived localities (see Figure 6.4). Smoking rates among the poorest groups in society have remained unchanged for more than a decade (Richardson and Crosier 2002). Indeed of all the lifestyle behaviours discussed in this book smoking has the simplest relationship with social class and is the only behaviour to demonstrate a totally linear relationship with class.

High levels of nicotine dependence have been reported in those lower SES groups and this may be related to the link between social disadvantage and financial and psychological stress (e.g. Marsh and McKay 1994) and the fact that many smokers consider their smoking to be stress related (Kouvonen et al. 2005). Hence, it may be that those in lower SES have more stress in their lives, smoke more heavily as a result and are thus more dependent. Alternatively, it may be that those in the lower SES have less social pressure to quit and less social support for quitting (Sorensen et al. 2002). Evidence suggests that those in the lower SES tend to commence smoking earlier (Droomers et al. 2002) and hence may be more hardened smokers than their higher SES counterparts. It is also evident that health promotion at a population level is differentially effective on different socio-economic groups and being less effective for those

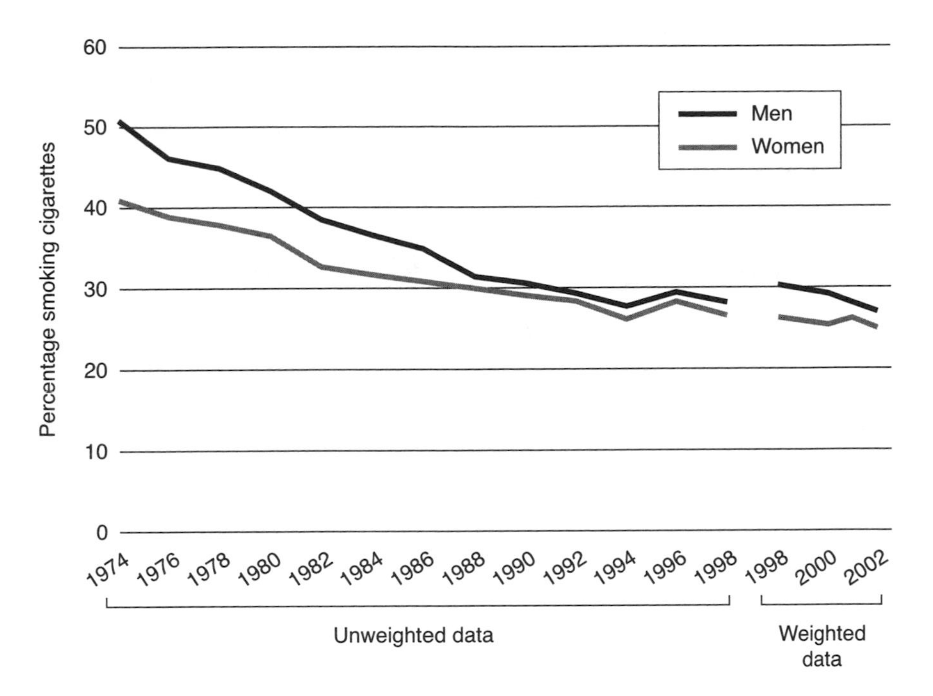

Figure 6.3 Smoking in men and women (McNeil et al. 2005)

in the lower social strata. Obviously, there are a number of explanations for this:

- The health promotion messages are not directed uniformly across the socio-economic groups (e.g. messages are not appropriate).
- Certain socio-economic groups *choose not* to act on the health promotion message (e.g. less peer pressure to quit, lower self-efficacy).
- Certain socio-economic groups *cannot* act on the health promotion message (e.g. more dependence, less access to support).

Studies have also found smokers from poorer communities find it more difficult to quit (Bauld et al. 2003), perhaps related to the levels of addiction (Jarvis and Wardle 1999). The resistance of disadvantaged groups to anti-smoking advice remains high even in areas where there are substantial smoking cessation services (e.g. Chesterman et al. 2002). Lawlor et al. (2003) suggest that this is a valid lay epidemiology whereby smoking can be deemed a rational response to everyday reality involving a clear assessment of risk in relation to life chances as well as being a health-promotion mechanism in itself.

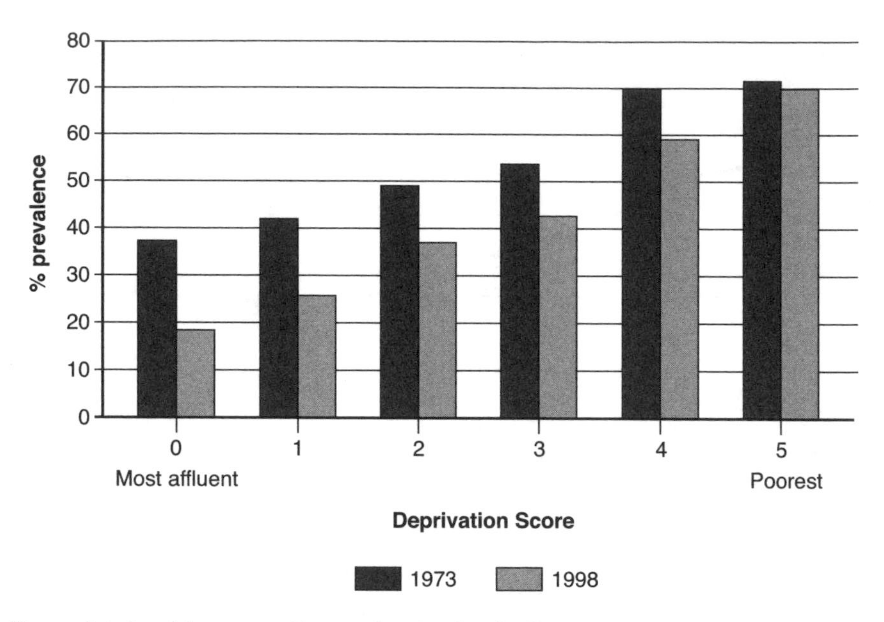

Figure 6.4 Smoking according to deprivation indices (McNeil et al. 2005)

Low income smokers may have lower access to pharmacotherapy and other treatments that improve cessation (Chesterman et al. 2005). It may be that the disparity in smoking cessation among the social classes may be related to differences in the use of smoking cessation resources (Honjo et al. 2006), whether these be at home, work or with peers.

Many studies have indicated that the provision of cessation services within deprived areas can be more limited than in better-off areas (Bauld et al. 2002; Thorndike et al. 2002) as MacIntyre (2001: 55) suggests: 'well-intentioned health promotion policies may actually increase, rather decrease inequalities in health'. It has been argued that the current smoking cessation initiatives have tended to reinforce health inequalities, since quit rates are most frequent among the most affluent (Jarvis and Wardle 1999).

Hence, targeted interventions are essential in order to reduce the disparity in smoking cessation rates and may have to stress the smoking cessation services on offer, and the design of the advertising campaigns. Importantly, however, smoking cessation resources have to be free and widely available so those in the lower SES can engage in the smoking cessation services.

The Department of Health (2001) has emphasised the need to reach the needs of this group and stressed the importance of developing services for these groups. The exact relationship between SES and smoking cessation has not been fully articulated, there is some indication that there is a link between SES and nicotine dependence, and self-efficacy (Siahpush et al. 2006). However, a number of approaches have been employed in the quest to improve cessation rates in deprived neighbourhoods (Pound et al. 2005):

- smoking cessation advisers in primary care venues in deprived areas
- advertising the service in deprived areas
- use of community venues in deprived areas
- training local people from poorer areas as smoking cessation advisers.

More recent research suggests that there has been some success in these approaches with smoking support being reported as 'excellent' in these deprived neighbourhoods. The Healthcare Commission (2007) reports that almost half of the primary care trusts (PCTs) in deprived areas are rated as excellent (i.e. the highest ratio of quitters to smokers) compared to only 20 per cent in the more affluent areas. However, the obvious caveat to this in the way in which the data were collected, analysed and reported. It is of interest that the quitting was calculated on the basis of a four-week abstinence (and not in accord with the Russell Standard outlined earlier) and makes the point that 'The review shows a weaker picture of quit rates among those specific groups of the population with the highest levels of smoking' which are those in the lower SES. So, there does appear to be some confusion in the overall message presented.

Warning labels

One of the major attempts to reduce smoking has been the introduction of graphic warning labels on cigarette packets or on posters and billboards.

Such warnings are popular with politicians and policy makers (Ruiter and Kok 2005) and the European Union has advised its member states to accompany warning text with graphic illustrations of the dangers of smoking (Official Journal of the European Union 2003) which the UK has subscribed to (Davis 2007). However, how successful have these messages been? Unfortunately, there is very little evidence of the success of this form of approach. When politicians are asked for the evidence of such approaches there is much filibustering and some reference to dated research which does not stand up to scrutiny (Ruiter and Kok 2005). For example, Hammond et al. (2004) reviewed the evidence on cigarette warning labels and suggested that they did have an aversive effect and that policy makers should introduce such labels. However, they used no control group, post-test only design with self-report being the outcome measure. There are obviously a number of problems with such a design (National Cancer Institute 2000) and the evidence can be described as, at best, insubstantial.

However, as we have described elsewhere (see Chapters 9 and 10) the literature on fear arousing communication (e.g. Job 1988; Ruiter et al. 2001) suggests that those most at risk from these messages react most defensively. After watching fear-arousing messages, smokers suggest that these are more effective than non-fear-arousing messages and they say that they are more likely to quit after such messages. However, when asked about their priorities these have changed little (Ruiter 2004) and the consequent behaviour change is minimal, especially those that are most at risk (Taubman Ben-Ari et al. 2005). It can be suggested that such messages promote a defensive reaction as fear-arousing messages and promote a sort of 'psychological immune system'. In conclusion, Ruiter and Kok (2005: 329) suggest that 'Policy makers should thus be reluctant to introduce cigarette warning labels and should instead focus on more effective interventions and policies'.

Individual level issues

The simplest individual interventions are those brief interventions that most health care professionals can engage in without any specific training: the Five As model (Coleman 2004) presented in Table 6.5 is one that is promoted for all health care professionals, but GPs in particular.

Table 6.5 The Five As model for facilitating smoking cessation

Five As	*Example*
Ask about tobacco use	Include questions about smoking in all consultations
Advise smokers to quit	Clear, strong and personalised advice
Assess smokers willingness to quit	Determine motivation to determine the next step
Assist the patient	Help the patient make a quit plan
Arrange follow-up	Follow-up should occur

Although this model is stressed in both the United States and the UK as a primary method for promoting smoking cessation, it has been argued that this does not fit with what GPs see as their role and as what patients need (McEwen et al. 2001; Aveyard and West 2007) and may damage the doctor–patient relationship (Butler et al. 1998).

Obviously, the 'Assist stage' can vary and many of these interventions (but not all) can improve smoking cessation rates efficaciously (e.g. Fiore et al. 2000). Among these therapies are self-help methods, physician advice, telephone counselling, cognitive behaviour therapy, nicotine replacement therapy (NRT) and non-nicotine medication such as bupropion (Willemsen et al. 2006).

But do patients get to know about these treatment options? Although a majority (some 60 per cent) of smokers do use methods (Hyland et al. 2004), not all of these are efficacious and evidence based (Willemsen et al. 2006) with Zeegers et al. (2005) reporting that some two-thirds of smokers who attempt to quit do not use efficacious methods. Why this is the case is difficult to determine but a number of methods have been suggested to increase uptake, for example, free smoking cessation services, but these tend to be underused (Britton 2004).

It can be argued, of course, that in the so-called 'hard to reach' groups, individuals are more likely to relate to the advice of those living in similar circumstances rather than those health care professionals perceived as an authority figure with different cultural norms (Springett et al. 2007). These health care professionals may find it difficult to move from their traditional role as an expert to a facilitator (Abrahamsson et al. 2005) and 'patients from less privileged backgrounds may react to their position of powerlessness by becoming non-compliant, uncooperative and helpless' (Lupton 1995: 75). However, the UK National Cancer Plan (DoH 2000b) lays great emphasis on having fully trained health care professionals to help support people who want to stop smoking.

One attempt at overcoming these concerns was by the introduction of a new health worker, the health trainer, an innovative attempt at increasing the adoption of healthy lifestyles and facilitating the use of preventative services by socio-economically deprived groups. Health trainers were promoted in *Improving Health*, which offers tailored advice, motivation and practical support to individuals who want help to adopt healthier lifestyles (DoH 2004c). The idea was that the health trainer would be recruited from the local community and work in local organisations, and would hence be the 'facilitator' rather than the trainer, supporting from the side, rather than giving advice from on high. It is envisaged that these trainers will be known and trusted by people in their community and have experience and understanding of what it means to live, or be part of, that community:

> In keeping with a shift in public approaches from 'advice from on high to support from next door', health trainers will be drawn from local communities, understanding the day-to-day concerns and experiences of the people they are supporting on health.
>
> (DoH 2004c: 103)

Health trainers should be visible and accessible to local people, proactively engaging individuals through the settings they work in. It is hoped that the role will enable them to receive and access referrals from professional groups, and direct people to local services through their knowledge of the local area. These trainers will employ evidence-based interventions that have their foundations in psychological theory (e.g. DoH 2004c).

Smokers will be informed of the strategies available for smoking cessation and the effectiveness of these. Evidence suggests that those that know more about smoking cessation methods and their effectiveness are more likely to use such methods.

However, unfortunately, many smokers have misconceptions about the efficacy and safety of NRT and other quit techniques (e.g. Bansal et al. 2004). Methods have been devised (see Willemsen et al. 2006) for the promotion of choice of appropriate cessation methods. These methods results in an increased chance of a quit attempt being made, and of that method being successful. These are related to their stage of change, with those in the contemplation stage (not surprisingly) benefiting the most. This is in line with the transtheoretical model, which states that people in the contemplation stage are most open to consciousness-raising techniques. That is, they seek new information and try to gain understanding and feedback about the problem behaviour (Prochaska et al. 1992). This model will be explored subsequently in more detail.

Pharmacological treatments

Pharmacological treatments are popular nowadays and include five forms of nicotine replacement therapy (NRT: gum, patch, nasal spray, inhaler, lozenge) and bupropion sustained release (Hughes 1999) (see Table 6.6). A recent review (Cofta-Woerpel et al. 2007) has suggested that these therapies can be considered a 'vital component' (Cofta-Woerpel et al. 2007: 47) of smoking cessation programmes and should be available to all. *The Guidelines* (Fiore et al. 2008) suggest that NRT can result in a doubling of abstinence rates at five months plus. On first examination it might be assumed that there was little psychology involved in NRT and that it was a pharmacological treatment of a physical problem. However, this would be a simplistic assumption and the psychological factors involved in NRT use are considerable. Indeed, without the motivation it can be argued that the success of NRT would be limited. Of course it could be argued that the use of NRTs undermines the value of the individual's will-power and seeks to medicalise a lifestyle behaviour although they have a value in reducing smoking rates.

Marks (1998) highlights that the use of NRT has a low efficacious rate in GP settings and, more importantly, deals with physiological dependence and *not* psychological dependency on tobacco. Hence, NRTs may not be entirely efficacious over the long term because the sensory and psychomotor aspects of smoking are inadequately addressed in cessation treatments (Rose and Behm 1995). Furthermore, investigators have suggested that simply focusing on NRTs is 'doomed to failure' because nicotine is only part of the explanation for smoking behaviour. Consequently, they suggest that use of either behavioural techniques or de-nicotinised cigarettes are required in order to deal with the sensory-motor activities

Table 6.6 Pharmacological interventions for smoking cessation

Medication	*Advantage*	*Disadvantage*	*Quit rates (%)*
Bupropion	Non-nicotine Easy to use Can be used with NRT	Can cause insomnia, dry mouth, headache, tremors, nausea or anxiety	21–30
Nicotine gum	Over the counter Flexible Quick delivery Different flavours	No food or drink 15 minutes beforehand Frequent use required Jaw pain, mouth soreness, dyspepsia Low compliance Underdosing is common	7–10
Nicotine inhaler	Flexible dosing Mimics hand-to-mouth action of smoking Few side-effects Comes in menthol flavour	Frequent dosing necessary May cause mouth and throat irritation Low compliance Underdosing is common	23
Nicotine lozenge	Over the counter Flexible dosing Quick delivery Oral administration	Frequent dosing necessary No food or drink 15 minutes beforehand May cause mouth soreness or dyspepsia Low compliance Underdosing is common	24
Nicotine patch	Over the counter Daily application Overnight use	Less flexible dosing Slow delivery of nicotine May cause skin irritation or sleep problems Not good at treating acute cravings	8–21
Nicotine nasal spray	Flexible dosing Fastest delivery Reduces craving within minutes	Frequent dosing necessary May cause nose and eye irritation Most addictive of the NRTs	30

associated with smoking (e.g. Rose and Behm 1995; Rose, Behm and Levin 1993). It is, of course, possible that the use of NRT will increase psychological dependence and actually increase the potential problem.

Although NRTs are successful in assisting people to quit smoking, NRTs have not been as influential as would be predicted (Cummings and Hyland 2005). Some have suggested that NRT merely encourages quit attempts by less motivated smokers who are less likely to succeed (Pierce and Gilpin 2002; Thorndike et al. 2002). Thus, although the usage rates and quit attempts may increase this is offset by an increase in relapse rates among those who are less committed to making a quit attempt (e.g. Pierce and Gilpin 2002). Consequently, the use of NRTs has not removed the need for psychological input into smoking cessation, rather it has increased it. Data support this view and there are a large number of studies that highlight that some type of in-person or telephone behavioural support with NRT increases quit rates, especially those using nicotine gum (Fiore et al. 2000; MacLeod et al. 2003; Shiffman et al. 2001; Silagy et al. 2002). This support works by increasing motivation for quitting and remaining tobacco-free. However, most quitters attempt to stop smoking by use of NRTs alone and overlook the behavioural and psychological support required to enhance and maintain the necessary motivation (Cummings and Hyland 2005; Zhu et al. 2000).

Psychological approaches

Psychological approaches to smoking cessation are important – either alone or in conjunction with pharmacological approaches and this has been recognised since the publication of the Surgeon General's report on smoking and health in 1964 (Office of the Surgeon General 1964). There are, of course, a number of psychological methods to the interventions whether this be at a behavioural or cognitive derived approach, or whether it be based on social cognition models or more complex psychological models. Table 6.7 summarises the effectiveness of particular psychosocial treatment contents (adapted from Piasecki 2006).

Table 6.7 Psychosocial content and abstinence rates

Psychosocial content	*Estimated abstinence rate (95% CI)*
No counselling	11.2
Relaxation	10.8 (7.8, 13.8)
Contingency contracting	11.2 (7.8, 14.6)
Cigarette fading	11.8 (8.4, 15.3)
Intratreatment social support	14.4 (12.3, 16.5)
Extratreatment social support	16.2 (11.8, 20.6)
Other aversive smoking	17.7 (11.2, 24.9)
Rapid smoking	19.9 (11.2, 29.0)

Behavioural approaches

Behavioural approaches to smoking cessation are usually based on the relapse prevention model of Marlatt and Gordon (1985) which suggests that common cognitive, behavioural and affective events can lead to high-risk situations that threaten abstinence. Consequently, it is suggested that individuals can prevent relapse by anticipating these events and learning to cope with them. This model has been taken up enthusiastically and has been exported to the community level (e.g. Moore et al. 2002). Such interventions do promote quitting but have indicated that they are generally akin to other programmes – the majority of smokers relapsing in the long term (Irvin et al. 1999). Furthermore, some have been quite explicit and stated that the evidence to date does not support the adoption of skills training interventions to prevent relapse (Lancaster et al. 2006).

Another method much favoured in the past was aversive smoking – for example, rapid smoking and rapid puffing (Danaher 1977). These methods involve intensive smoking to the point of discomfort, nausea or vomiting. Evidence indicates that such techniques can be successful and can be used with smokers who have not succeeded with other techniques (Vidrine et al. 2006). However, there are of course associated health risks and consequently aversive smoking interventions are rarely used in current practice.

Furthermore, such clinical approaches have one major drawback – the time taken to implement such programmes. Most emphasise the intensity of support required for successful quitting and there appears to be a greater chance of success with an increased input. However, public health interventions, despite their lower success rates, have a numerical advantage since they reach a broader spectrum of people.

Transtheoretical model of change (TTM) and stages of changes

There are a number of health promotion models (see Table 6.8) and health behaviour change models (see Chapter 2).

However, the most influential psychological model that has been used in smoking cessation has been the 'transtheoretical model of change' or 'stages of change' (Prochaska and DiClemente 1983). The model suggests that change proceeds through six stages summarised in Figure 6.5. Importantly, relapse can occur at any stage, and can mean that the individual goes back to the very first stage: it is not a linear model of simple progression from one stage to another and then relapse means that you simply revert to the previous stage: you can revert to *any* previous stage.

How can we use the stages of change model in the promotion of health and to assist individuals to quit smoking? The model is important because it allows professionals to identify where individuals are in their behaviour and then develop interventions – including computer and media based – founded of this information (e.g. Etter 2005; Cobb et al. 2005). For example, an individual smokes and has no intention of giving up and, as a consequence, the intervention to be developed will be different than that of the individual that is preparing to give up. In the first example then our obligation should be to try and get quitting into the person's thought processes. We want to try to get the individual to consider giving up smoking: we want

Table 6.8 Summary of the main theories of health promotion

Level	*Theory*	*Focus*	*Key concepts*
Individual	Stages of change model	Individual's readiness to change or attempt to change toward healthy behaviours	Pre-contemplation Contemplation Decision/determination Action Maintenance
	Health belief model	Perception of the threat of a health problem and appraisal of recommended behaviour(s) for preventing or managing the problem	Perceived susceptibility Perceived severity Perceived benefits of action Cues to action Self-efficacy
Interpersonal	Social learning theory	Behaviour is explained via a three-way, dynamic, reciprocal theory in which personal factors, environmental influences and behaviour continually interact	Behaviour capability Reciprocal determinism Expectations Self-efficacy Observational learning Reinforcement
Community	Community organisation theories	Emphasises active participation and development of communities that can better evaluate and solve health and social problems	Empowerment Community competence Participation and relevance Issue selection Critical consciousness
	Organisational change theory	Concerns processes and strategies for increasing the chances that healthy policies and programmes will be adopted and maintained in formal organisations	Problem definition (awareness stage) Initiation of action (adoption stage) Implementation of change Institutionalisation of change
	Diffusion of innovation theories	Addresses how new ideas, products and social practices spread within a society or from one society to another	Relative advantage Compatibility Complexity Trialability Observability

to shift them from the pre-contemplation stage to the contemplation stage. The most common method in this approach is a simple consciousness-raising exercise: increasing information about the problem and how it can

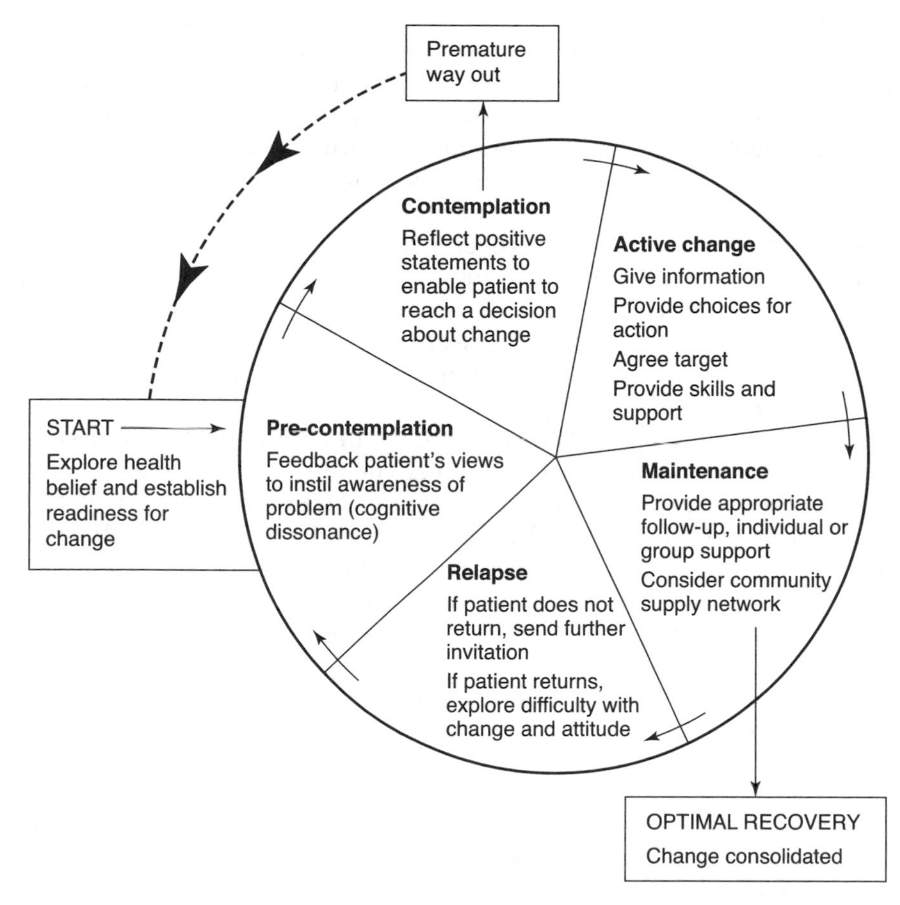

Figure 6.5 Stages of change model

affect the individual concerned. So at this stage it would simply be a case of getting them to realise that smoking is health damaging and that it can affect them individually, and then spelling out the individual health problems that they either are facing or could be facing because of their behaviour. Interventions based on the stages of changes model usually incorporate two key elements. First, it is necessary to identify accurately an individual's stage of change (or readiness to change), so that an appropriate intervention can be designed and applied. Second, the stage of change needs to be reassessed frequently, and the intervention modified in light of this assessment. In this way, stage-based interventions evolve and adapt in response to the individual's movement through the stages. It is suggested that such interventions are better than the 'one size fits all' model and that the intervention will be more efficient and effective than such models.

Velicer et al. (1993) have developed self-help interventions, based on the transtheoretical model (TTM), designed as substitutes for skilled smoking cessation counselling. These courses achieved quit rates equivalent to those achieved using smoking cessation counselling and nicotine replacement therapy (NRT). The intervention included a stage-based manual, which gives a detailed description of where individuals are in the stopping process, and provides exercises that engage the appropriate processes of change to move forward. This was supplemented by an expert system letter. Hence, the theoretical basis underlying the intervention appeared to be of benefit to quitting smoking.

The TTM has been primarily applied to smoking (West 2005 reported that 33 per cent of all TTM studies dealt with smoking, compared to only 13 per cent for alcohol, cocaine, heroin, opiates and gambling) and has been *the* model for developing interventions. Indeed, surveys have suggested that the stages of change model and motivational interviewing were the main topics covered in training courses, as well as the primary theory used to explain behaviour change (McEwen and West 2001). Prochaska and Goldstein (1991), proponents of the model, argue that the model has revolutionised health promotion, suggesting that interventions that are tailored to the particular stage of the individual improve their effectiveness (Prochaska and Velicer 1997). The stages of change model has been popular with practitioners as a practical intervention guide for clinicians, and as an example of how to apply complex theories of behaviour change in an approachable and understandable form. From a research perspective, however, there is less value placed on it with the efficacy relatively low in smoking cessation (West 2005), suggesting that TTM does not account for much of the variance. A systematic review exploring the value of staged based interventions has been completed by Riemsma et al. (2003) and they concluded that 'Despite the widespread and uncritical use of stage based interventions in smoking cessation, we found only limited evidence for their effectiveness' (p. 5). Similarly, Michie and Abraham (2004) report that 'despite the popularity of this model, the psychological processes described by TTM are not well supported by available data' (p. 34).

A number of eloquent critiques of the model have been presented (e.g. Etter and Perneger 1999; Bunton et al. 2000; Whitelaw et al. 2000; Sutton 2001; Etter and Sutton 2002; Littell and Girvin 2002). There is a considerable body of research that explores the stage of change but many have used sub-optimal designs (Riemsma et al. 2003) and consequently the evidence is somewhat limited. However, despite these limitations the proponents of the TTM argue that the model has revolutionised health promotion, that the interventions tailored to the particular stage of the individual improve their effectiveness (Prochaska and Velicer 1997).

West (2005) argues that the TTM is nothing more than a security blanket for both researchers and clinicians for a number of reasons (although there are repudiations by both Prochaska 2005 and DiClemente 2005). At the outset, it provides a perception that the assessment and intervention is objectively accurate and scientific and that a form of diagnosis is being made. Furthermore, he argues that there are scientific labels attached to meaningless behaviours. Hence, the model describes people as a 'precontemplator' which is actually somebody who is not planning on making any change (i.e. somebody who wishes to carry on as they are normally). Thus this medicalisation and 'scientification' of the model actually suggests more than it can offer. Furthermore, when they are in this stage the suggestion is that individuals should be offered support and strategies to help them move along the model into understanding the benefits of change. Yet, some people may simply jump this stage straight into action if something appeals to them which is novel to them (e.g. with Zyban being offered as a smoking cessation aid: Zwar and Richmond 2002).

So what should be the next step? West (2005) argues that a new model of behaviour change is clearly needed. Obviously there are many such models available (see Chapter 2) but these need to include decision-making processes, motivational processes, habits, labels and other such psychological factors that are not necessarily under conscious control. For example, an individual may label themselves as 'a smoker' and this comes with a set of values, and motivational processes. Alternatively, they may label themselves as a 'non-smoker' which may motivate the smoker to exercise restraint when temptation to smoke arises. Any model consequently needs to assess both state and trait factors and how these interact to promote the stage of change of the individual (West 2007).

Motivational interviewing

At an individual level, the concept of the TTM can be used clinically to work with smokers. Miller and Rollnick (2002) concluded that motivation is fundamental to change and they suggest motivational interviewing is the appropriate approach. Motivational interviewing can be defined as 'a client-centred, directive method for enhancing intrinsic motivation to change by exploring and resolving ambivalence' (Miller and Rollnick 2002).

Motivational interviewing has as its goal the simple expectation that increasing an individual's motivation to consider change rather than showing them how to change should be the key step. If a person is not motivated to change then it is irrelevant if they know how to do it or not. However, if a person is motivated to change then the interventions aimed at changing behaviour can begin.

Motivational interviewing (MI) is a technique based on cognitive-behavioural therapy which aims to enhance an individual's motivation to change health behaviour. The whole process aims to help the patient understand their thought processes and to identify how their thought processes help produce the inappropriate behaviour and how their thought processes can be changed to develop alternative, health-promoting behaviours.

Motivational strategies include eight components that are designed to increase the level of motivation the person has towards changing a specific behaviour. It is important to note that the motivation is specific to one behaviour, thus being motivated to quit smoking does not simply transfer to being motivated to reduce alcohol consumption. The eight components are:

- giving advice (about specific behaviours to be changed)
- removing barriers (often about access to particular help)
- providing choice (making it clear that if they choose not to change that is their right and it is their choice; the therapist is there to encourage change but not insist on change)
- decreasing desirability (of the ambivalence towards change or the status quo)
- practising empathy
- providing feedback (from a variety of perspectives – family, friends, health professionals – in order to give the patient a full picture of their current situation)
- clarifying goals (feedback should be compared with a standard (an ideal), and clarification of the ideal can provide the pathway to the goal)
- active helping (such as expressing caring or facilitating a referral, all of which convey a real interest in helping the person to change).

'Hardcore' or 'hardened' smokers

There has been considerable advance in the number of smokers quitting but there still remains a large group of individuals who will not or cannot give up. Although there is no agreed definition of a 'hardcore smoker' it is suggested that some 16 per cent of all smokers may be of such a type (Jarvis et al. 2003) and there may be some link with nicotine dependence, lower SES and being male (MacIntosh and Coleman 2006).

Although there has been a decline in smoking over the decades, the rate of decline has flattened considerably and therefore the smoking population remaining may be the hardened smoker. This 'hardening hypothesis' has been the focus of debate because it is based on correlation data that are open to varied interpretations (Warner and Burns 2003). However, there needs to be careful monitoring of the situation and appropriate interventions devised and implemented to deal with this diminishing population of smokers (Piasecki 2006).

Relapse

Cigarette smoking is a behaviour that is relatively difficult to change. Despite the health risks associated with smoking, relatively few smokers succeed in their attempts to quit (Piasecki 2006). The definition of 'lapse' and 'relapse' has been debated in various forums (e.g. Velicer et al. 1992) but simply a 'lapse' is a slip into smoking behaviour, whereas 'relapse' refers to long-term failure.

Most smokers who attempt to quit do so through self-quitting (Fiore et al. 2000) but the rates of success are very low with reports suggesting that only about 3–5 per cent of those self-quitting attain long-term abstinence at 6–12 months (Hughes et al. 2004). More recently, self-quitters have been aided by being able to purchase over the counter NRT and although this can double the rate of success this is still a paltry 6–10 per cent success rate.

Even with successful treatment, relapse can occur quickly, with many smokers not even attaining 24 hours of continuous abstinence (Spanier et al. 1996; Piasecki 2006) with the majority abandoning their quit attempts within 5–10 days. In order to explore relapse, researchers have explored psychological processes such as withdrawal, urge and craving, and negative affect. The rate of attempts to stop is high: 78 attempts per 100 smokers in the UK, with many smokers making more than one attempt a year (West 2006). Although the majority of smokers want to stop smoking and predict that they will have stopped in twelve months, only 2–3 per cent actually stops permanently a year (Taylor et al. 2006).

Factors associated with successful cessation

Although the majority of smokers want to stop smoking, and some 41 per cent of current smokers have tried to quit in the previous twelve months (Centers for Disease Control and Prevention (CDC) 2004) the success rate is low (Taylor et al. 2005). A number of studies have been undertaken exploring factors associated with successful quitting and these were often inter-related. For example, Derby et al. (1994) found that for women not living with another smoker was of key importance, but for men it was an increased age. Similarly, a successful quitter was reported to be an older male with higher income and smoking fewer cigarettes with having previous quit attempts (Hymowitz et al. 1997). Furthermore, the environment was also found to be important – being in daily contact with other smokers, for example, is associated with less success whether this be in the workplace (e.g. Moher et al. 2005) or at home (e.g. Gourlay et al. 1994).

In terms of behaviours, switching to low-tar cigarettes has found to be both useful and not (e.g. Kozlowski et al. 1998) and a gradual reduction in cigarette smoking compared to 'cold turkey' has been reported as being more successful (e.g. Cinciripini et al. 1995).

However, many of these studies have explored factors in one-off settings and have not appreciated the dynamic nature of smoking and its cessation as highlighted in the TTM. The dynamic nature of the quitting process was explored by Lee and Kahende (2007), who report a number of factors associated with successful quitting and these are presented in Table 6.9.

Table 6.9 Factors associated with successful smoking cessation.

Positive	*Negative*
Smoke-free home	Multiple previous attempts
No smoking policy at work	Switching to low tar products
Aged 35+	
Having university education	
Being married or co-habiting	
One previous attempt at quitting	
Social support	

Conclusion

Smoking is the major preventable killer of individuals in the world and hence has attracted considerable funding, research and debate on how best to promote smoking cessation. One the one hand, smoking is a behaviour which is avoidable: society and civilisation would not suffer considerably if it was banned across the country.

The consequences of smoking are severe and the health impacts considerable. As a result any psychological interventions should be efficacious, but need they be efficient? How successful have the psychological approaches to explaining smoking been? And what about smoking cessation, how successful have the psychological approaches been? What next for the psychological approaches to smoking cessation? However, as we have emphasised throughout this text any lifestyle behaviour cannot be seen in isolation and neither can the intervention. Although it is trite to stress the multi-method approach to smoking cessation, it can be concluded that NRTs, pharmacological or psychological approaches used in combination will have a higher rate of success than when any one is used in isolation. Furthermore, although psychological and physiological factors may be important the social context of the behaviour cannot be ignored and can be considered of key importance.

Summary points

- Cigarette smoking remains the single most avoidable cause of death and disability in the UK and the Western world.
- There are differences in prevalence rates of smoking across England, Wales, Scotland and Northern Ireland.

- Although the number of people smoking has decreased considerably, this is mainly due to the established smoker giving up – the number of young people starting to smoke remains, broadly, the same.
- Smoking has been linked to a whole host of diseases and chronic conditions including heart disease, cancer, peripheral vascular disease, premature and low weight babies, bronchitis, emphysema, sinusitis, peptic ulcers, dental hygiene problems and can worsen the effects of asthma, and infections.
- Despite knowledge of the health risks associated with smoking, people continue to smoke and display unrealistic optimism regarding the impact of their smoking behaviour.
- Clinical smoking cessation includes (either alone or in combination) behavioural and pharmaceutical interventions and they range from brief advice and counselling to intensive support, and administration of medications that contribute to reducing or overcoming dependence.
- Population level interventions appear to be less effective with lower SES groups. These groups may have restricted access to individual level interventions.
- The most influential model used in smoking cessation is the Transtheoretical or Stages of Change Model. This suggests that people move between different stages of "readiness" for change. People can move forwards or backwards and relapse can occur at any time. There is limited evidence that smoking cessation programmes based on the TTM are effective however.
- Motivational interviewing can be used to attempt to increase a smoker's motivation to quit.
- Lapse and relapse rates are high in smokers attempting to quit. Contact with other smokers, age, gender and previous quit attempts can all impact on the likelihood that a quit attempt will be successful.

7 Sex

I practice safe sex – I use an airbag.

Garry Shandling

At the end of this chapter you will:

- appreciate how 'sex' and 'safe sex' have been defined by professionals and the lay public alike
- understand the nature of sexually transmitted diseases and their health consequences, along with their extent nationwide
- appreciate some of the explanations for the increase in levels of sexually transmitted diseases and the relationship between unsafe sex and other lifestyle behaviours
- evaluate the psychological determinants of sexual behaviour and safe sex practices
- explore the broader influences on sexual behaviour
- reason how the social cognitive models have been used to predict safe sex practices (in particular condom use) and how they can be employed to develop appropriate interventions.

Definitions

A simplistic definition of 'sexual behaviour' could refer to all actions and responses that make fertilisation possible. In order to effect a fertilisation a male and female have to perform a specific series of actions and physiological responses. However, a more pragmatic definition refers to any behaviour that involves a 'sexual response' of the body. In this way the physical actions associated with sexual behaviour do not have to result in fertilisation. The definition covers all types of human sexual activity (sexual self-stimulation, heterosexual and homosexual intercourse, and sexual contact with animals), but it does not imply any hierarchical order among them. Moreover, it leaves each of these activities open to interpretation. In short, the above definition does not equate sex with reproduction or any other particular purpose. It merely calls attention to a certain physical response common to a variety of activities.

A final definition includes all actions and responses related to pleasure seeking. This is a modern, very wide definition which can be traced to Sigmund Freud and his psychoanalytic theory. Thus, in this view 'the sex drive' came to stand for the human pursuit of pleasure in all its forms. 'Sex' was the underlying motive of every life-enhancing activity. As we can see, when used in this fashion, the term 'sexual behaviour' becomes quite inclusive. The only question in all of these cases is one of motivation. If the behaviour is somehow motivated by the wish for pleasure, if it is prompted by an individual's inner need for self-fulfilment, if it satisfies or gives the individual comfort, if it heightens the sense of being alive, then it is clearly sexual.

Most sexual researchers use the second of these definitions. The definition does not equate sex with reproduction or any other particular purpose. It merely calls attention to a certain physical response common to a variety of activities. Obviously this definition is important for health researchers, when asking members of the population if they engaged in 'sex', 'dangerous sexual behaviour' or 'safe sexual behaviour' it is important to clearly define what this covers.

In contrast to these formal, academic definitions, the majority of UK adults obtain their sexual health information from media such as television, newspapers and magazines (National Statistics Omnibus Survey (NSOS) 2007). It is therefore essential that the information available is correct, consistent and easily accessible. Not only in terms of 'sexual behaviour' but also and more importantly *safe* sexual behaviour.

Government public health campaigns aimed at raising awareness of safe sex via the media are relatively infrequent. The last of these was in 2004 (DoH 2004b), although a campaign during 2007 and 2008 on the risks associated with unsafe sex has also been widespread. A succinct safe sex message is not, however, easily accessible in the media nowadays. Furthermore an online search of 'safe sex' into a popular search engine fails to return a full explanation of safe sex from UK websites. When available, the message from the majority of sexual health sites, including institutions such as the Family Planning Association (FPA 2007), was 'when having sex, wear a condom at all times' (Faculty of Family Planning and Reproductive Healthcare 2007; Likeitis 2007; RUThinking 2007; Society of Sexual Health Advisers (SSHA) 2007).

The concept of safe sex was derived in response to the HIV/AIDS epidemic and consequently it originally focused on male homosexuals, the community where the outbreak originated, with the earliest reference to this professional term being in 1984 (Morin et al. 1984). A governmental definition of 'safe sex' involves taking precautions during sex that can keep you from getting a sexually transmitted disease (STD), or from giving an STD to your partner. These diseases include genital herpes, genital warts, HIV, Chlamydia, gonorrhea, syphilis, hepatitis B and C, and others. In 1985, the Coalition for Sexual Responsibility drafted safe sex guidelines to promote the distribution and use of condoms 'to eliminate the exchange of body fluids during anal intercourse or oral sex' (Lindsey 1985), and subsequently health promotion officials extended the definition to heterosexual adolescents: 'judicious selection of sexual partners, the use of mechanical and chemical barriers during intercourse, and avoidance of sex practices such as those in which bodily fluids are exchanged' (Slevin and Marvin 1987). Following on from these American developments, the concept of 'safe sex' began to be promoted in the UK with the 'tombstone' HIV/AIDS campaign in 1986 leading on to a number of high-profile safe sex (demonstrated through condom use) campaigns.

Abstinence is an absolute answer to preventing STDs. However, abstinence is not always a practical or desirable option. Next to abstinence, the least risky approach is to have a monogamous sexual relationship with someone that you know is free of any STD. Condoms can be used to avoid contact with semen, vaginal fluids or blood. Both male and female condoms dramatically reduce the chance that individuals will get or spread an STD (Collins 1985).

However, although the 'official' and 'educational' definitions of 'sex' and 'safe sex' are well known and agreed, there is a paucity of literature on how the general public (and those at risk in particular) define 'safe sex' (Moskowitz et al. 2006). A Californian study reported that most defined safe sex in terms of condom use (with 26.3 per cent suggesting this alone was 'safe sex'). Condom use in conjunction with other common methods (e.g. abstinence, safe partner, or monogamy) was mentioned by two-thirds of respondents. Definitions of safe sex varied across socio-demographic groups. For example, males were more likely to mention monogamy and less likely to mention abstinence. Condom use was mentioned most often by adults aged 18–24 years and tended to decrease with age. Adults aged 25–64 years were most likely to mention monogamy, and those aged 45–64 years were most likely to mention safe partner (Moskowitz et al. 2006).

However, what is not clear from the above is what people understand by 'sex'. According to a study of undergraduates, approximately 60 per cent of them did not regard oral sex as 'sex' (Chambers 2007). Supporting this is the finding that between 10 and 30 per cent of virgins have engaged in oral sex as a means of maintaining virginity (Bruckner and Bearman 2005). It is possible that individuals who engage in oral sex, but do not consider it 'sex', may not associate the acts with the potential health risks they can bring (CDC 2006a; Chambers 2007). In fact, anecdotal evidence suggests that teenagers may engage in oral sex as a means for reducing sexually transmitted infections and HIV risk (Barrett 2004). Furthermore, some reports have suggested that 10 per cent of students did not consider anal sex as 'sex'.

One website that provides an excellent safer sex definition is actually a Department of Health website (www.condomessentialwear.co.uk). The message is clear, anyone who is having sex can contract an STI: 'whether young or old, straight or gay, do it once in a while or all night every night'. The website defines safer sex as 'any sex that does not allow an infected person's blood, semen, pre-ejaculatory fluid or fluid from the vagina to get inside the other person's body'. The site goes further to describe a number of regular and more extreme sexual practices which can place an individual at increased risk of infection before imparting advice on when it may be safe to agree to stop using condoms. This single website, accessed only after a reasonable amount of time spent searching, seems to be one of the very few information sources offering a full, comprehensive definition and advice concerning safer sex. It is clear that much more could be done to encourage safer sex practices. It is of particular concern that the only safe sex message available in the media is on the internet, as it has been reported that very few UK residents of any age obtain their sexual health information via this method (NSOS 2007).

Recent surveys indicate that the general public's knowledge about sexual health, in particular human immunodeficiency virus (HIV), has deteriorated by a significant amount (National AIDS Trust 2006; UNAIDS 2006). In London, the area with the highest prevalence of HIV in the UK, 30 per cent of people did not know HIV could be transmitted through unprotected sex (National AIDS Trust 2006; UNAIDS 2006). Generally knowledge about how the disease is transmitted is poor, with more than one in ten 18–24 year olds thinking it can be passed on through kissing, and about one in ten people believing it can be passed through sweat and sharing cutlery (Terrence Higgins Trust (THT) 2007). Many young adults also believe that there is a cure despite the fact that HIV has killed over 17,000 people in the UK since 1982 and is the UK's fastest growing serious health condition (National AIDS Trust 2006; UNAIDS 2006).

The National Survey of Sexual Attitudes and Lifestyles (Wellings et al. 1994) examined the sexual behaviour of over 18,000 men and women across Britain and produced considerable data on factors such as age of first intercourse, sexual behaviour and contraception use. The report indicates that for men and women aged 16–24 the most popular form of contraception was condom use (see Figure 7.1). It was rather worrying, however, that many young adults in this age group reported using either no contraception at all, or potentially unreliable methods, such as withdrawal or the 'safe period'. In terms of safe sex, health care professionals should try to encourage condom use to prevent sexually transmitted diseases along with potentially unwanted pregnancies.

Other reports have investigated the views of both men and women. In general, men tend to report a number of negative attitudes towards condom use including reduction in spontaneity of behaviour and reduced

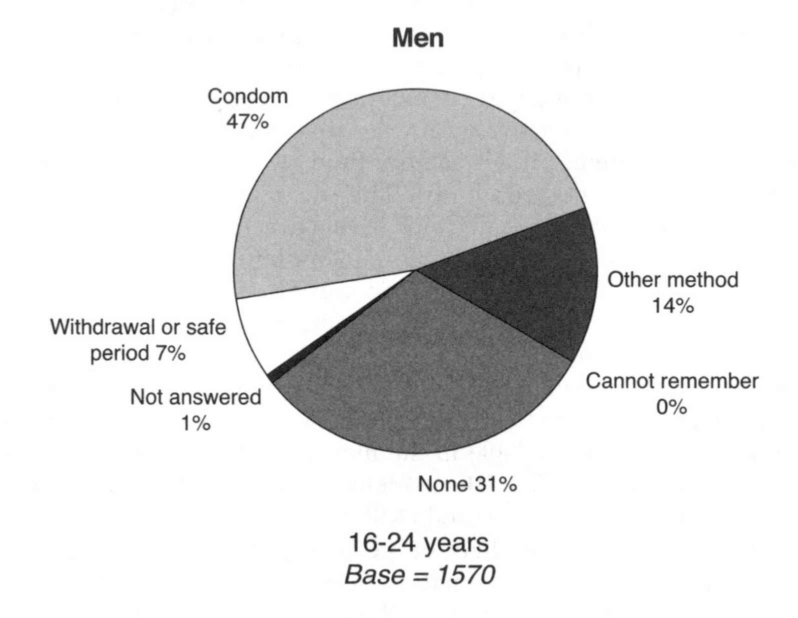

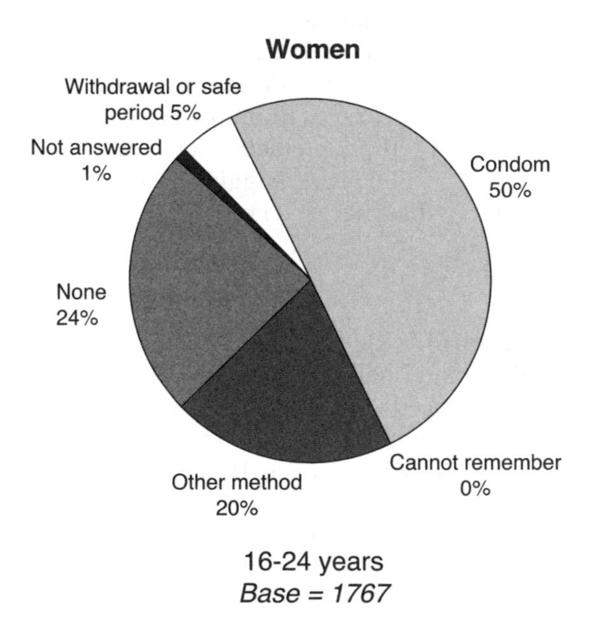

Figure 7.1 Forms of contraception used by both men and women

sexual pleasure. Surveys of young women suggest they also hold these negative attitudes. However, they also tend to hold unrealistically optimistic estimates of personal risk of infection with STD or HIV (Bryan et al. 1996, 1997). There are a number of other negative attitudes held by women that can potentially hinder condom use and these include:

- anticipated male objection to a female suggesting condom use (denial of their pleasure)
- difficulty or embarrassment in raising the issue of condom use with a male partner
- worry that suggesting use to a potential partner implies that either themselves or their partner is HIV+ or has another STD
- lack of self-efficacy or mastery in condom use.

Evidence of the problem

In 2006 there were almost 40 million people worldwide living with HIV and 4 million new cases the same year (UNAIDS 2006). In Eastern Europe and Central Asia there has been a twenty-fold increase in people living with HIV in less than a decade (EuroHIV 2006). In Western Europe and North America the number of people living with HIV continues to increase, partly due to the life-prolonging effects of antiretroviral therapy in addition to the continuing new diagnoses. The UK has seen the largest increases in Western Europe where annual new HIV diagnoses have doubled since 2000 (Health Protection Agency (HPA) 2007a). Three-quarters of new diagnoses in heterosexual men and women were among people originating from countries outside the UK, mainly from sub-Saharan Africa. People infected in sub-Saharan Africa are now the group most affected by HIV in the United Kingdom, slightly more so than men who have sex with men (HPA 2007a).

An increasing proportion of HIV infections are thought to be occurring through unprotected sexual intercourse (EuroHIV 2006). Consequently, women, many younger than 25, bear a growing part of the HIV burden. Almost two-thirds of HIV infections diagnosed among men in 2004 were attributable to unsafe sex with other men (CDC 2007a) and several studies have reported evidence of an increase in unsafe sexual behaviour in this population group (CDC 2007a).

The latest statistics on AIDS and HIV in the UK were published in August 2007 by the Health Protection Agency. As can be noted from Table 7.1 the number of women diagnosed with HIV has increased in recent years and in 2007 it was some 40 per cent of the total (compared to 10 per cent of all diagnoses in 1990). Table 7.1 also shows that the annual number of AIDS diagnoses and deaths among HIV-positive people rose during the early 1990s but then dropped dramatically after the widespread introduction of highly active antiretroviral therapy (HAART) in 1996–97.

Table 7.2 shows that 92 per cent of UK HIV diagnoses have been made in England (around 84 per cent of the UK's population lives in England).

Table 7.1 UK HIV diagnoses, AIDS cases and deaths by year of diagnosis and sex

Year of diagnosis	HIV			AIDS			Deaths[a]		
	Male	Female	Total[b]	Male	Female	Total	Male	Female	Total[c]
1991 or earlier	17,365	2,137	19,536	5,791	391	6,182	4,107	246	4,355
1992	2,200	546	2,747	1,406	173	1,579	1,164	89	1,253
1993	2,109	531	2,641	1,551	238	1,789	1,405	164	1,569
1994	2,050	539	2,590	1,626	227	1,853	1,527	182	1,709
1995	2,089	576	2,665	1,489	283	1,772	1,503	223	1,726
1996	2,130	595	2,725	1,174	270	1,444	1,258	224	1,482
1997	2,085	678	2,764	863	217	1,080	599	149	749
1998	2,102	760	2,863	599	195	794	417	97	514
1999	2,178	969	3,149	569	193	762	391	81	472
2000	2,491	1,393	3,884	589	245	834	386	98	484
2001	3,120	1,980	5,101	495	243	738	359	118	477
2002	3,614	2,652	6,266	562	331	893	413	107	520
2003	4,090	3,245	7,335	525	411	936	407	165	572
2004	4,380	3,174	7,556	498	375	873	347	149	496
2005	4,528	3,134	7,662	499	291	790	399	140	539
2006	4,257	2,835	7,093	385	281	666	356	141	497
Until June 2007	1,314	736	2,050	112	50	162	137	46	183
Total	62,102	26,480	88,627	18,733	4,414	23,147	15,175	2,419	17,597

a Includes all deaths of people diagnosed with HIV, with or without a reported AIDS diagnosis.
b Includes 44 HIV diagnoses with sex not stated on the report (which results in some of the totals not matching).
c Includes three deaths with sex not stated on the report.

Table 7.3 highlights the proportion of individuals diagnosed with various STIs across the UK.

Table 7.2 HIV infected persons by country and year of HIV diagnosis

Year of diagnosis	*England*	*Wales*	*N. Ireland*	*Scotland*	*UK total*	*Channel Isles/Isle of Man*
1991 or earlier	17,461	276	96	1,703	19,536	28
1992	2,547	50	12	138	2,747	1
1993	2,408	40	12	181	2,641	2
1994	2,373	45	15	157	2,590	8
1995	2,460	45	12	148	2,665	1
1996	2,503	35	17	170	2,725	6
1997	2,542	46	9	167	2,764	8
1998	2,661	29	9	164	2,863	6
1999	2,943	35	15	156	3,149	0
2000	3,661	45	19	159	3,884	1
2001	4,837	63	19	182	5,101	5
2002	5,938	76	27	225	6,266	7
2003	6,916	108	32	279	7,335	4
2004	7,041	107	62	346	7,556	4
2005	7,115	122	63	362	7,662	4
2006	6,595	154	57	287	7,093	2
Until June 2007	1,849	64	13	124	2,050	0
Total	81,850	1,340	489	4,948	88,627	87

Table 7.3 Rates per 100,000 of population of STI diagnoses by country (2006)

	Gonorrhea	*Syphilis*	*Chlamydia*	*Genital warts*	*Genital herpes*
England	35	5.0	197	141	38
Wales	16	1.1	126	125	22
Northern Ireland	11	1.7	115	125	22
Scotland	17	3.7	170	135	27
UK	32	4.6	189	139	36

Young people aged over 15 accounted for 40 per cent of new HIV infections in 2006 (UNAIDS 2006). This may be because young people fail to integrate their general knowledge regarding HIV risk into their sexual interactions and may perceive high safety and little risk for infection, despite inconsistent condom use (O'Sullivan et al. 2006). Young people under 16 have also seen the largest increase in Chlamydia; the largest prevalence rates are in those aged between 16 and 24 (ONS 2006b). Chlamydia and gonorrhoea are the two most common STIs and both are the key cause of preventable infertility among women; along with other STIs they make the acquisition and transmission of HIV between three and five times more likely (Barry and Klausner 2006).

Sexually transmitted infections can be prevented by condom use, but surveys indicate that individuals rarely use condoms for this preventative purpose (ONS 2006b). For example, 95 per cent of 16–24 year olds who use a condom do so in order to prevent pregnancy whereas only 71 per cent report using a condom in order to prevent infection. Furthermore, less than half (48 per cent) of men and only 37 per cent of women report using a condom 'always'. The potential for sexually transmitted diseases arising from this lack of knowledge and appropriate usage has to be stressed.

It is apparent from the evidence presented here that the combination of deteriorating STI knowledge, and rapidly increased prevalence rates underlines the urgent need to educate and strengthen the safe sex message in the public domain. However, the majority of adults report making no changes to their behaviour as a result of what they hear regarding sexual health (NSOS 2007). This was reflected in a more positive manner when recent changes in the UK law which made emergency hormonal contraception available over the counter have been found to have had no impact on its usage levels, and has not led to an increase in unprotected sex (Marston et al. 2005). However, with regard to the safe sex message it is clear that information and awareness campaigns are ineffective in achieving their goal and other strategies must be implemented

Consequences of unsafe sex

STIs remain an important cause of morbidity throughout the world despite being some of the simplest infections to treat (Barry and Klausner 2006). Having multiple sexual partners characterises a risk behaviour for sexually transmitted infections and HIV (Howard and Qi Wang 2004). As the number and variety of new sexual partners increases, so does the risk of exposure to individuals infected with STIs. Many societies and cultures are intolerant of sex outside marriage and much is made of the effect on sexual health as a result of sex outside of wedlock (Wellings et al. 2006). However, marriage does not protect against sexually transmitted disease and it has been found that the sexual health benefits of marriage for women can be counterbalanced by lower rates of condom use, higher rates of intercourse and their husbands' risk behaviour (S. Clark 2004).

Marriage cannot be relied upon to ensure safer early sexual experiences (Wellings et al. 2006).

Unsafe sexual practices can result in any one or more of the most common STIs as presented in Table 7.3 (Barry and Klausner 2006). Evidence on the use of condoms to prevent STI transmission is limited by poor study design (Warner et al. 2006); there is some evidence to suggest a reduction in STI transmission when consistent and correct use of condoms is employed. For example, the more consistently women's male sex partners use condoms, the less likely women are to acquire genital human papillomavirus (HPV) infection (Winer et al. 2006). Similarly Wald et al. (2005) found that participants reporting more frequent use of condoms were at lower risk for acquiring Herpes Simplex Virus-2 than participants who used condoms less frequently. However, even with consistent and correct use, condoms may not completely eliminate the risk of STI transmission. Despite this the correct use of condoms in this manner is highly recommended to offer protection against many of the following STIs (Warner et al. 2006; FFPRCH 2007).

- *Chlamydia trachomatis:* this may be transmitted in vaginal or seminal fluids. An estimated 2.8 million new infections occur each year. Chlamydia is most often asymptomatic. Untreated infections can progress to pelvic inflammatory disease (PID) and approximately 40 per cent of women with PID later have decreased fertility (CDC 2007c).
- *Gonorrhoea:* this is transmitted via seminal and vaginal fluids and easily transmitted through sexual activity. Gonococcal urethritis causes painful urination and discharge, although approximately 25 per cent of men have no symptoms. Among women, gonorrhoea can cause cervicitis with vaginal discharge, pain with intercourse, or painful urination; however, approximately half of infected women are asymptomatic. Gonorrhoea can infect the rectum and throat. Infections at these sites are predominately asymptomatic but can cause pharyngitis. Rectal infections increase the risk for HIV acquisition, if a person is exposed through receptive anal sex. Pharyngeal infections usually have minor clinical consequences but can be transmitted to male partners through oral sex (HPA 2007b).
- *Nongonococcal urethritis:* NGU is the most common clinical sexually transmitted syndrome among men and is characterised by painful urination with or without discharge (CDC 2006c)
- *Syphilis:* clinical manifestations of syphilis are varied, and its natural history is complex. Syphilis Treponema pallidum can be transmitted through sexual intercourse or direct contact with syphilitic sores or rash. Infected individuals may be asymptomatic (CDC 2004; HPA 2005).

- *Herpes:* genital herpes is the most common ulcerative STI in the UK (HPA 2007c). There is no cure, and as with other STIs, herpes simplex virus (HSV) infection facilitates the transmission and acquisition of HIV infection. Transmission of HSV can occur with unprotected sex or direct contact with genital ulcers or in the absence of clinical lesions when the virus is shed in asymptomatic men and women. There is an especially high risk of transmission when those infected have an active genital sore or an active oral cold sore (HPA 2007c).
- *Hepatitis B virus:* HBV can be passed via seminal and vaginal fluids and is approximately 100 times more transmissible than HIV. About one-fifth of all new HBV infections occur among men having sex with men (MSM) and people are often unaware of their status. Vaccination is the most effective strategy against HBV (HPA 2007d).
- *Hepatitis C virus:* HCV can be transmitted through seminal and vaginal fluids, however the risk of sexual transmission is low (HPA 2007e). It is likely that if condoms are used consistently then sexual transmission of hepatitis C will be avoided (HPA 2007e).
- *Hepatitis A:* this is spread via the faecal–oral route but usually via food, water or by close (non-sexual) contact (CDC 2006d).
- *Human papillomavirus (HPV):* in total, 40 types of HPV can infect the genital tract. HPV-16 or -18 cause over 70 per cent of cervical cancers worldwide, whereas HPV-6 or -11 cause over 90 per cent of genital warts. HPV infection is extremely common. At least 50 per cent of sexually active men and women acquire genital HPV infection at some point in their lives and may develop warts. The disease can be transmitted through unprotected sex or direct contact with genital warts (HPA 2007f).
- *Human immunodeficiency virus:* the risk of sexual transmission of HIV is difficult to quantify due to confounding variables such as viral load, coexisting STIs, and the presence of ulcers or menstrual blood (Nandwani 2006). An uninfected individual is most at risk of acquiring HIV from receptive anal or vaginal sex (Nandwani 2006). The risk of acquiring HIV from one act of unprotected receptive vaginal intercourse with an infected male partner is approximately one in a thousand (Nandwani 2006).

Why do people practise unsafe sex?

In addition to the inconsistent general knowledge surrounding STIs and the risky sexual practices associated with substance misuse, there are a number of other reasons why STI rates are increasing. For example, a 2006/07 NSOS survey of adults in the UK revealed that of all the people who had had two or more sexual partners in the past twelve months, less than half had used a condom consistently. About 10 per cent of adults were having concurrent sexual relationship between 1999 and 2001 (ONS

2006b). Women aged 16–19 were least likely to be using contraception despite almost two-thirds of teenagers having had intercourse by age 13 (CDC 2007b). This is perhaps due to the lack of recent public health campaigns. However, people in this age group who were using contraception were more likely to use condoms than any other age group. Regarding marital status, only 10 per cent of divorced women used condoms compared to 50 per cent of single women. This is an area for concern as individuals over a certain age may have been in monogamous relationships with the arrival of HIV/AIDS and may have missed the safe sex message. These people now may be dating and engaging in sexual relationships. It is estimated that the majority of HIV carriers will be over age 50 by 2015 and currently about 15 per cent of new infections occur in this age group (CDC 2006e). In addition, postmenopausal women may be at an elevated risk of being infected with blood-borne diseases like HIV or Chlamydia because their thinner vaginal lining can more easily tear during penetrative sex (Kotz 2007).

Ignorance may be another reason for the spread of STIs and HIV. It has been found that the majority of individuals who know that they have genital herpes either abstain from vaginal sex or always use condoms when they have symptoms. However only one-fifth do so when they are free of symptoms, yet asymptomatic shedding and thus transmission can occur (Rana et al. 2006). Regarding HIV it is estimated that one-quarter of people living with the disease do not know that they have it and are therefore at risk of transmitting the virus to others (CDC 2006e). Anecdotal evidence suggests that adolescents engage in oral sex as a means of reducing STI and HIV risk (Barrett 2004). However, the major viral and bacterial STIs can be transmitted via oral sex, including human papillomavirus, herpes simplex virus, hepatitis B, gonorrhoea, syphilis, Chlamydia and chancroid (CDC 2006a; Chambers 2007). In addition, whereas herpes simplex virus type 2 has traditionally infected the genital region, herpes simplex virus type 1, most commonly found in the region of the mouth, is now appearing in the genital region, with oral sex identified as the main culprit (Cherpes et al. 2005). Barrier methods, such as the male condom and dental dams, have been endorsed as protection during oral sex (Palo Alto Medical Foundation 2005). In terms of incidence and frequency, it appears that oral sex among university students is rising (Grunseit et al. 2005). Similarly sexual encounters between women in Britain have also risen since the 1990s (National Survey of Sexual Attitudes and Lifestyles (Natsal) 2000), indicating elevated opportunities for oral transmission of STIs despite the fact that sex between women has traditionally been thought to be low risk (Mercer et al. 2007). Data from Natsal (2000) showed that women who have sex with women and men were significantly more likely to report adverse sexual behaviours and health outcomes than women who exclusively have sex with either men, or women (Mercer et al. 2007). Although there may be health risks of oral sex, over 20 per cent of young adults were unaware of the health risks, and there was even greater confusion surrounding methods of protection (Chambers 2007) indicating a need for greater information regarding this practice.

Another reason for the cited increase in STIs may be because many MSM are practising safe sex less consistently (Jefferson et al. 2005; Schwarcz et al. 2007). A sense of security afforded by antiretroviral drugs, combined with increasing drug use, increases the likelihood of unprotected sex in HIV negative men occurring fourfold (CDC 2007a). Similarly it has been found that HIV-positive MSM report unprotected sex with multiple serodiscordant partners (Hirshfield et al. 2004). This indicates a continued risk of spreading HIV and other sexually transmitted diseases.

A group at high risk for acquiring and spreading HIV are bisexually active men. Bisexual activity may be considered a bridge for the transmission of HIV from homosexual to heterosexual populations. Bisexual men have been shown to engage in high rates of unprotected anal intercourse with men and women, as well as unprotected vaginal intercourse (Agronick et al. 2004; Jeffries and Dodge 2007). As HIV prevention methods have tended to focus on gay men, bisexually active men may be a relatively hidden population. Bisexual men have been found to report higher rates of intravenous drug use (Dodge and Sandfort 2007; Jeffries and Dodge 2007) compared to heterosexual males – an activity associated with the spread of HIV (UNAIDS 2006). Furthermore, bisexual men may live in cultures that view homosexual practices in a negative light so identify as heterosexual and eschew gay and bisexual identities (Agronick et al. 2004; Millett et al. 2005). Consequently, these men may view their same-sex behaviours negatively, resulting in elevated levels of internalised homophobia and possible increases in substance use and the associated sexual risk behaviours associated with this (Parsons et al. 2004). However, the evidence is inconclusive and bisexual men have been found to use condoms more consistently than heterosexual men when considering their last female encounter (Jeffries and Dodge 2007).

Lack of any intention to use condoms can also contribute to the rise in STIs. In a study of African American males, over half of the men planning to have sex in the forthcoming month had no intentions of using condoms during these interactions (Kennedy et al. 2007a), however African American youth condom intentions and use were higher than white males (Davis et al. 2007). Despite the level, or lack, of intention to use condoms, use was inconsistent in both groups (Davis et al. 2007; Kennedy et al. 2007b).

Lifestyle behaviours and sexual health

Epidemiological research suggests that all of the leading causes of mortality in Western societies are behavioural; that is, that many deaths are preventable if behaviours are changed (Marks et al. 2005). Sexual behaviour is no exception and there are various factors that can influence the decision to have safer sex or not.

The pharmacological effects of alcohol and various other non-prescription substances tend to have the effect of reducing inhibitions, boosting confidence, intensifying emotions and increasing the importance of immediate cues such as sexual desire, at the expense of more future-oriented considerations such as STIs. As a result, users have been shown to engage in more risky sexual behaviours (Colfax et al. 2004; Parsons et al. 2004; Ramisetty-Mikler et al. 2004; Rusch et al. 2004; McElrath 2005). Additionally, certain drugs such as amyl nitrites, MDMA and crystal methamphetamine may be used specifically to enhance sexual experiences (Hirshfield et al. 2004; Jefferson et al. 2005; McElrath 2005).

Methylenedioxymethamphetamine (MDMA) or Ecstasy produces both stimulant and psychedelic effects (Halley et al. 2007). Research indicates that among MDMA users there are two distinct groups – those who find it increases sexual desire, and those who say it produces feelings of sensuality but not sexuality (Levy et al. 2005; McElrath 2005). However, because many MDMA users also partake in alcohol, it is difficult to disentangle the effects of one over the other and there is conflicting evidence concerning whether alcohol used in conjunction with MDMA increases the likelihood of risky sex. Sexual risk behaviour fits within a cohort of MDMA users in that not using a condom denotes trust of each other, consistent with the 'loved up' trusting environment in which MDMA is often consumed (McElrath 2005).

Alcohol use is associated with multiple risks for disease transmission among both men and women (Weiser et al. 2006). Among heterosexual males the level of alcohol consumption by them and their female partners is related to higher rates of unprotected sex (Kalichman et al. 2007). However, it was found that among females, it was their partners drinking before sex that was related to higher frequencies of unprotected intercourse. This raises other concerns about the ability of females to enforce condom use with an intoxicated partner.

There has been a huge rise in the amount young people are drinking recently, and the amount consumed in a single-session is also increasing (Alcohol Concern 2007). Alcohol use and sexual activity often co-occur and more than one-quarter of sexually active teens used alcohol or drugs during their last sexual experience (CDC 2006b). There is evidence to suggest that adolescent alcohol use is associated with a variety of sexual risk-taking behaviours through impaired judgement (Ramisetty-Mikler et al. 2004) leading to subsequent regretted experiences (Coleman and Cater 2005). Being inebriated, compared to being sober, is associated with significantly less likelihood of using a condom at first intercourse (Dye and Upchurch 2006). However, in the same study it was found that girls who reported some alcohol use had higher probabilities of condom use than those who reported no alcohol use. This suggests that the pseudo confidence afforded by slight alcohol intoxication may have enabled the girls to feel empowered enough to insist on condom use from their partner. In contrast the lowest levels of condom use in boys was by those who had consumed some alcohol, rising with inebriation and again with being sober, however these findings were not significant (Dye and Upchurch 2006).

Research and epidemiological studies have reported noticeable increases in unprotected sex among gay and bisexual men (Wolitski et al. 2004). This may in part be due to the relationship between alcohol, substance use, and sexual risk behaviours (Parsons et al. 2004). HIV-positive MSM reported using alcohol to ensure easier interaction with others, both socially and sexually. A qualitative study revealed that MSM use alcohol within three sexual scripts: routine, spontaneous and taboo (Parsons et al. 2004). Routine users of alcohol did so with a clear intention of diminishing sexual inhibitions when purposefully seeking out sex. Spontaneous users ascribed their activities and partner selection as a result of the alcohol. Finally, in the taboo script alcohol enabled some MSM to overcome negative emotions such as guilt and fear surrounding some sexual behaviour (Parsons et al. 2004). The use of alcohol was associated with increased desire and assertiveness and therefore increased the likelihood of atypical sexual behaviour and unsafe sex, particularly unprotected anal intercourse (UAI) (Colfax et al. 2004; Hirshfield et al. 2004; Vanable et al. 2004; Parsons et al. 2004).

Further studies have found that using certain drugs increases the risk of engaging in UAI (Colfax et al. 2004; Halkitis et al. 2005) and that the risk of reporting UAI increases with the number of drugs used (Hirshfield et al. 2004). HIV-positive MSM have been found to partake in UAI more frequently than HIV-negative MSM during methamphetamine episodes (Halkitis et al. 2005) or when using amyl nitrites (Schwarcz et al. 2007). However, directional causation is not clear.

In order to design safe sex interventions, researchers and practitioners need to understand the contextual issues of using alcohol and other substances in venues such as at house parties or bathhouses (Parsons et al. 2004; Bimbi et al. 2006).

Interventions to promote safe sex

To combat the spread of sexually transmitted diseases (STDs) the UK government's message is to use a condom. Research evidence has supported the contention that consistent condom use is associated with reduced risk of STDs (e.g. Gallo et al. 2007) and use of condoms during each risky sexual encounter is the only efficient way to prevent the spread of most STDs (Carey et al. 1992). In one US study some 78 per cent of respondents declared they did not always use a condom during sexual intercourse (Choi and Catania 1996). In a European study, among the respondents having had more than one partner in the year preceding the study, only 52 per cent of the men and 41 per cent of the women declared having used a condom at least once (Guiguet et al. 1994). However, not only does the condom have to be used, but also it has to be used effectively (i.e. properly). Hatherall et al. (2007) report that a sizeable minority (between 12 and 40 per cent) applied a condom imperfectly. Given that imperfect use of condoms fails to maximise their effectiveness as a method of STI prevention, it is obviously important to address this through appropriate public health messages. Health promotion is an integral part of preventing the spread of STI infections and giving people sex-positive messages that build self-respect and self-knowledge.

Adolescents and young adults have a high risk of acquiring STIs as compared to those above the age of 25. Young people's sexual encounters are often unplanned, sporadic and sometimes the result of social pressure, coercion or alcohol (Lear 1995). Individuals tend to be unaware of the health risks of sexual intercourse (Buysse 1996). Since the late 1970s the number of sexual partners has increased, and the age of first intercourse decreased. Many of these adolescents do not use condoms consistently: in one study 22 per cent regarded acquiring a STI as an acceptable risk (Bakker and Vanwesenbeeck 2002).

Psychological research on the determinants of unsafe sexual practice has usually employed the social cognition models outlined in Chapter 2, including theories such as the health belief model (Rosenstock 1990), protection motivation theory (Rogers 1975), theory of reasoned action (Fishbein and Ajzen 1975) and the theory of planned behaviour (Ajzen 1985). Within this type of conceptualisation it is assumed that individuals are motivated to use a condom if the benefits of doing so outweigh the costs, and that they are able to perform the behaviour. Subsequently, the strength of the motivation or intention to use condoms is considered to be the most proximal determinant of having protected sex. Several studies have attested to the value of such approaches (e.g. Sheeran et al. 1999; Buhi and Goodson 2007).

Albarracin et al. (2001) suggest that intention is a significant determinant of condom use, the weighted average correlation between the two variables estimated as being in the range 0.45 to 0.58. However, research indicates that only approximately 19 per cent of the variance in condom use is explained by intentions (Sheeran and Orbell 1998). Overall, several studies have suggested that these models have limited explanatory power (e.g. Bennett and Bozionelos 2000; Albarracin et al. 2001; Gredig et al. 2006) and yield an insufficient explanation of the variance in condom use. Of course, this is not unexpected as Ajzen (1991:180) appears to recognise this as an issue with the TPB:

> The theory of planned behaviour is, in principle, open to the inclusion of additional predictors if it can be shown that they capture a significant proportion of the variance in intention or behaviour after the theory's current variables have been taken into account.

Thus, there is a substantial gap between the intention to have safe sex and the actual use of condoms (e.g. De Visser and Smith 2004) and the need to include additional variables in the appropriate models.

Of course different individual studies have identified additional variables that can contribute to the model. For example, self-efficacy, moral norm, perceived behavioural control, past behaviour, attitude, habits and so on (e.g. Godin et al. 2005). Indeed, self-efficacy drawn from the theory of Bandura (1977) probably plays a significant part in determining intention (as acknowledged implicitly by Ajzen 1991). Some studies have been reported to have found a significant relationship between self-efficacy and intention after perceived behavioural control is taken into account (e.g. Sniehotta et al. 2005). Similarly, Godin et al. (2005) and Buunk et al. (1998) support the value of self-efficacy in predicting condom use.

A review of potential risk factors identified eleven reports examining the empirical relationships between self-efficacy and sexual behaviour (Buhi and Goodson 2007). The majority of these studies indicated a protective effect of self-efficacy. For example, greater self-efficacy resulted in the ability to resist peer pressure to have sex (Dilorio et al. 2001), delay initiation of sexual intercourse (Santelli et al. 2004), avoid sexual activity or risky sexual behaviour (Robinson et al. 1998, 1999; Faryna and Morales 2000) and to remain abstinent (Collazo 2004). In contrast, however, there were five studies that reported no relationship between self-efficacy and sexual behaviour (e.g. Carvajal et al. 1999; Bachanas et al. 2002; Sionéan et al. 2002; Dilorio et al. 2001; Villarruel et al. 2004).

Another psychological variable implicated in the Godin et al. (2005) study was moral norm, which had been predicted previously by several researchers (e.g. Parker et al. 1995; Godin and Kok 1996; Godin et al. 1996, 1997) to predict sexual behaviour. This variable represents a measure of personal feelings of moral obligation or responsibility for adopting a given behaviour. This is perceived as a growing variable of importance in the health related domain and has implications for the development of appropriate interventions and media campaigns.

Other reasons why unprotected sex may occur is that there may be other goals besides health. For example, sharing intimacy, experiencing belongingness and increasing one's own self-esteem are some of the goals which may override thoughts of health in an immediate situation (e.g. Logan et al. 2003; Gebbhardt et al. 2006). These psychological functions served by sexual behaviour may impact on safe sex behaviour. For example, Browning et al. (2000) found within a sample of students, that pursuit of pleasure within a sexual relationship was negatively related to condom use.

Buhi and Goodson (2007) reviewed the predictors of risky sexual behaviour in adolescents and classified these factors under common themes (see Table 7.4).

Table 7.4 Summary of predictors of sexual behaviour

Theme	*Element*
Intention to have sex	• Initiation of sexual behaviour (+)
Environmental constraints	• Greater parental involvement (+/0) • High quality of relationship with parents (+/0) • Fewer rules/boundaries (–/0) • Increased parental support (+/0/–) • Greater parental monitoring/supervision (+/0) • Increased peer support (0) • Increased time home alone (without a parent) (–)
Norms	• Perceptions of peer sex behaviours (believing most peers have had sex) (–/0) • Perception of peer disapproval of sex or negative attitudes towards sex (+/0) • Perceived parental disapproval of engaging sexual intercourse (+) • Self-efficacy (+/0) • Pro abstinence self-standards (+) • Negative emotions regarding sex/positive emotions towards sexual abstinence (+/0) • Positive attitudes toward abstinence/fewer sexually permissive attitudes (+/0)

Note: (–) indicates this element is a risk factor, (+) indicates a protective factor, (0) indicates a non-statistically significant finding

A different approach was adopted by Marston and King (2006), who reported on a systematic review of qualitative studies exploring young peoples' sexual behaviour and revealed seven themes. First, young people assess the risk by deciding whether the partner is 'clean' or 'unclean' on the basis of how well they know their partner, their partner's appearance or other such 'indicators'. Second, sexual partners have an important influence in general: individuals might see sex as a way of strengthening a relationship while conversely, fear of physical violence can split up a relationship. The third theme identified was that condoms could be stigmatising and associated with lack of trust: they were perceived as undesirable and suggesting that their partner might be 'unclean' and demonstrating a lack of trust (e.g. Lear 1996; Hiller et al. 1999). Fourth, gender stereotypes were seen as important – men are expected to be highly heterosexually active, and women chaste (e.g. Holland et al. 1991). Fifth, the social rewards (i.e. penalties and rewards) influence behaviour. Complying with gender expectations can raise social status: for men by having many partners (e.g. Thianthai 2004) and for women by chastity to securing a stable relationship (e.g. de la Cuesta 2001). The sixth theme was that reputation and social displays of sexual activity or inactivity are important. Finally, these social expectations hamper communication.

Interestingly, Marston and King (2006: 368) suggested that 'sexual behaviour [is] strongly shaped by social forces, but those forces are surprisingly similar in different settings'.

A persuasive argument can be made for the inclusion of those additional variables in appropriate models, but on the other hand it might be suggested that the individualistic approach of the TPB demands a predictor concerning social and situational dimensions, without being holistic. Bengel (1993) argues that it is questionable to use a combination of socio-cognitive and macro-sociological variables. Socio-cognitive concepts form an integral part of TPB since they deal with subjective perceptions of social reality. Gredig et al. (2006) argue that a possible solution could be the concept of Bourdieu's habitus, which describes how incorporated social structure, generated in an individual's socialisation process, guides a person's action. In short, individuals sharing similar social conditions develop a system of dispositions that generate similar modes of practice (Bourdieu 1974, 1997).

Broader influences on safe sex

Cultures that are tolerant of early intercourse may be a breeding ground for sexual risk, as it is well documented that the earlier first sex occurs the less likely it is that contraception will be used (Dye and Upchurch 2006). Furthermore early sexual activity is associated with alcohol and drug use, intimate partner violence, pregnancy and inconsistent condom use, as well as multiple sex partners (Hahm et al. 2006). It is possible that the two decisions (young age of first sex and non-use of condom) are related and may be that younger teens are less able to negotiate condom use or that younger age at first sex is a marker for other underlying risk-taking propensities. Developmentally, adolescence is characterised by changes in biological, cognitive and social functioning. It is also the period during which various health behaviours are experimented with. It has been found that girls who fight, smoke cigarettes and binge drink were more likely to also have multiple sexual partners (Howard and Qi Wang 2004). Shafil et al. (2007) found that adolescents who use condoms at their sexual debut are more likely to engage in subsequent safe sex and experience fewer STIs than adolescents who do not use condoms at their sexual debut. Adolescents who have sex with casual partners tend to have riskier attitudes toward condom use than those who have only main partners and this tends to be associated with alcohol and marijuana use (Lescano et al. 2006).

Acculturation may also impact on sexual behaviour. Asian adolescents, particularly women, often live in a bicultural world where they experience contradictions between their heritage and culture and it has been found that the influence of Western cultural values on young Asian women's sexuality is greater than their influence on young Asian men (Hahm et al. 2006). From a sociocultural perspective this may be because Asian cultures convey different expectations about independence and sexual activity for young men and women. Acculturated Asian women may perceive sex as an assertion of independence and gender equality and they may place less importance on the cultural values of their heritage (Hahm et al. 2006).

Within different cultures, barriers exist to prevent help-seeking behaviour regarding sexual health (Cottew and Oyefeso 2005). For example, in some countries condoms are available to young people in schools; in others, for example in parts of Indonesia, possession is a criminal offence (Simon and Paxton 2004). AIDS prevention research has demonstrated that culturally sensitive prevention programmes have been able to induce changes in sexual behaviour and condom use (Levinson et al. 2004). Programmes were developed through the application of theories of behaviour change to the specific behavioural domain of condom use (e.g., social learning theory, the health belief model, and self-efficacy theory). The programmes were tailored to address cultural beliefs and practices and to help the target groups develop a set of social skills relevant for their requirements. HIV prevention programmes and condom use interventions that have been successful in one country may not be so effective in another. Levinson et al. (2004) used the Condom Self-Efficacy Scale with Brazilian teenagers to investigate the interpersonal interactions, meta-cognitions and behaviours that influence their sexual negotiations and behaviours, within the framework of self-efficacy theory. Results revealed inconsistent and illogical rationales surrounding when the participants perceived condom use to be necessary and when use actually occurred. The Brazilian boys found the idea of girls taking an active role in condom use distasteful; girls were expected to be gatekeepers regarding sex and they admitted pressurising girls into sex as this was expected of them as a man. There was a great deal of confusion about masturbation, which was considered not a socially acceptable practice. Among the Brazilian girls a clear sense of powerlessness arose in many facets of communication about using and acquiring condoms. Despite knowing the risks of unprotected sex both sexes continued to engage in risky sexual behaviours. The reasons for this are convoluted, but may include cultural definitions of gender roles and expectations (Levinson et al. 2004). The powerlessness of the girls to enforce condom use in this study is not a unique situation and gender differences in relational power (Millett et al. 2005) may result in women engaging in unprotected sex. In one qualitative study HIV-positive women with a single primary partner of a serodiscordant status engaged in unprotected sex at the continued insistence of their more dominant male partner, despite fears of being responsible for transmitting the disease and causing their partners' illness (Stevens and Galvao 2007).

Additional factors that may predict condom use include past experience and behaviours. Patel et al. (2006) found that adolescents made decisions about safe sex that were congruent with their beliefs and past behaviour and experiences. Individuals at low risk for unprotected sex focused on cues in sexual scenarios relating to "risks of unprotected sex" and were found to have well-established and stable belief structures. Individuals at high risk of having unprotected sex were more inconsistent regarding their sexual behaviour and their decisions were dependent on context, and emotions during sexual encounters. Mental health problems may also play an important role in the development and maintenance of sexual risk behaviour. Significantly higher rates of risky sexual behaviour, STIs and HIV have been found in psychiatric populations (Donenberg et al. 2006). Depressive symptoms (Donenberg and Pao 2005; A. Brown et al. 2006) and unemployment (A. Brown et al. 2006) are associated with unprotected sex and it may be that they act as a barrier to individuals taking responsibility for their health and behavioural change.

It is important to understand how and why young people make decisions about health behaviours. Van Empelen and Kok (2006) examined the differences in planning, preparation and willingness to engage in condom use in young people. It was found that in steady sexual relationships, condom use may be more of a planned approach and therefore preparatory behaviours seem to be important mediators of the intention–behaviour relationship. Furthermore the study found that when condom use has become habitual, future behaviour can be explained directly by habitual patterns. Risk willingness is likely to play a less prominent role in a steady relationship because of the increased opportunities for intercourse. When considering casual sex, condom use may depend on the availability of condoms, intention strength and opportunities. Behavioural willingness also was found to play a role in the context of casual sex and condom use (van Empelen and Kok 2006).

Possibly the most powerful influences on sexuality are the social norms that regulate its expression. Morals, taboos, laws and religious beliefs of countries and societies worldwide restrict and determine the sexual behaviour of their inhabitants. Since the late 1990s, the international policy arena has increasingly focused its attention on sexual rights. As a result, new standards are being devised for the creation and maintenance of sexually healthy societies; encompassing values of dignity, respect and choice (Miller and Vance 2004).

Interventions

With the diversity of sexual behaviour, a range of strategies are needed to protect sexual health. In view of the importance of the broader determinants on sexual behaviour, approaches focusing exclusively on attempting to alter individual behaviour change are unlikely to produce significant improvements in sexual-health status. They are especially inappropriate to poor countries, where sex is more likely to be tied to survival (Barnett and Parkhurst 2005) and where individual agency is restricted. In wealthier countries, personal choice is greater than in poorer countries, yet power inequalities persist (Millett et al. 2005; Stevens and Galvao 2007). Numerous calls have been made for public health interventions to pay greater attention to the social context within which sexual interaction occurs (Barnett and Parkhurst 2005; A.B. Roberts et al. 2005). Interventions encouraging adoption of risk reduction practices remain a cornerstone of sexual-health promotion, but the evidence shows that they need to go beyond mere provision of information to be effective (NSOS 2007). Young people are most commonly targeted in schools and the evidence is that curriculum-based sex education does not increase risky sexual behaviour as many fear (Kirby et al. 2006). Reviews have shown that school-based sex education leads to improved awareness of risk and knowledge of protection strategies, and increases intention to adopt safer sex behaviours. It has also been found to delay sexual debut (Kirby et al. 2006).

Strategies to achieve behaviour change using mass-media communication have proved effective in reducing high-risk behaviour (Bertrand et al. 2006). Furthermore, approaches that target individuals based on their lifestyles and values are superior to those targeting based on demographic characteristics alone (Chapman 2004; Grier and Bryant 2005). Tailoring interventions to individual requirements and circumstances is obviously essential to respect diversity and preserve individual choice. Issues which appear to have rarely been discussed, such as mutual masturbation in the place of penetrative sex, or advice on the best protection when engaging in oral sex (Chambers 2007) need to be tackled in the fight for sexual health.

Within the UK, the Department of Health suggested that there were a number of actions that needed to be put in place, the first of which was to develop a national campaign aimed at younger men and women to ensure that they understand the real risk of unprotected sex and persuade them of the benefits of using condoms to avoid the risk of STIs or unplanned pregnancies (see, for example, www.condomessentialwear.co.uk). Second, there was a longer-term strategy to ensure that children and young people were on the right path towards improving their sexual health by reducing teenage pregnancy, alcohol and illicit drug consumption. This was followed by developments of new resources for the health service (e.g. FIT magazine, confidential email service, websites such as www.RUthinking.co.uk or www.teenagehealthfreak.org and the development of interactive learning material for specific groups).

The interventions aimed at risky sexual behaviour have concentrated on promoting condom use. These interventions have been theoretically inspired, as well as atheoretical. Indeed, many of the early interventions were found not to be effective and this may have been a consequence of their atheoretical nature (Fisher and Fisher 1992; Oakley et al. 1995). Fisher and Fisher (1992) concluded that the lack of success of such interventions was primarily due to their atheoretical nature. This view is supported by published reviews (e.g. Kirby et al. 1980). This is unfortunate given that 'Our review indicates that the theories of reasoned action and planned behaviour are highly successful predictors of condom use' Albarracin et al. 2001: 14). Although some would not necessarily agree with this statement (as demonstrated earlier in this chapter), another key message is to use the appropriate elements of the TRA in any developed intervention.

Such interventional programmes aimed at promoting condom use have used a range of strategies and media, including among others, lectures, leaflets, interactive games and websites, films, role-modelling and posters. Public health campaigns have employed poster campaigns, TV, newspaper and cinema advertising, interactive computer and web programmes and health promotion leaflets (see websites above; Fisher et al. 1994; Kirby et al. 1997; Dunn et al. 1998; Jemmott et al. 1998, 1999; Sanderson 2000).

The theoretically derived interventions have concentrated on social cognition models approach to safer sexual behaviour. These models have suggested that a knowledge about STDs and beliefs about infection, risk and symptom severity are weaker correlates of condom use than action-specific cognitions, such as attitudes towards condom use, perceived self-efficacy in relation to condom use, the social acceptability of condom use and condom use intentions (e.g. DiClemente 1991; Jemmott and Jemmott 1991; Fishbein et al. 1995; Krahe and Reiss 1995; Bengel et al. 1996). A meta-analysis of studies applying the theories of reasoned action (Fishbein and Ajzen 1975) and planned behaviour (Ajzen 1991, 2001) to condom use confirmed the utility of these theories as models of the cognitive antecedents of condom use (Albarracin et al. 2001). Sheeran et al. (1999) reported a comprehensive meta-analysis of 121 empirical research studies into cognitive and behavioural correlates of heterosexual condom use. The study identified key measures associated with modest correlations with condom use. These were: (1) attitudes towards condoms; (2) descriptive norms in relation to condom use (i.e. perceptions that others approve of and use condoms); (3) pregnancy motivation (e.g. the belief that condoms should be used for contraceptive purposes as well as STI protection); (4) intentions to use condoms; (5) carrying condoms; (6) ensuring condoms were available; and (7) communication with sexual partners about condoms. Sheeran et al. (1999: 126) conclude that these results 'provide empirical support for conceptualising condom use in terms of . . . an extended Theory of Reasoned Action' and suggest that these correlates specify potentially useful targets for safer sex promotion.

On the basis of this meta-analysis Abraham et al. (2002) investigated whether this had been taken into account when developing health education practice. They reported that leaflets focused mainly on the provision of information, highlighting risk, encouraging professional contact and confirming efficacy of condom use. Unfortunately few of these measures was strongly correlated with condom use (Sheeran et al. 1999) and as Abraham et al. (2002) state: 'the cognitions targeted most frequently by the majority of leaflets are not those found to be most strongly correlated with condom use'.

Only a few instances of interventions have been found in research studies that highlight abstaining from or delaying sexual intercourse (Kirby et al. 1997; Thomas 2000; Schaalma et al. 2004). This is surprising given there is a growth of such a movement within the United States (e.g. The Silver Ring Thing: www.silverringthing.com/) and smaller movements within the UK. It may be that health educators fear that their audience will be unwilling to contemplate delaying sexual intercourse.

Individual-based interventions also need to address social norms that work against individuals having safer sex. Any effects brought about by interventions will be transient if individuals do not return to practice new behaviours within supportive environments. There is evidence to indicate that information received through social networks is more likely to lead to behaviour change, than that portrayed by more impersonal agencies (McIntyre 2005). For example, interventions that utilise naturally occurring social networks have reduced risky behaviour in homosexual men in Russia (Amirkhanian et al. 2005), increased condom use in sex workers in India (Dandona et al. 2005) and have proved more effective in changing norms than more conventional approaches to portraying sexual health messages. The broader structural determinants of sexual behaviour, such as poverty and unemployment, are significantly much slower to change than individual behaviours (Halperin et al. 2004; Adimora and Schoenbach 2005; Lesch and Kruger 2005). Nevertheless success has been achieved in challenging social attitudes, such as those of young men towards fatherhood and contraception (Verma et al. 2005). Addressing structural determinants, particularly poverty, requires the involvement of social and health sectors.

Evidence has suggested that although condom use has increased significantly over the previous years (Anderson et al. 2003), the majority of adolescent mothers still do not use them and are therefore putting themselves at risk from both sexually transmitted diseases and the possibility of further pregnancy. A number of studies have indicated that there is a range of factors which influence condom use and these have indicated that the predictors derived from social cognitive models are important (Jemmott and Jemmott 2000). In consequence, it is important to develop safe sex interventions for women of this age and to use the variables from the social cognitive methods outlined previously.

Such interventions, for this age group, require good, accurate information, capture the audience's attention and promote changes in both attitudes and behaviour. Shrier et al. (2001) explored whether an individual intervention based on various psychological models, including the stages of change (Prochaska and DiClemente 1983) and implemented through motivational interviewing (Miller and Rollnick 2002) could improve condom use. The intervention began with a seven-minute video in which popular entertainers and sports figures discussed and dramatised condom names, buying condoms, and negotiating condom use and two female adolescents demonstrated condom use to their peers. Condom use was portrayed as normative behaviour.

In addition to this, a series of female health educators were employed and trained in various theories and were taught to use a standardised intervention manual that outlined key points to cover, activities to perform and the motivation strategies to employ. At the outset, participants were asked about how much they needed and wanted to change their sexual risk behaviour (on a so-called 'wheel of change'). The intervention ensured that the same information was provided to all participants but the educator tried to individualise the session based on the stage of change. On the basis of this intervention there was an improvement in condom use. The stages of change model, as used in this particular clinical example, was successful in implementing change in condom use.

The greatest challenge to sexual-health promotion in almost all countries comes from opposition from conservative forces to harm-reduction strategies. Policy-makers need to be able to show that the effect on sexual health status of providing services to unmarried young women, supplying condoms, decriminalising homosexual activity, and prosecuting people who commit sexual violence is likely to be beneficial rather than detrimental. Furthermore, to do otherwise will force stigmatised behaviours underground leaving the most vulnerable people unprotected. Sexuality is an essential part of human nature and its expression needs to be affirmed rather than denied if public health messages are to be heeded. Strategies used should enable people to make their own choices, rather than have them imposed on them.

Conclusion

Sexual behaviour is a natural behaviour that has, at its root, a fundamental physiological purpose. However, it serves a range of other cultural, emotional, psychological and social purposes which have to be considered when attempting to promote safe sexual behaviour. The promotion of a safe sex message is important given the rise in sexually transmitted diseases both nationally and worldwide. Psychological factors contribute to whether people engage in safe sex or not, and social cognitive models have proved modestly successful in predicting condom use. A number of models and variables have been identified that can be used to develop and implement appropriate interventions, but with as with other lifestyle behaviours discussed this has not always been the case.

Summary points

- Researchers generally define sexual behaviour as any behaviour that involves a sexual response of the body.
- Safe sex is hard to define but involves taking steps to reduce the chance of contracting or transmitting STIs. Most people associate this with condom use and/or monogamy.
- The UK has seen the largest rise of HIV cases in Western Europe since 2000 and cases of other STIs, such as Chlamydia and gonorrhoea, are also increasing.
- Evidence suggests that consistent and correct condom use is associated with reduced STI transmission. Despite this, many people in the UK are not consistently practising safe sex.
- The increase in STIs has been attributed to a lack of safe sex practices, lack of knowledge regarding STIs and their transmission, low rates of condom use in high-risk populations and lack of intentions to use condoms.
- Alcohol and illicit drug use are associated with risky sexual behaviours.
- Social cognition models have been shown to predict at least some of the variance in safe sex practices. Including additional variables, such as self-efficacy, can increase the predictive power of these models.
- Wider cultural and social factors have also been shown to impact upon sexual behaviour.
- Interventions to reduce unsafe sex include providing sex education in schools and mass media campaigns. Interventions have been shown to be more effective when they are targeted to a specific audience, theoretically derived and address wider social norms as well as individual behaviour.

8 Illicit drug misuse

> Drugs are a bet with your mind.
>
> Jim Morrison

At the end of this chapter you will:

- understand the problems associated with defining substance abuse
- understand the extent of illegal drug misuse in the UK and worldwide at present
- have explored the consequences of illegal drug misuse in the UK including health consequences for the user and wider implications for society
- appreciate the complexity in assessing what factors increase risk of drug taking and which factors are protective against illicit drug use
- have an awareness of current UK government policy to reduce illicit drug use and the guiding principal upon which such policy is based
- have identified various clinical approaches to the prevention and treatment of illicit drug use.

Definitions

There are many definitions of 'drug abuse'. The *Handbook on Drug and Alcohol Abuse* (Winger 1992) defines drug abuse as 'non-medical use of drugs, both drugs that have and those that do not have generally accepted medical value'. It should be emphasised that the current terminology is now 'substance abuse' rather than drug abuse, as this recognises that the abuse can be more than drugs and could include, for example, the misuse of alcohol or glue.

The World Health Organisation (2007a) provides a comprehensive definition and explanation of 'abuse'. In particular, they relate to the DSM-IIIR (*Diagnostic and Statistical Manual of Mental Disorders*, 3rd edition, revised: American Psychiatric Association (APA) 1987) criteria of a maladaptive pattern of use indicated by . . . continued use despite knowledge of having a persistent or recurrent social, occupational, psychological or physical problem that is caused or exacerbated by the use [or by] recurrent use in situations in which it is physically hazardous.

The more recent criteria for harmful use (ICD-10) and substance misuse (DSM-IV) are presented in Table 8.1. The two diagnostic systems differ substantially:

- DSM-IV (APA 1994) emphasises the negative social consequences of the substance use.
- ICD-10 (WHO 1992b) specifically excludes socially negative consequences and emphasises physical and mental consequences.

The result is that the ICD-10 definition of harmful use is a more socially stable syndrome that applies across different cultures (Finch and Welch 2006).

Table 8.1 ICD-10 (1992b) and DSM-IV (1994) criteria for harmful use and substance abuse

ICD-10: criteria for harmful use	*DSM-IV: criteria for substance abuse*
A pattern of psychoactive substance abuse that is causing damage to health, either physical or mental. The diagnosis requires that actual damage should have been caused to the mental or physical health of the user. Socially negative consequences, or the disapproval of others are not in themselves evidence of harmful use.	• Recurrent substance use resulting in a failure to fulfil major role obligations at work, school or home • Recurrent substance abuse in situations in which it is physically hazardous • Recurrent substance-related legal problems • Continued substance use despite having persistent or recurrent social or interpersonal problems caused or exacerbated by the effects of the substance

The term 'abuse' is sometimes used disapprovingly to refer to any use at all, particularly of illicit drugs, and hence to avoid the pejorative connotations and vague concepts the terms 'misuse', 'harmful use' or 'hazardous use' are employed. In other contexts, abuse has referred to non-medical or unsanctioned patterns of use, irrespective of consequences. Thus the definition published in 1969 by the WHO Expert Committee on Drug Dependence was 'persistent or sporadic excessive drug use inconsistent with or unrelated to acceptable medical practice'. Spooner (1999) makes a key distinction between drug use and drug abuse, suggesting that those who use drugs do not necessarily become continual users (although see review of gateway hypothesis p 223) and they do not necessarily become addicts. Hence, we should talk about 'use', which refers to any use including experimentation, 'misuse', which refers to problematic or very heavy use and 'addiction', which refers to a chronic relapsing condition characterised by compulsive drug seeking and abuse. 'Substance' refers to alcohol, illicit drugs and volatile substances.

Government recommendations

In the UK there are three classes of drugs (A, B, C) that are termed as controlled substances under the Misuse of Drugs Act 1971, with Class A being considered the most harmful (see Table 8.2). Illegal drug misuse is socially constructed: it is those drugs defined by the government to be illegal and the most harmful. For example, cannabis was until 2001 a Class B drug but has since been classified as Class C. Two other drugs – alcohol and tobacco – are not currently defined as illegal drugs in the UK, although of course they have been at different times and in different cultures.

Table 8.2 Penalties for possession and dealing

		Possession	*Dealing*
Class A	Ecstasy, LSD, heroin, cocaine, crack, magic mushrooms, amphetamines (if prepared for injection)	Up to seven years in prison or an unlimited fine or both	Up to life in prison or an unlimited fine or both
Class B	Amphetamines, Methylphenidate (Ritalin), Pholcodine	Up to five years in prison or an unlimited fine or both	Up to 14 years in prison or an unlimited fine or both
Class C	Cannabis, tranquillisers, some painkillers, Gamma hydroxybutyrate (GHB), ketamine	Up to two years in prison or an unlimited fine or both	Up to 14 years in prison or an unlimited fine or both

Most cultures have some form of law associated with the misuse of drugs. In the UK the Misuse of Drugs Act 1971 states that it is an offence to:

- possess a controlled substance unlawfully
- possess a controlled substance with intent to supply it
- supply or offer to supply a controlled drug (even where no charge is made for the drug)
- allow premises you occupy or manage to be used for the purpose of drug taking.

Drug trafficking attracts serious punishment, including life imprisonment for Class A offences. To enforce this law the police have special powers to stop, detain and search people under the 'reasonable suspicion' that they are in possession of a controlled drug.

Evidence of the problem

The World Health Organisation (2007a) highlights the global burden of psychoactive substance use in terms of health, social and economic consequences. The WHO estimated the extent of worldwide psychoactive substance use to be 2 billion alcohol users (for more on this see Chapter 5), 1.3 billion smokers (see Chapter 6) and 185 million drug users. As can be noted, the major substances used are alcohol and tobacco (see Chapters 5 and 6), with drug use (or substance, more correctly) being a distant third (Figure 8.1).

The World Health Organisation estimated that the global burden of disease related to tobacco, alcohol and illicit drugs contributed to a total of 12.4 per cent of all deaths worldwide in the year 2000. Looking at the percentage of total years of life lost due to these substances, it has been estimated that they account for 8.9 per cent (see Table 8.3).

The sex ratio for deaths attributable to psychoactive substance use varies from 80 per cent male for tobacco and illicit drug use and 90 per cent for alcohol. One of the differences between these three categories of

Table 8.3 Mortality and morbidity related to substance misuse worldwide

	Mortality (% of all deaths worldwide)	*DALYs (% of total years of life lost)*
Tobacco	8.8	4.1
Alcohol	3.2	4.0
Illicit drugs	0.4	0.8

(World Health Organisation 2007)

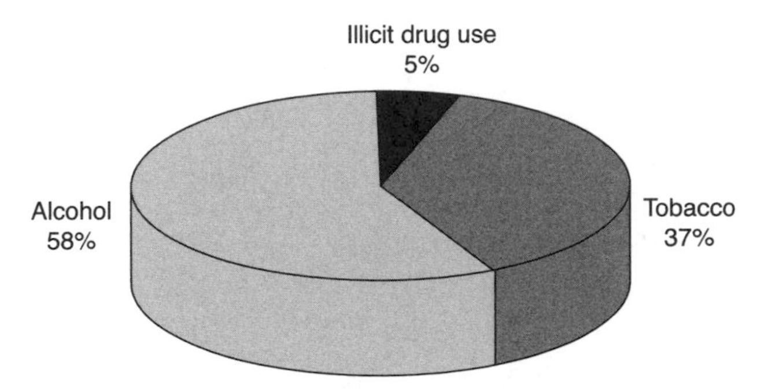

Figure 8.1 World extent of psychoactive substance use (World Health Organisation 2007a)

psychoactive substances is the fact that they inflict their disease burden on different age groups. Illicit drug use inflicts its mortality burden earliest in life, alcohol also mainly (65 per cent) before the age of 60, while 70 per cent of the tobacco deaths occur after the age of 60.

Drug use in the UK

Some 10 per cent of the UK population reports having taken illegal drugs in the preceding year (see Table 8.4). This rate is almost half to one-third the rate of tobacco use but the figures do vary according to age. People aged between 16 and 24 years are more likely than older people to have used drugs in the last year and in the last month: 28 per

Table 8.4 The proportion of 16–59 year olds reporting to having used drugs in the previous year (2006–07).

Drug	*Percentages*
Class A	
Any cocaine	2.6
Cocaine powder	2.6
Crack cocaine	0.2
Ecstasy	1.8
Hallucinogens	0.7
LSD	0.2
Magic mushrooms	0.6
Opiates	0.2
Heroin	0.1
Methadone	0.1
Class A/B	
Amphetamines	1.3
Class B/C	
Tranquillisers	0.4
Class C	
Anabolic steroids	0.1
Cannabis	8.2
Ketamine	0.3
Not classified	
Amyl nitrite	1.4
Glues	0.2
Total	
Class A	3.4
Any drug	10.0

(British Crime Survey 2007)

cent of 16–24 year olds had used at least one illicit drug in the year. The use of Class A drugs in the last year among 16–24 year olds has remained stable since 1995 and stands around 8 per cent. However, the number of youngsters taking drugs is relatively high with some 1.6 million having taken illicit drugs in the previous twelve months (see Table 8.5). Other figures indicate that over one-third of 16–59 year olds has 'ever' used an illegal drug, and currently there are estimated to be about 4 million users of illicit drugs in the UK (Condon and Smith 2003). The National Treatment Agency (2005) estimates that about 250,000 people in England and Wales will develop serious problems associated with their drug use every year.

Comparing individual countries within the UK reveals some differences. The figures for Wales, for example, show that 11 per cent of adults (aged 16–59) and almost one-third of young adults (16–24) in Wales reported using drugs in the last year. This figure is higher than other regions in the UK (see Figure 8.2). In the Scottish 2004 survey, it was estimated that 7.7 per cent of the adult population (aged 16–59 years) had used illicit drugs during the previous year, compared with 9.5 per cent in 2003. The most commonly reported illicit drug in Scotland used was cannabis, with 8 per cent of adults surveyed in 2003 and 6.3 per cent in 2004 reporting cannabis use within the last year.

Results from the Northern Ireland survey suggest that one-fifth (20 per cent) of the Northern Ireland adult population aged 15–64 have used illegal drugs. Overall lifetime prevalence rates for the use of any illegal

Table 8.5 Estimate of last year drug use in 16–24 year olds

Drug	*Number of users*
Cocaine	270,000
Crack	27,000
Ecstasy	312,000
LSD	49,000
Magic mushrooms	99,000
Heroin	12,000
Methadone	9,000
Amphetamines	216,000
Tranquillisers	47,000
Cannabis	1,497,000
Amyl nitrite	247,000
Glues	29,000
Class A	474,000
Any drug	1,629,000

(British Crime Survey 2007)

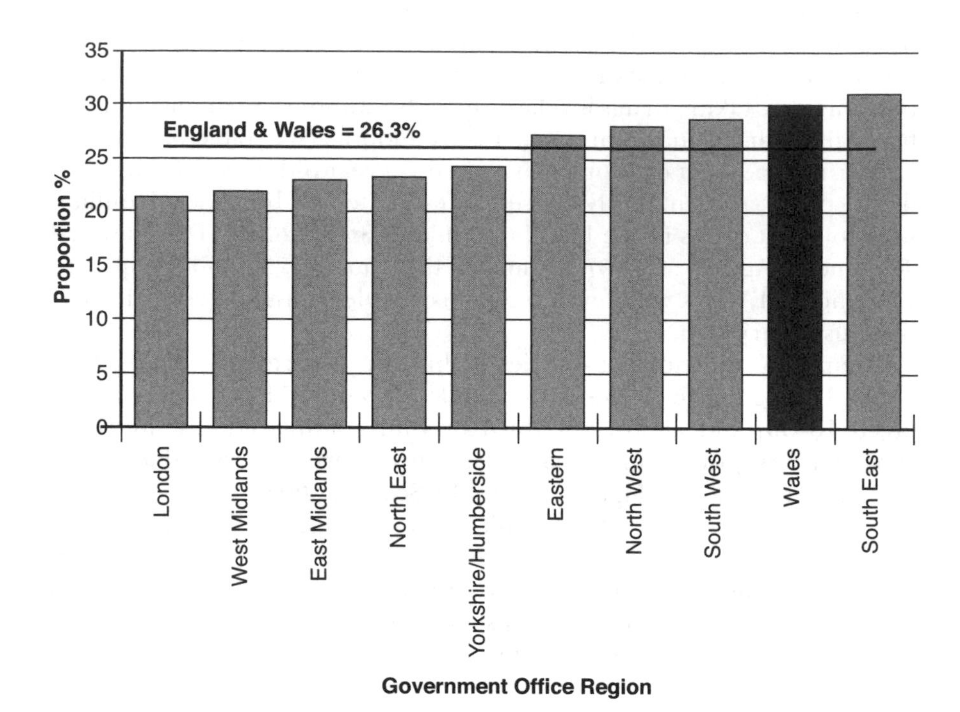

Figure 8.2 Proportion (%) of 16–24 year olds reporting having used any drug in the past year
(Home Office 2005)

drug were highest among younger age groups, with nearly one-third (31 per cent) of young adults aged 15–34 reporting use: there was little difference between those aged 15–24 (29 per cent) and those aged 25–34 (33 per cent) in this regard. For older age groups prevalence rates were lower: 18 per cent for those aged 35–44 falling to 4 per cent for those aged 55–64. Male respondents reported higher prevalence rates than females – almost twice as many men (27 per cent) than women (14 per cent) reported ever using an illegal drug (DHSSPNI 2007).

Consequences of illicit drug use

It goes without saying that those individuals that take illicit drugs face potential health risks – the drugs taken are not controlled or supervised by health care professionals and those that are sold 'on the streets' are of variable quality, strength and origin. As well as the immediate health risks, drugs can also lead to long-term addiction and health damage.

The Drug Harm Index (DHI) (Home Office 2006) has been developed by the Home Office to measure one of the aims of the Drugs Strategy:

'reduce the harm caused by illegal drugs including substantially increasing the number of drug misusing offenders entering treatment through the criminal justice system'. The DHI captures the harms generated by the problematic use of any illegal drug by combining robust national indicators into a single-figure, time series index. There are 19 harms included in the DHI that include drug-related crime, community perceptions of drug problems, drug nuisance, and the various health consequences that arise from drug abuse (e.g. HIV, overdoses, deaths). The DHI captures the economic and social costs associated with drug use. Any change in the DHI will be due to the level or volume of harms (e.g. the number of new HIV cases) and the change in their economic or social cost (e.g. change in cost per new HIV case). The value of the DHI fell from 104.8 to 87.9 between 2003 and 2004, a 16 per cent decrease (the latest figures available) thereby suggesting that the health impact of drug abuse is being minimised, although the individual health consequences of illicit drug use are still both severe and considerable.

Drug-related deaths

Drug-related deaths often attract a great deal of political and media attention and these are used to illustrate the harm that drugs can cause and to promote the drug abuse message (see, for example, the death of Rachel Whitear). With these individual case studies, statistics are often produced on drug-related deaths, and these along with anecdotes from individual cases, are often used to illustrate the harm that drugs can cause and to defend prohibitionist policies.

The Office for National Statistics (ONS) produces mortality statistics for drug-related deaths based upon information on death certificates (see Table 8.6). All deaths that mention drugs on the death certificate are counted, which includes deliberate poisonings (homicides and suicides). The ONS produces data for alcohol-related deaths, but the definition is different from that used for other drugs, as it includes only deaths regarded as being most directly due to alcohol consumption. This excludes homicides and suicides but does include deaths for chronic liver disease and cirrhosis, even when alcohol is not specifically mentioned on the death certificate.

Although these statistics can be used to provide one indication about how harmful drugs are, they are an overly simplistic indicator of harm. Most drug-related harm is non-fatal, and drug-related deaths are not proof that a certain drug is inherently harmful, since harm to an individual is determined by how the drug is used (dose, frequency, poly drug use, method of use, and so on).

In Wales between 2002 and 2004 there were on average 112 deaths resulting from drug related conditions. Overall for every woman who died from drug-related conditions, three men died. The number of deaths

Table 8.6 Number of UK deaths related to substance misuse (as recorded on death certificate) 2005

Drug	*Deaths*
Heroin and morphine	842
Methadone	220
Cocaine (including crack)	176
All amphetamines	103
(*of which MDMA/ecstasy*)	58
Cannabis	19
Gamma-hydroxybutyrate (GHB)	4
All benzodiazepines	190
Zopiclone/Zolpidem	48
Barbiturates	14
All antidepressants	401
Paracetamol (including compound formulations)	466
Codeine (non-compound formulation)	44
Dihydrocodeine (non-compound formulation)	106
Aspirin	19
Tramadol	53

peaks in 20–34 year olds (Childs 2007). In 2005, there were 336 drug-related deaths in Scotland, down from 356 in 2004 again with a similar sex ratio (Scotland Public Health Observatory 2007).

These deaths are, of course, relatively low and significantly less than those caused by either alcohol or smoking (see Chapters 5 and 6). Nonetheless, they are avoidable and significant to the individual families and friends concerned. Obviously, the health consequences of substance misuse are not restricted to death, but there may be some health impact that differs dependent on the drugs being used (see Table 8.7).

Hospital admissions

During 2005/06 there were 8,113 finished consultant episodes (FCEs: a period of admitted patient care under one consultant within one healthcare provider) in England with a primary diagnosis of a drug-related mental health and behavioural disorder. This number has remained relatively stable since 1996/97. Over 40 per cent of these episodes were for people aged between 25 and 34 years of age and males were twice as likely to be admitted to hospital with the diagnosis of drug-related mental health. In 2005/06, there were 5,015 admissions to acute general hospitals in Scotland with a diagnosis of drug misuse, and in most of these episodes the patients had been admitted as emergencies.

Table 8.7 Illicit drug use and health consequences

Drug	*Consequences*
Heroin and morphine	Short-term effects include a surge of euphoria followed by alternately wakeful and drowsy states and cloudy mental functioning. Associated with fatal overdose and (particularly in users who inject the drug) infectious diseases such as HIV/AIDS and hepatitis.
Cocaine (including crack)	A powerfully addictive drug, cocaine usually makes the user feel euphoric and energetic. Common health effects include heart attacks, respiratory failure, strokes and seizures. Large amounts can cause bizarre and violent behaviour. In rare cases, sudden death can occur on the first use of cocaine or unexpectedly thereafter.
Club drugs (the most common club drugs include, GHB, Rohypnol, ketamine, methamphetamine)	Chronic use of MDMA may lead to changes in brain function. GHB abuse can cause coma and seizures. High doses of ketamine can cause delirium, amnesia and other problems. Mixed with alcohol, Rohypnol can incapacitate users and cause amnesia.
Cannabis	Short-term effects include memory and learning problems, distorted perception, and difficulty thinking and solving problems.
LSD	Unpredictable psychological effects. With large enough doses, users experience delusions and visual hallucinations. Physical effects include increased body temperature, heart rate, and blood pressure, sleeplessness, and loss of appetite.
Ecstasy	Short-term effects include feelings of mental stimulation, emotional warmth, enhanced sensory perception and increased physical energy. Adverse health effects can include nausea, chills, sweating, teeth clenching, muscle cramping and blurred vision.
PCP/Phencyclidine	Many PCP users are brought to emergency rooms because of overdose or because of the drug's unpleasant psychological effects. In a hospital or detention setting, people high on PCP often become violent or suicidal.

Among clients younger than 18 years, the most frequently reported main problem drug was cannabis (67 per cent) while 14 per cent reported heroin as the main problem drug. For clients aged 18 years or over, the most frequently reported main problem drug was heroin (67 per cent) with 7 per cent reporting cannabis.

Financial costs

According to estimates from the NHS Information Centre (2007), the total economic and social cost of Class A drug use in 2003/04 was around £15.4 billion. This equates to £44,231 per year per problematic drug user. Drug-related crime accounts for 90 per cent of this cost (£13.9 billion), drug-related deaths 6 per cent (£924 million), health service use 3 per cent (£488 million) and social care 1 per cent (£69 million).

Why do people take illicit drugs?

There have been a large number of studies that have explored the risk factors associated with drug use. There is, not surprisingly, no 'definitive list' of risk factors that is agreed and supported by research evidence. There is, however, general agreement that there is no one single factor and that the origin of substance misuse is multifactorial. Various psychosocial factors have been identified as significant correlates of substance use and these can vary across the lifespan (see Table 8.8).

Table 8.8 Factors associated with illicit drug use

Risk factor	*Example*	*Example studies*
Personal factors	Gender	Young et al. (2002)
	Age	Young et al. (2002)
	Ethnicity	Olsson et al. (2003)
	Life events	Turner (2003)
	Self-esteem	Hoffman and Cerbone (2002)
	Hedonism	Ljubotina et al. (2004)
	Depression/anxiety	Hoffman and Cerbone (2002)
	Mental health factors	Hofla et al. (1999)
	Learning disabilities	Fischer and Barkley (2003)
	Genetic	Lynskey et al. (2002)
Personal factors: behavioural or attitudinal	Early onset of substance use	Von Sydow et al. (2002)
	Other substance use	Von Sydow et al. (2002)
	Perceptions of substance use	McCambridge and Strang (2004)
Interpersonal relationships	Young parents	Reinherz et al. (2000)
	Large families	Reinherz et al. (2000)
	Parental divorce	Lynskey et al. (2002)
	Low discipline	King and Cassin (2004)
	Family cohesion	Hoffman and Cerbone (2002)
	Parental monitoring	Case and Haines (2003)
	Family substance abuse and psychiatric conditions	Merikangas and Avenevoli (2000)
	Peer behaviour and use	Li et al. (2002)
Structural-environmental and economic	Socio-economic	Poulton et al. (2002)
	Education, school performance and school management	Hallfors et al. (2002)
	Drug availability	Von Sydow et al. (2002)

From Table 8.8 it is clear that there are a considerable number of putative factors associated with illicit drug taking, from the prenatal environment (including maternal behaviours) through to genetic factors and to wider social influences including school and socio-economic issues. These factors are those which are important and have been empirically derived through appropriate data analysis.

The role of psychological factors as potential risk factors has been widely studied. For example, Sareen et al. (2006) report that anxiety is related to lifetime heroin use and Fergusson et al. (2006a) report on the importance of social interaction with substance-using peers and conduct problems in adolescence in the development of illicit drug use. They also report the importance of appreciating other lifestyle behaviours such as cigarette smoking and alcohol consumption, indicating the importance of the interplay and clustering of lifestyle behaviours. Finally, they also report on psychological factors such as risk-taking and novelty-seeking behaviours. The continual use of the conjunction indicates the difficulty in identifying the role of risk factors: the numerous potential risk factors and the interplay and identification of further factors ensures that research is continually incomplete.

These two studies are two among many and hence there is a necessity to review the range of studies systematically and this realisation has led to the completion of many systematic reviews from both a European and a US perspective. For example, Lloyd (1998) outlined the complex nature of the evidence and the interplay between various factors and identified key high-risk groups such as the homeless, those looked after by local authorities, prostitutes, truants, those excluded from school, young offenders, children from families with substance abusing parents or siblings, and young people with conduct or depressive disorder. As highlighted earlier, a distinction between user, abuser and addict has to be made (Spooner 1999) as does the distinction between individual aetiologies. Spooner suggests that the aetiological factors for drug use may be more social, whereas those for abuse may be more likely to be psychological. Frischer et al. (2007) stress that the evidence suggests that alienation needs to be countered before positive behavioural changes can be initiated (Calabresa and Adams 1990), and that conventionality predicts health-related behaviour (Donovan et al. 1991). Hawkins et al. (1992) identify seventeen major factors that influence drug abuse risk, of which four are broader sociocultural factors (i.e. laws and norms favourable towards the behaviour, drug availability, extreme economic deprivation, and neighbourhood disorganisation).

The most recent British review was sponsored by the Home Office and produced by Frischer et al. (2007), who report a systematic review of the factors associated with illicit drug initiation. They report that of the studies reviewed, 27 per cent explored personal factors that are difficult to change (e.g. biological, psychological and demographic), 24 per cent explored other psychological factors (e.g. behavioural or attitudinal), 33 per cent interpersonal relationships and 16 per cent structural-environmental and economic factors. Some of these factors, along with key references, are presented in Table 8.9. What is apparent is that the factors are considerable, extensive and include both individual basic elements (e.g. genetics) and more diverse and socially constructed elements (e.g. socio-economic status).

What is not evident from the figure but should be emphasised is that these risk factors are not discrete entities and their complex interactions are difficult to analyse and comprehend. Indeed, literature indicates that these factors are additive (or multiplicative) and are the result of complex interactions. Comprehensive reviews have been written attempting to identify empirically derived risk factors for drug problems (Thomas 2007). Although the bulk of aetiological research has concentrated on testing the main effects of models of drug use, a smaller number have examined the interactions between these (Epstein et al. 2007). For example, Stacy et al. (1992) reported that a number of personality variables (e.g. liberalism, self-acceptance and extraversion) moderated the effect of social influences to use drugs on individual drug use measures of marijuana and cocaine use.

A further complication can be added to the already complex picture. Although the factors outlined in Table 8.9 are extensive, interactive in an additive or possibly multiplicative manner, they also are differentially important dependent on the timeline. As an example of this, Table 8.9 denotes some of the potential risk factors and their importance dependent on the age of the individual concerned.

Table 8.9 Risk factors for illicit drug use among young people

	Explanation	*Pre-natal*	*Birth*	*0–2 years*	*3–8 years*	*9–11 years*	*12–18 years*	*Adult*
Prenatal environment	Maternal smoking, maternal drug use	✓	✓					
Genetic	Genetic relationship	✓	✓	✓	✓	✓	✓	✓
Family	Parental discipline, family cohesion, parental substance use, parental monitoring, sibling drug use, early life trauma			✓	✓	✓		
School	Truancy, educational attainment, problems at school, school rules				✓	✓	✓	

Table 8.9 Risk factors for illicit drug use among young people (continued)

	Explanation	*Pre-natal*	*Birth*	*0–2 years*	*3–8 years*	*9–11 years*	*12–18 years*	*Adult*
Friends	Friends' drug use, friends' antisocial behaviour						✓	
Psychological traits	Low self-esteem, hedonism, ADHD, phobia, depression, anxiety, aggressive behaviour					✓	✓	
Psychological explanations	Get intoxicated, escape from negative moods						✓	
Socio-economic	Low household income, lack of neighbourhood amenities							✓
Early use of other drugs	Gateway hypothesis						✓	✓
Protective factors	In addition to the above there are also factors such as not considering drugs as part of lifestyle, not being exposed to drugs, adherence to conventional values, involvement in religion or sport, strategies to resisting peer pressure, positive future plans which protect from drug use							✓

However, these life-course transitions do not occur in isolation. Merikangas (2000, 2002) provides an explanation for drug abuse as the result of a complex dynamic interaction among characteristics of the host, environment and drug agent (see Figure 8.3). Despite the recognition that drug abuse is a multifaceted problem, there is a general focus on individual factors at the expense of an understanding of the interaction of broader and interrelated factors within a social context. The social environment can be conceptualised as a sphere that encompasses many factors interacting with the individual's psychological and personal characteristics. Orford (2001) suggests that

> the origins of excess are likely to lie as much in social norms and group pressure as in character and attitudes; that the uptake of new behaviour does not occur in a psychological vacuum but as part of a constellation of changing beliefs, preferences and habits of thought, feeling and action; and that appetitive behaviour cannot be divorced from the demands, both biological and social, of the stage of the life-cycle at which a person finds him or herself.
>
> (Orford 2001: 141)

Orford thus stresses the environment, the personal and the timeline.

This material presents two areas for further discussion. First, there is the need to consider the wider social context rather than simply concentrate on the individual personal characteristics. A blame culture can exist that suggests the health problems – including illicit drug use – is an individual choice but this cannot be divorced from the socio-political environment (Whitehead et al. 2002; Marks et al. 2005). There is, therefore, a need to ensure that illicit drug use research includes an examination of individual susceptibility interacting with social and biologic environments, both as main effects and as effect modifiers, and the accumulation of risk and how these determinants differentially impose risk across time and generations (Thomas 2006). Concepts of how social group, neighbourhood and community, culture (familial, group), or the environment influence drug abuse will remain unfocused if only individual-level risk factors

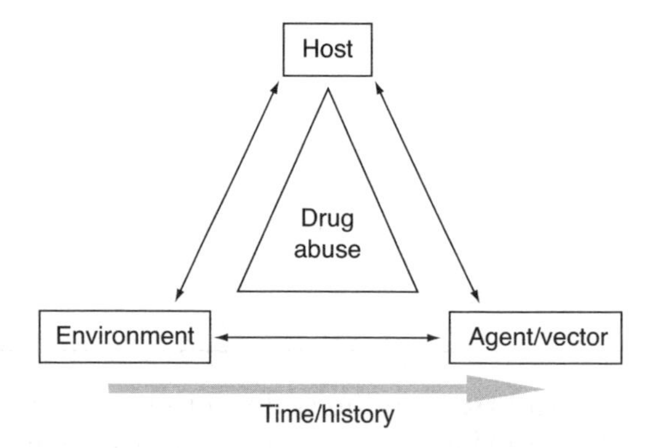

Figure 8.3 Epidemiological triangle
(Adapted from Merikangas 2000)

are addressed. The perceived drug norms of the social peer group and family play a tremendous role in adolescent drug use through social learning (Bandura 1977).

The psychological peer cluster theory views the peer group as critical in adolescent drug use (Oetting and Beauvais 1986, 1987). Adolescents become less reliant on parental influences in making drug use decisions and turn instead to friends and peers (Miller et al. 2000). Reviews of research on the development of drug use all report that drug use of peers and friends is a major risk factor for adolescent drug use (Belcher and Shinitzky 1998) and that perceived peer norms tend to be the strongest predictor of gateway drug use in middle school and high school (Jenkins 1996).

Second, the time course of these factors and their relative importance across the life span needs to be clearly articulated. For example, risk factors have been identified by the Home Office and have been used within the Offending Crime and Justice Survey (2003) data set. This data set has been analysed, using Logistic regression modelling, to determine which factors were associated with drug taking. The model for the 10–16 year olds group showed that, of the factors under consideration, eight were associated with taking drugs (Dillon et al. 2006):

- serious antisocial behaviour
- weak parental attitude toward bad behaviour
- being in trouble at school (including truanting and exclusion)
- having friends in trouble
- being unhelpful
- early smoking
- not getting school meals
- minor antisocial behaviour.

In contrast, a different set of factors was important in the 17–24 age group. The key findings for the 17–24 year olds showed that just six variables were associated with taking any drug:

- antisocial behaviour
- early smoking
- being in trouble at school
- being impulsive
- being insensitive
- belonging to few or no social groups.

The factors presented previously are those that are associated with increased risk of drug taking. In contrast, but of equal interest, are the factors that may protect against drug use. Indeed, research has now had a shift from the focus on risk factors to one that incorporates the skills individuals need to meet environmental challenges (Norman 1994). These two research themes complement one another. A pure risk factor approach has as its aim eliminating, reducing or mitigating risk factors. In contrast, a resiliency approach emphasises prevention by enhancing behavioural factors that protect against vulnerability. Taken together this approach suggests that both risk factors and vulnerability significantly contribute to a model of adolescent drug use and furthermore, that resilience moderates the effects of individual vulnerabilities and environmental hazards (Epstein et al. 2007).

A number of protective variables have been identified. Psychological protective factors in particular are important in shaping the design and implementation of drug protection methods. Specifically such programmes should highlight that some individuals despite being exposed to a social environment where drugs are present, as are other risk factors, decide not to use drugs. Exploring such individuals leads to a range of protective factors including:

- lifestyle aspirations and relationships (other people's disapproval, legal consequences, role as parent, career aspirations)
- practicalities of being a user (availability of time, financial cost)
- physical and psychological consequences of drugs (personal experience with drugs, current health conditions, fear of effect on health, fear of addiction, fear of losing control)
- perceived benefit of using drugs (sources of 'buzz', sources of support/coping mechanism).

The summary of factors young people identified as facilitating or impeding resilience to drug use is presented in Table 8.10 (Dillon et al. 2006).

Dillon et al. (2006) also explored the youngsters' strategies for avoiding or refusing drugs. The strategies fell into two types of refusal:

- active refusal strategies, saying no
- avoidance-based refusal strategies.

In refusing offers of drugs young people wanted to minimise the risk of repercussions from their refusals. These were in terms of damaging friendships and causing arguments or fights. If possible they did not want to offend the person making the offer, at times emphasising that they respected other people's decisions to use drugs while hoping they in turn would respect their decision not to use. Being confident about their decision not to use and the context in which the offer was made, supported by the people they were with, and feeling able to deal with the threats in terms of the consequences a refusal would have, all facilitated an easier refusal process.

Table 8.10 Factors associated with resilience to drug use

Other people's motivation to use	*Contextual risk factors*	*Factors making it easier or more difficult to refuse offers*	*Motivations not to use*
• Following example of others • To fit in • Peer pressure • Alleviate boredom • The buzz • Curiosity about effects • Escape problems • Ease physical pain • To look hard • To feel more confident	• In trouble with the police or school • Alcohol use • Boredom • Familial substance use • Mental health issues • Problematic family relationships	• Reputation as resilient to drug use • Type of drug offered • Reputation as a smoker or drinker • Age • Happy to be the odd one out • Being drunk • Offered by friends or strangers	• Other people's disapproval • Fear of effect on health • Fear of addiction • Alternative sources of support/ coping mechanisms • Current health conditions • Fear of losing control • Career aspirations • Role as a parent • Availability of time • Financial cost • Personal experience with drugs

An implicit, and often explicit, explanation for the resilience shown by individuals is that they show an effective sense of self-efficacy. As previously discussed, self-efficacy can be conceptualised as people's beliefs about their capabilities and their ability to put their decisions into practice (Bandura 1977, 1986).

The relationship between strong self-efficacy and effective self-management behaviours, such as assertiveness, and functional problem-solving skills have been explored. The findings from such reports generally demonstrate certain strategies that resilient young people use to refuse drugs. For example Epstein et al. (2007) suggested that young people used a range of assertive strategies that were constantly tested by friends and peers persistently offering drugs. Concurrently, there also appears to be an effective rational problem solving skill required. For example, balancing the benefits of refusing drugs (e.g. health, finances) with the need to maintain friendships and the negative consequences that may occur as a result of refusal. Consequently, individuals reported that they were the 'odd one out' but were the 'bigger person for saying no'. Success was measured in two ways: continuing to refuse drugs but not compromising their friendships or relationships. Again, the link to self-efficacy is seen in such individuals: the strength of well-being and mastery are increased with such a position.

Epstein et al. (2007) found that refusal assertiveness significantly mitigated the impact of friends' use on drug use, whereas those with low refusal assertiveness showed the highest incidence of drug use. This study highlights how important the critical relationship between risk and protective factors is. In this study, social risk factors like friends' smoking and friends' drinking can be mitigated by competence skills such as refusal assertiveness and decision-making skills – a finding supported by other longitudinal studies (Botvin 1998; Epstein and Botvin 2002). The interplay between the psychological (self-efficacy) and the social (peer relationships and behaviours) is once again stressed.

The crucial role of the family in the development of antisocial or delinquent behaviours has been long emphasised both by practitioners and in academic research (Sullivan and Wilson 1995; Repetti et al. 2002). The quality of parenting has been found to interact with psychosocial variables such as well-being, stress and social support in predicting many such antisocial behaviours including substance use and misuse (Yoshikawa 1994). On the basis of such studies, many interventions have been designed and implemented suggesting that the delinquent behaviours which lead to substance misuse (e.g. National Institute on Drug Abuse (NIDA) 1997) have arisen from maladaptive socialisation and therefore interventions aimed at improving parenting and socialisation can result in fewer antisocial behaviours.

As with all correlation-based studies, causal relationships cannot be deduced and hence questions remain. For example, does conflict with parents increases the likelihood that a young person will misuse substances, or is it that those who misuse substances have other antisocial behaviours which results in greater levels of familial conflict. Particular personality characteristics may encourage certain young people to spend more time with their family and may, at the same time, encourage the avoidance of behaviours such as drug or alcohol use.

However, there are numerous studies that attest to the importance of the family. Forney et al. (1989), Ary et al. (1993), Olsson et al. (2003), S. Clark (2004) and Wood et al. (2004), have all highlighted the strength of parental influence (via both behaviour and attitudes) on young people commencing substance use. Social factors that affect early development within the family, such as a chaotic home environment, ineffective parenting, and lack of mutual attachment, have been shown to be crucially important indicators of risk (NIDA 1997). The strongest social predictor of both drug and alcohol use has been shown to be use by parents and friends (Challier et al. 2000). Velleman and colleagues (e.g. Velleman et al. 2005) have argued that there are seven areas in which the family context could influence the child's substance use behaviour: family relations versus structure, family cohesion, family communication, parental modelling of behaviour, family management, parental supervision and parent or peer influences. In a comprehensive review Velleman et al. (2005) conclude that:

> There is considerable evidence that family factors are important in increasing risk and also in protecting young people in relation to their taking up of the use of various substances, and in the development in some of those young people of problematic substance use.
>
> (Velleman et al. 2005: 103)

Marijuana use and the gateway hypothesis

Cannabis is a relatively 'new' recreational drug that first began to be used by large numbers of young people in developed societies during the 1970s. Marijuana or cannabis is the most commonly used illicit drug with approximately 50 per cent of secondary school students in the United States indicating having used marijuana (Johnston et al. 2003). The figure for the UK is of a similar level (Webb et al. 1996). Experimentation with substances usually takes place during adolescence when tolerance is lower and risk of dependence is greater than in adulthood (Chen et al. 1997).

In recent decades there has been a growing interest in the effects of cannabis use on mental health and adjustment (e.g. Fergusson et al. 2006a; Hall 2006) with some evidence suggesting a link between cannabis use and psychosis (e.g. Fergusson et al. 2006b) although this is not a definitive. One aspect of this concern has been the contention that cannabis acts as a 'gateway drug' which leads to the use of other 'harder' drugs such as cocaine, methamphetamine and heroin at a later time (e.g. Kandel 2003). The gateway hypothesis assumes that there is a link between cannabis use and the onset of other illicit drug use and that the use of cannabis increases the likelihood of using other illicit drugs. Three explanations are often suggested for these patterns: first, that users of cannabis are more likely to use other illicit drugs because they obtain cannabis from the same black market and hence have more opportunities to use other illicit drugs; second, that those who use cannabis at an early age are more likely for other reasons to use other illicit drugs; and third, that the pharmacological effects of cannabis increase an adolescent's propensity to use other illicit drugs. Each of these hypotheses has been explored and reviewed (e.g. Cohen 1972; Goode 1974; Fergusson and Horwood 2000; Hall 2006), yet there still remains a lack of clarity.

There is a strong association between regular and early cannabis use and other illicit drug use and this has persisted across a number of different studies. Nonetheless, the gateway hypothesis remains controversial because it is difficult to exclude the hypothesis that it is due to the common characteristics of those who use cannabis and other drugs. A number of well-controlled longitudinal studies suggest that selective recruitment to cannabis use does not wholly explain the association between cannabis use and the use of other illicit drugs (Hall 2006).

Interventions to reduce illicit drug use

The UK government's Drug Strategy has the overarching aim of 'reducing the harm that drugs cause to society, including communities, individuals and their families'. To achieve this, the government has set the objective to 'reduce the use of Class A drugs and the frequent use of any illicit drug among all young people under the age of 25 especially by the most vulnerable young people'.

The UK government's updated Drug Strategy (2002) built on the findings of the previous ten-year strategy: *Tackling Drugs to Build a Better Britain* (1998). This was the first strategy designed to tackle drugs in an integrated way. In November 2004 the UK government published *Tackling Drugs*, an update on the progress of the strategy.

The government's strategy is to reduce the harm that drugs cause by persuading potential users not to use drugs: prevention is better than the cure. Hence, the strategy is aimed at reducing the prevalence of drugs on our streets and reducing the number of current drug users by the use of effective treatments. Consequently, the broad aims of the strategy were:

- preventing young people from using drugs by maintaining the prohibition of the drugs which deters use
- providing education and support for those most vulnerable to drug taking
- reduce the prevalence of drugs on the streets: tackling supply at all levels
- reduce drug-related crime: providing support to drug misusers and communities on the dangers of drug-related social and crime issues
- reduce the demand for drugs by reducing the number of problematic drug users.

Given that 99 per cent of societal costs from drug misuse are due to problematic drug users and that for every £1 spent on treatment at least £9.50 is saved in crime and health costs then there is a proportionate investment in this area. To prevent the current generation from becoming tomorrow's drug users, a series of government actions to reduce access to drugs have been implemented: to deliver high quality drug education and information, to develop key interventions with young people and families, and to provide treatment for young people before the drug problems escalate. The evidence base for education and treatment investments is poor, but certainly the strategy suggests that they are of greater cost effectiveness compared to the use of the legal system (the £9.50 saved for every £1 invested is a commonly cited consequence). As Maynard (2001) states, however, there is a need for the evidence base to be evaluated and reviewed and to prioritise appropriate investment in trials: 'While there is significant academic enthusiasm for such work . . . government shows little inclination to invest appropriately' (Maynard 2001: 7).

It is of note that the strategy is an integrated one and there are a range of government departments that are involved in the drug strategy including health, education and the home office. For example, the needs of young people are addressed in *Every Child Matters: Change for Children, Young People and Drugs* strategy guidance, a cross-government approach to the development of services to prevent drug harm. This has been developed in support of the drugs strategy and to support the Be Healthy aim of the overall *Every Child Matters: Change for Children* programme. This strategic guidance sets out a comprehensive approach to young people and drugs including: 'Ensuring provision is built around the needs of vulnerable children and young people; more focus on prevention and early intervention with those most at risk' (HM Government 2005: 2).

Social cognition models and illicit drug misuse

The theory of planned behaviour (TPB) and theory of reasoned action (TRA) have been applied to the use of illicit drugs (Petraitis et al. 1995) as have other such models, although perhaps not as widely as with other lifestyle behaviours (Michie and Abraham 2004). McMillan and Conner (2003) report just three studies applying the theory of planned behaviour to illicit drug use, with cannabis (Armitage et al. 1999) and ecstasy (Conner et al. 1998; Orbell et al. 2001). The theory of reasoned action proposes that an individual's substance abuse behaviours are based on intentions, which in turn are determined by attitudes and perceived social norms regarding substance use (see Chapter 8). Furthermore, the TRA suggests that attitudes are determined by perceived costs and benefits and the affective value placed on those consequences (Petraitis et al. 1995). Numerous studies have supported the predictive ability of TRA in substance-use contexts (e.g., Ajzen et al. 1982; Laflin et al. 1994; Morrison et al. 2002), although not all are focused on illicit drug misuse (McMillan and Conner 2003).

Intervention campaigns that have targeted key TRA variables have proven successful in preventing substance use (Flynn et al. 1994). On this basis, media campaigns have been developed that influence attitudes and perceived norms regarding substance misuse. The strength of these media campaigns can be maximised if social marketing principles are used within this theoretical context.

Social marketing, FRANK and drug use

Social marketing is the application of commercial sector marketing tools to the resolution of a number of social and health problems. The idea dates back to 1951 when Wiebe asked the question 'Can brotherhood be sold like soap?' (Wiebe 1951–1952). During the subsequent two to three decades there was a refinement of the thinking and social marketing began to inform family planning and disease control programmes (Manoff 1985). Social marketing thinking is now located at the centre of many government health improvement programmes, including reducing illicit drug use. A distinguishing feature of social marketing is that it goes beyond mere education and awareness-raising and focuses instead on behaviour. Although outcomes have traditionally been conceptualised in terms of behaviour change, more recent work has expanded this conceptualisation to include the prevention of certain behaviours such as the use of illicit substances (Andreasen 2006).

More recently there has been a growth in interest, research and practice in social marketing by policy makers, practitioners and health professionals in the UK (Gordon et al. 2006b). Indeed, the White Paper, *Improving Health* (DoH 2004c), advocates the use of 'the power of social marketing' and 'marketing tools applied to social good'. This has led to the development of the DoH-backed National Social Marketing Strategy (NSMS) for Health, in order to 'help realise the full potential of effective social marketing in contributing to national and local efforts to improve health and reduce health inequalities' (Consumer Council and Department of Health 2005).

One key feature of social marketing is that it is 'fanatically customer-driven' (Andreasen 2002: 7) and employs extensive formative research to ensure that the target audience will perceive the 'product' as highly appealing, valuable, and capable of influencing individual behaviour. The formative research process is guided by the '4 Ps' (product, price, promotion and place). While social marketers have offered varying definitions of 'product' ranging from the tangible tools of the social marketing effort to the desired end behaviour (see Peattie and Peattie 2003, for a discussion), one definition that appears congruent with substance-abuse prevention is that the 'product' is the package of benefits that accompanies the recommended behaviour (Andreasen 2006).

Social marketing is not a theory itself but is a framework that draws from many other bodies of knowledge including psychology, sociology, anthropology and communications theory to understand how to influence people's behaviour (Stead et al. 2007b). Although there are a number of definitions of social marketing, the most quoted is that of Andreasen (2002):

> Social marketing is the application of commercial marketing technologies to the analysis, planning and execution and evaluation of programs designed to influence the voluntary behaviour of target audiences in order to improve their personal welfare and that of society.
>
> (Andreasen 2002: 4)

In light of this definition, Andreasen (2002) suggested six essential benchmarks for a 'genuine' social marketing intervention (see Table 8.11).

Table 8.11 Andreasen's benchmark criteria

Benchmark	*Explanation*
1 Behaviour change	Intervention seeks to change behaviour and has specific measurable behavioural objectives
2 Consumer research	Intervention is based on an understanding of consumer experiences, values and needs. Formative research is conducted to identify these intervention elements and pre-test with the target group.
3 Segmentation and targeting	Different segmentation variables are considered when selecting the intervention target group. Intervention strategy is tailored for the selected segment(s).
4 Marketing mix	Intervention considers the best strategic application of the 'marketing mix'. This consists of the four Ps: Product, Price, Place and Promotion. Other Ps might include Policy change or People (e.g. training is provided to intervention delivery agents). Interventions which use only the Promotion P are social advertising and not social marketing.
5 Exchange	Interventions consider what will motivate people to engage voluntarily with the intervention and offers them something beneficial in return. The offered benefit may be intangible (e.g. personal satisfaction) or tangible (e.g. rewards for participating in the programme and making behavioural change).
6 Competition	Competing forces to the behaviour change are analysed. Intervention considers the appeal of competing behaviours (including current behaviour) and uses strategies that seek to remove or minimise this competition.

(Adapted from Stead et al. 2007a)

Studies of effectiveness of social marketing have been conducted, including a number of reviews (e.g. Gordon et al. 2006b; Stead et al. 2007b). In terms of illicit drug use, a total of thirteen studies have been reviewed. Twelve of the studies examined short-term impact, of which eight reported some positive significant impact. Unfortunately, the study that explored impact in the long term (two years or more) did not report sustained effects (Ellickson and Bell 1990).

The most recent social marketing strategy in the UK is Project FRANK. Project FRANK is reported as being successful (Home Office 2007) and as having established itself as an informed and trusted source of help and information and has worked at both a national and local level. It has received over three-quarter of a million telephone calls and responded to millions of hits on its website (talktofrank.com). It has made nearly 40,000 referrals to treatment and services and received over 300,000 visits to the treatment pages of the website. The formal review of the FRANK campaign suggested that:

> As the strategy to 'Experience' FRANK through 2006–2007 comes to an end, it's apparent that FRANK continues to be a credible and reliable source of information on all drug-related matters. With its innovative use of media and continued support for stakeholders, FRANK is well placed to contribute to the government's goal of improving the lives of children and young people by helping them to choose a positive and healthy future.
>
> (Home Office 2007: 3)

However, the review was focused on the marketing perspective rather than the strategy's effectiveness in reducing drug taking (which of course is a more long-term impact).

The state of evaluation of the drug prevention programmes is currently poor (McGrath et al. 2006). Although no formal evaluation of the FRANK programme's effectiveness of drug reduction has been published, Sumnall and Bellis (2007) suggest that it may be little different from the other social marketing campaigns in the United States and UK.

Sumnall and Bellis (2007: 930) propose that such campaigns may have a negative impact on health, and that since the campaigns regularly suggest that taking cannabis results in mental health difficulties and affects the 'brain' or 'mind', individuals may begin to believe they are experiencing such effects. Consequently, they suggest that cannabis users may suffer 'amotivation, memory loss or even paranoia, not as a direct result of the drug, but through psychological mechanisms induced through high-profile social-marketing campaigns that effectively "sell" such negative effects'. Of course there is no evidence of such an impact at present (although research has documented that exposure of ecstasy users to suggestions of drug-induced brain damage and memory loss is related to them performing worse on memory tests: Cole et al. 2006) it does present an interesting dilemma about the use of 'fear' in health promotion (see also Chapter 6 on smoking and the use of fear-inducing messages on cigarette packets and the concept of the 'worried well'). Consequently it is important that any of the new 'social marketing' campaigns are robust in their documentation of evidence and that they consider both the positive and negative consequences of any intervention campaign.

Recent trends in both commercial and social marketing have seen a move into relational rather than transactional thinking. It has been stressed within the business community that retaining customers is the key factor these days rather than continually seeking out new ones. Social marketing has adopted similar thinking, recognising the potential for people who are delighted with one aspect of health improvement to become more committed to health improvement in general (Hasting and McClean 2006). This ties in with the Wanless concept of 'full engagement' being the only way to bring about a step change in health improvement.

Social marketing 'theory' (or rather the principles underpinning social marketing) assumes that the purpose of an intervention is aimed at 'marketing' behaviour change using a mix of marketing techniques. Therefore, the behaviour is viewed as primarily the responsibility of the individual rather than society as a whole. However, as we have previously noted, the reasons for illicit drug use are many and varied and not simply a consequence of individual choice. It can be noted that the validity of the assumptions behind social marketing rests on a number of analogies (Rayner 2007). First, it assumes that the products to be marketed – behaviour, behaviour change or the benefits of behaviour change – are equivalent to goods and services marketed commercially. This is unlikely, giving up cannabis will have benefits in the long term, but a new pair of shoes or a bar of chocolate will have immediate gratification. Second, social marketing assumes that the target audience for the interventions act as 'consumers' of the behaviour change. But people do not 'consume' behaviour the way they do goods. Third, social marketing assumes an exchange (e.g. in purchasing a book or food there is an exchange of money for goods) but does this occur in social marketing? Indeed, Rayner (2007: 198) gives a damning indictment of social marketing: 'It is essentially a psychological theory with a few theoretical assumptions borrowed from organisational theories'.

Clinical approaches

There are a number of psychological approaches to assessing and preventing substance misuse and treating people with such problems. A summary of the psychological interventions is presented in Table 8.12. Many approaches are cognitive, behavioural or a mixture of the two in origin.

A number of such cognitive-behavioural approaches have developed an evidence base for treating substance misuse and these include such interventions as those described in further detail below.

Table 8.12 A brief summary of the main psychological therapies used in treating substance misuse

Behavioural therapy (BT)

A structured therapy focusing on changing behaviour and the environmental factors that trigger maladaptive behaviour. Includes:

Cue exposure treatment (CET)

A structured treatment involving exposure to drug-related cues that have been associated with past drug use without consumption of the drug. This is intended to lead to a reduction (or habituation) of reactivity to drug cues and hence to a reduced likelihood of relapse.

Community reinforcement approach (CRA)

A behavioural approach that focuses on what the client finds rewarding in his/her social, occupational and recreational life. It aims to help him/her change their lifestyle and social environment to support long-term changes in behaviour whereby using substances is less rewarding that not using them.

Contingency management (CM)

Also known as voucher-based therapy, this aims to encourage adaptive behaviour by rewarding the client for attaining agreed goals (e.g. no use of illicit drugs as checked by urine screens) and not rewarding them when these goals are unmet (e.g. illicit drug use). Vouchers can usually be exchanged for consumer goods.

Cognitive therapy (CT)

A structured therapy using cognitive techniques (e.g. challenging a person's negative thoughts) and behavioural techniques (e.g. behavioural experiments; activity planning) to change maladaptive thoughts and beliefs.

Cognitive behavioural therapy (CBT)

A combination of both cognitive and behavioural therapies.

Relapse prevention (RP)

Uses several CBT strategies to enhance the client's self-control and prevent relapse. It highlights problems that the client may face and develops strategies he/she can use to deal with high-risk situations.

Motivational interviewing (MI)

A focused approach aiming to enhance motivation for changing substance use by exploring and resolving the individual's ambivalence about change.

Motivational enhancement therapy (MET)

A brief intervention based on MI which also incorporates a 'check-up' assessment and feedback.

Twelve-step approaches

Interventions used by self-help organisations like Alcoholics Anonymous. They are based on a philosophy that adopts an illness model and sees substance use as stemming from an innate vulnerability. An individual must acknowledge their addiction and the harm it has caused to themselves and others; they must also accept their lack of control over use and thus the only acceptable goal is abstinence.

Other approaches

The involvement of partners and family through marital and family therapy builds on the known social context of substance use. There are also various forms of counselling, group therapy and milieu therapy.

Contingency management therapies

Contingency management is one form of behavioural therapy in which patients receive incentives for achieving specific behavioural goals. These approaches are based on operant conditioning whereby appropriate behaviour is rewarded with positive consequences and therefore more likely to be repeated. These forms of intervention have particularly strong and robust empirical support. For example, allowing a patient the privilege of taking home methadone doses, contingent on the patient's providing drug-free urine specimens is associated with significant reductions in illicit drug use (Stitzer et al. 1992). Similarly, Budney and Higgins (2006) demonstrated the efficacy of vouchers redeemable for goods and services, contingent on the patient's providing cocaine-free urine specimens, in reducing targeted drug use and enhancing retention in treatment.

There are, of course, some limitations to contingency management interventions. For example, the effects of the intervention tend to reduce after the contingencies are reduced. Second, there are costs involved and sometimes these are an impediment to their introduction (Crowley 1999). Finally, not all those users of illicit drugs are responsive to contingency management and there is consequently a need to explore individual differences in responses to behavioural treatment (Carroll and Onken 2005).

Cognitive behaviour and skills training therapies

Cognitive behaviour approaches, such as relapse prevention, are grounded in social learning theories and principles of operant conditioning. A number of meta-analyses and literature reviews have established the value of cognitive-behavioural approaches in drug-using populations (e.g. Irvin et al. 1999). Indeed, several research studies have indicated that CBT is demonstrably effective in the treatment of cocaine-dependent outpatients (e.g. Rohsenow et al. 2000). Another study involving 450 marijuana-dependent individuals demonstrated that a nine-session individual approach that integrated cognitive behaviour therapy and motivational interviewing was more effective than a two-session motivational interviewing approach, which was in turn more effective than a delayed-treatment control condition (MTP Research Group 2004).

Motivational interviewing

Motivational interviewing approaches have strong empirical support for use in treating alcohol users and smokers (see Chapter 5), with several studies showing significant and durable effects (Dunn et al. 2001; Burke et al. 2003). Marijuana-dependent adults who received motivational interviewing had significant reductions in marijuana use, compared to a delayed treatment control group (Stephens et al. 2000). However, the research has not always been positive and equivocal results have been found. For example, Miller et al. (2003) did not support the efficacy of motivational interviewing.

Couples and family treatments

The defining feature of couples and family treatments is that they treat drug-using individuals in the context of family and social systems in which substance use may develop or be maintained. The engagement of the individual's social networks in treatment can be a powerful predictor of change, and thus the inclusion of family members in treatment may be helpful in reducing attrition (particularly among adolescents) and addressing multiple problem areas (Liddle et al. 2001). Reviews of such treatments, including meta-analyses, have indicated that these approaches are effective (e.g. Deas and Thomas 2001).

The National Institute for Health and Clinical Excellence issued guidelines on psychosocial interventions for drug misuse in July 2007. NICE made recommendations for the use of psychosocial interventions in the treatment of people who misuse opioids, stimulants and cannabis in the healthcare and criminal justice systems. There were several key priorities for implementation:

- *Brief interventions:* opportunistic brief interventions focused on motivation should be offered to people in limited contact with drug services (for example, those attending a needle and syringe exchange or primary care settings) if concerns about drug misuse are identified by the service user or staff member.
- *Self-help:* staff should routinely provide people who misuse drugs with information about self-help groups. These groups should normally be based on twelve-step principles.
- *Contingency management:* drug services should introduce contingency management programmes. The programme should offer incentives (usually vouchers that can be exchanged for goods or services of the service user's choice, or privileges such as take-home methadone doses) contingent on each presentation of a drug-negative test (for example, free from cocaine or non-prescribed opioids).
- *Contingency management to improve physical healthcare:* for people at risk of physical health problems (including transmittable diseases) resulting from their drug misuse, material incentives (for example, shopping vouchers of up to £10 in value) should be considered to encourage harm reduction.

Conclusion

Illicit drug use is a behaviour that is, in comparison to the other negative health behaviours discussed in this text, relatively rare. However, it comes with serious consequences for an individual's health and well-being and society as a whole. Risk factors associated with illicit drug use involve a complex interaction of individual biological and psychological variables within the social milieu and the individual's timeline. Conversely, factors associated with resilience can be identified and many of these have a self-efficacy basis. Interventions to increase resilience may be successful. Other interventions within a TRA framework and with underlying social marketing principles have been employed by government to try and reduce substance misuse. Clinical interventions to prevent and/or treat illicit drug use are mainly based on cognitive and behavioural therapies or a combination of the two. Evaluation studies have generally supported the efficacy of such programmes in reducing illicit drug use.

Summary points

- Substance misuse is now the generally accepted term for illicit drug use. There is no one generally accepted definition. Different definitions cover the purpose of drug taking, whether the behaviour is persistent and the consequences of the behaviour.
- Most cultures have laws associated with the misuse of drugs. What constitutes misuse and the seriousness of a particular transgression is culturally bound and varies across time and between cultures.
- The WHO estimated that there were 185 million drug users worldwide in 2007. Ten per cent of the UK population report having taken illegal drugs in the preceding year and one third of adults admit to having ever taken an illegal drug.
- Health consequences of illicit drug use include death and a variety of medical complaints dependent upon drug used. For example, cocaine use can result in heart attack, respiratory failure, stroke or seizures.
- Illicit drug use carries a significant financial cost. The HPA estimated that Class A drug users cost the UK economy £15.4 billion in 2003/2004.
- Multiple risk factors have been identified that increase the probability that an individual will engage in illicit drug use. Psychological risk factors include anxiety, risk-taking and novelty seeking tendencies. Socio-cultural factors include drug availability, economic deprivation and peer group substance use. Demographic characteristics have also been implicated, and have genetic factors. There are complex interactions between these and other factors, and their influence varies over the lifespan.

- Protective variables such as parental responsibilities, career aspirations, lack of funds, fear of effects on health, negative personal experiences and self-efficacy have been identified as reducing the probability of illicit drug use.
- The gateway hypothesis proposes that use of 'softer' drugs (e.g. cannabis) is associated with the use of 'harder' drugs (e.g. cocaine, heroine) at a later time. There is evidence that the two are linked, although the causal mechanisms have not been identified.
- Social cognition models of illicit drug use suggest that drug use is determined by intention to perform the behaviour which is in turn influenced by such things as attitudes, social norms, perceived control and self-efficacy. Studies have supported the predictive ability of social cognition models and interventions based upon them have been successful.
- Social marketing, using commercial marketing strategies to solve social and health problems, has been used in a number of other interventions, for example, FRANK. Studies investigating the effectiveness of such interventions have shown some support for a reduction of illicit drug use over the short term, but there is no evidence of a long-term effect as yet.
- There are a number of psychological interventions available to treat people with substance misuse problems. These include cognitive behavioural therapy, contingency management and motivational enhancement therapy. There is support for the efficacy of these approaches.

9 Evaluating lifestyle psychology

At the end of this chapter you will:

- be aware of any potential patterns of lifestyle choices
- recognise how social cognitive models can improve lifestyle change interventions
- understand the generic psychological concepts that are of relevance across all lifestyle behaviours.

The aim of this chapter is to evaluate the relevance of lifestyle psychology to promoting healthy lifestyles. In order to do this, there are two key questions that have to be considered. First, are there any distinct relationships between lifestyle choices that could be employed to develop more effective lifestyle interventions? De Bourdeaudhuij and Van Oost (1999) have argued that if congruence in health behaviours exist then public health interventions could be made more effective, less expensive and less time consuming. Lifestyle diseases are never influenced in their aetiology, or their progression, by a single lifestyle behaviour, rather a number contribute to the overall risk of disease. Effecting positive changes in more than one behaviour would have greater health benefits than achieving a change in only one (De Bourdeaudhuij and Van Oost 1999).

Second, are there common psychological principles for effective behavioural change that can be applied across all lifestyle behaviours? If common principles exist then health professionals could be trained in a set of generic techniques. Developing a generic set of psychological skills would enable health professionals to deal with the range of behavioural issues that may arise in their case load. It may not only be primary care professionals who could benefit from developing generic psychological skills. Health professionals, who are traditionally specialists in one lifestyle area, are not averse to such ideas. Anderson (2002) has argued that it is time for public health nutrition practitioners to add recommendations about physical activity to their portfolio, given that they are both key factors in the onset of obesity, diabetes and other lifestyle disorders.

Lifestyle patterns

Blaxter (1990) was one of the first to consider the relationship between lifestyle behaviours by analysing patterns of eating, drinking, smoking and exercising in the 9,003 adults who participated in the Health and Lifestyle Survey, carried out in 1984 and 1985. Before the Health and Lifestyle Survey the only reported link between lifestyle behaviours was that between drinking alcohol and smoking (Wilson 1980; Burke et al. 1997). However, Blaxter (1990) reported that smoking and diet, not smoking and alcohol, were the most highly correlated behaviours in her study: those who smoked were far more likely to report a poor diet than those who did not. The relationship between smoking and drinking, although present, was not as strong. In fact, ex-drinkers were the most likely of all drinking categories to be heavy smokers. These are positive correlations, in that someone who smokes is more likely to report drinking or a poor diet and positive habits predict positive habits. However, not all the relationships described by Blaxter (1990) were positive. In some cases negative habits in one behaviour predicted positive habits in another. For instance, alcohol consumption was negatively correlated with exercise; drinking predicted exercise and non-drinking predicted lack of exercise.

Blaxter (1990) found that 10–11 per cent of her sample reported all good behaviours, and 7 per cent of men but very few women reported all bad behaviours. Although there is a caveat here in that she described non-drinking as good and the evidence is that moderate drinking, especially for men, is not deleterious and can be beneficial for health (Room et al. 2005; French and Zavala 2007). Blaxter (1990) then went on to consider patterns of mixed behaviours. There were many different combinations of behaviours but five mixed patterns of interest emerged. Two were all good behaviours with one bad habit. All good habits but a lack of exercise was a common pattern in men aged over 60 and in women from middle age and older. All good habits apart from drinking was common in younger men in professional occupations. Young men from the lower end of the socio-economic scale were more likely to report all bad behaviours apart from high activity. The other two prominent patterns were poor diet and lack of exercise combined with no smoking or drinking, which was common among elderly people. In comparison, poor diet and drinking, while not smoking and taking exercise, was common among young people.

Interpreting these patterns is not straightforward. Cross-sectional data such as these can tell us nothing about whether young people will change their habits as they age or whether these are generational effects. It is clear that in the 1980s drinking and taking exercise were youthful habits, which tended to reverse in older people. Similar patterns are reported in cross-sectional data from the more recent national English,

Welsh, Scottish and Northern Irish surveys (respectively DoH 2003; Welsh Assembly Government 2007; Scottish Executive 2005; Department of Health, Social Services and Public Safety 2001). This adds weight to the argument that lifestyle behaviours change over the life course. It is intuitively logical that levels of activity would decrease with ageing, given the increased likelihood of life impairing conditions associated with advancing age, however only a longitudinal study of lifestyle habits would confirm this hypothesis.

Evidence suggests that young men are more active than young women because they play more sport (Scottish Executive 2005). It seems plausible that lifestyle choices in young men who play sport are determined by their sport of preference and the culture associated with it. The behavioural patterns described by Blaxter (1990) of young men with all good behaviours bar drinking or all bad behaviours bar exercising indicate that sports participation may underpin the adoption of certain lifestyle patterns. High activity is an inevitable outcome for young men participating in sport but post-match drinking is also a normative behaviour for the majority of sporting activities (Burke et al. 1997). The impact of diet and smoking on sport performance is now well understood and it is possible that different sports may place a different emphasis on importance of these behaviours and could support either bad or poor diets and smoking or non-smoking. Burke et al. (1997) found that post-match drinking and smoking was common in Australian young men but in some contexts it may only be drinking that is normative post-match behaviour. Consequently, the sports arena, traditionally associated with exercise, may also be a useful place in which to reach and influence other lifestyle behaviours. Although young men are the most physically active group in society, their activity levels decline rapidly as they age and men are no more active than women by the time they are in their sixties (DoH 2003; Welsh Assembly Government 2007; Scottish Executive 2005; Department of Health, Social Services and Public Safety 2001). Maintaining activity through the life course is key to reducing risk of chronic conditions so consideration need to be given to how activity in men can be maintained through the life course.

Unfortunately, in the years since Blaxter (1990) raised the idea of identifiable lifestyle patterns, relatively few studies have explored this idea. The lack of research in this area is probably due to a number of different factors. It may reflect the discipline-specific nature of academic study with dieticians, addiction specialists and exercise professionals each focused on their own field of expertise. It probably also reflects the complexities of investigating four different behaviours in one study. Longitudinal studies of lifestyle choices are indicated but such studies are rare, due to their cost and their failure to deliver immediate outcomes. Another possibility is that studies have taken place but few meaningful relationships or distinct lifestyle patterns have emerged and there have not been publications associated with the research. For whatever reason, lifestyle patterns have been relatively unexplored.

De Bourdeaudhuij and Van Oost (1999) used cluster analysis to explore relationships between lifestyle behaviours in their sample of 2400 adults. Unlike Blaxter (1990) they found no evidence that one positive lifestyle behaviour inclined people to practice other positive lifestyle behaviours. Indeed, they postulated that certain positive health habits may be practiced to compensate for other negative habits.

Burke et al. (1997) found that smoking was related to deleterious eating and drinking in all of their sample of 18 year old Australians and furthermore was also associated with lack of exercise, but only in women. They argued that smoking was a gateway to other deleterious lifestyle choices. Interestingly, Burke et al. (1997) implicated sport as a determinant of lifestyle choices. They argue that sporting culture is the reason why smoking fails to predict lack of exercise in young men. They reflect that binge drinking and smoking are common post-match activities in Australian young men. Burke et al. (1997) argue that smoking is the behaviour that can most powerfully indicate adverse health choices but that patterns of clustering differ between men and women, potentially because of the cultural patterns of behaviour practised by sporting young men. Other authors agree that smoking can be a gateway behaviour into other deleterious behaviours such as drinking and drugs (Orford 2001). However, Burke et al. (1997) can only hypothesise about the traits that underlie the associations between the decision to smoke and how it influences other lifestyle choices. They postulate that unconventionality or rebelliousness may underpin smoking behaviour but whether it is smoking per se that leads to other adverse behavioural choices or the same underlying facets of unconventionality or rebelliousness is not evident.

In conclusion it would seem that there is little evidence for a set of distinct lifestyle patterns in the population with the only clear contender for a specific lifestyle being that of a sporting young man. Sport could be argued to support a distinct lifestyle among its male participants. Another key emerging factor in lifestyle choice is progression through the lifecourse. Cross-sectional studies indicate that lifestyle choices change through the lifecourse (Blaxter 1990; DoH 2003; Welsh Assembly Government 2007; Scottish Executive 2005; Department of Health, Social Services and Public Safety 2001). It may be that certain points during the lifecourse are significant for the direction of lifestyle choices. The cross-sectional studies that indicate that lifestyle choices change as people move through the life course, delineate between different stages in the life course using chronological age. It is possible that grouping people in terms of key life events for instance becoming a parent or retiring may reveal even clearer patterns of lifestyle choice linked to role and role expectations.

Traditionally sex has been a key factor in lifestyle choices. One of the most interesting aspects of sex-related lifestyles is the decreasing difference in male and female choices. When Blaxter (1990) looked at lifestyle behaviours in men and women in the 1980s, men drank more, smoked more and ate a poorer diet but took more exercise. However, the percentages of women and men smoking are now much more similar as more men than women have given up smoking. Similarly, women have started to drink more and percentages of women drinking dangerously are much closer to male percentages than they were in the late 1980s (Blaxter 1990; DoH 2003; Welsh Assembly Government 2007; Scottish Executive 2005; Department of Health, Social Services and Public Safety 2001).

Socio-economic factors are commonly understood to predict lifestyle choices but in actuality it is only for smoking that a clear linear relationship between class and behaviour exists. Poor diet is also linked socio-economic position, though not as strongly and for exercise and drinking socio-economic relationships are complex and probably not useful in public health.

Psychological principles of lifestyle behaviours

Perception of risk

It was argued in Chapter 2 that risk perception is an essential component of any theory of behavioural change and that all social cognitive models of behavioural change include it. The central notion is that in order to promote positive change an individual must recognise the risk in the first place. The underlying principle is that the better risk is understood the more likely an individual is to adopt a preventative behavioural strategy. Belief in the benefit of the preventative strategy works in tandem with the concept of risk. If you perceive yourself to be at risk and believe that the proposed behavioural change will reduce that risk then this should increase your likelihood of adopting the healthy behaviour. However, risk perceptions and belief in the effectiveness of risk prevention strategies consistently fail to predict lifestyle behaviours (Floyd et al. 2000; Milne et al. 2000; Ruiter 2004; Taubman Ben-Ari et al. 2005; Blue 2007).

The failure of risk perception or belief in the benefits of risk reduction strategies to predict health behaviour is one that many health professionals fail to or refuse to recognise (Minugh et al. 1998; Blue 2007). Indeed, some authors have argued that the methodology for measuring risk perceptions must be flawed if it cannot predict behaviour (Blue 2007). Consequently, fear drive messages about the dangers of particular behaviours continue to be a popular health promotion strategy (Ruiter et al. 2001; Ruiter 2004). Warnings about the dangers of excess drinking, lack of physical activity or unsafe sex are commonplace.

Health promotion messages have been successful in communicating the risks of unhealthy lifestyles and the majority of people can competently cite what they should do to lessen their risk of future ill health (Blaxter 1990; Lawton 2002). Despite this, the majority of people continue to drink heavily, remain sedentary or perform unsafe sex (DoH 2003; Scottish Executive 2005; Welsh Assembly Government 2007; Department of Health, Social Services and Public Safety 2001; CDC 2007b). Social cognitive explanations of behavioural change cannot provide an adequate explanation of why perception of risk does not predict behavioural choices. However, if you consider the situation from a lifestyle perspective then the failure of individuals to respond to risk messages is more comprehensible.

First, a health risk message requires the audience to consider the behaviour and its outcomes solely in terms of health. However, lifestyle behaviours all have other social outcomes that may have more resonance than health outcomes for many people. Consequently, their personal cost-benefit analysis, if they do one, may include non-health factors such as peer approval or pleasure.

Second, health messages are predominantly focused on long-term health outcomes. This requires individuals to be future-orientated and many people are focused in the present where many of the positive outcomes of unhealthy behaviours are experienced (Lawton 2002). Risks objectify a potentially dangerous future but the anxiety they evoked is immediate. Thirlaway and Heggs (2005) found that faced with a health risk message about the relationship between alcohol and breast cancer, many women described feeling anxious and worried. Worried women used a wide range of defensive strategies to alleviate the anxiety; altering the risky behaviour was only one of these strategies and it was not the most popular. The most popular strategy was to decide that their own behaviour did not put them at risk. Many women stated that although they drank, they did not drink enough to be at risk. It was common for women in this study to rationalise that they were not at increased risk because they kept to the government weekly guidelines of 14 units per week. This is despite the very clear statement in the risk message that drinking only 7 units a week increased the risk of breast cancer and that drinking 14 units would increase it still further. This could be interpreted as unrealistic optimism. Another popular strategy to offset anxiety was to dismiss the message by deciding the source of the message was untrustworthy. Women variously reported distrusting statistics, scientists and journalists. All of the defences utilised dealt effectively with the anxiety in the 'here and now' while failing to decrease the future risk. Lawton (2002) has argued that few studies have considered how people in their daily lives anticipate their futures. In her qualitative study of how people think about their future health she found that the majority of people did think about the future but perceived it extremely optimistically. She argued that only when people actually experience ill health in the present are they inclined to consider the future more negatively, consequently the uptake of preventative lifestyle change was therefore more likely to be reactive rather than proactive. Interestingly Lawton (2002) found that although older people were more likely to be health conscious, there was considerable overlap between different age groups, with many older people remaining unconcerned about their health. It was the experience of ill-health rather than chronological age that best predicted increased health consiousness, concern and consequently lifestyle adaptation. However, not everyone who has experienced ill health can be reliably predicted to make preventative lifestyle changes. There are many studies that report continued adverse lifestyle choices in people experiencing lifestyle diseases that are adversely influenced in their aetiology and continued progression by lifestyle behaviours (HM Government 2007).

Perhaps we should be encouraging people to view their health in the future more realistically and possibly more negatively. As predictive genetic testing for increasing numbers of diseases becomes available, efforts to prevent the development of disease through lifestyle change could be tailored to the individual. However, it is not clear that providing people with clearer indications of their own personal risk will actually increase their adoption of healthy lifestyle choices. People who are known to be at risk of various genetic conditions such as breast and bowel cancer, with acknowledged lifestyle components to the aetiology and progression of disease, do not report significantly different lifestyle choices (Marteau and Lerman 2001). Perceptions of genetic risks as 'fixed' are common in the population (Bates 2005). It is equally plausible that being informed of a genetic risk of disease may increase fatalistic thinking and encourage more adverse lifestyle choices.

One of the negative effects of the increasing emphasis on preventing ill health and the associated plethora of health promotion campaigns is the associated increases in anxiety among low risk individuals. A concern is that these campaigns attract only the 'worried well' and induce anxiety in otherwise healthy individuals (Northern Ireland Executive 2000; Addley et al. 2001).

Finally, it is likely that many established health behaviours have become habitual and are not controlled by cognitive thought but by automatic responses to external stimuli (Aarts et al. 1997). When behaviours are considered within this lifestyle perspective the failure of risk messages is not surprising. The common factors to all lifestyle behaviours identified in Chapter 1 and elucidated here can provide a convincing explanation for the failure of risk messages to result in positive lifestyle choices.

There is evidence that providing people with information about new unknown risks can encourage behavioural change (Murgraff et al. 1999). However, risks of unhealthy lifestyle behaviours are generally well known and understood so repetition of familiar risks are unlikely to change the behaviour of people who have not already responded to the risk. It is well documented that stand alone educational strategies about the risk of unhealthy and the benefits of healthy lifestyle choices do not effect lifestyle change. Nevertheless, it is still a popular, if not the most popular, health promotion strategy in the UK and other countries (Kahn et al. 2002; Plant and Plant 2006). Risk messages may be appropriate to set the scene for a behavioural change intervention and to reaffirm the appropriateness of behavioural change but are unlikely to engineer a change in behaviour in isolation.

It was argued at the start of Chapter 2 that risk messages may be a necessary but not sufficient factor to cause behavioural change. However, given the multiple outcomes from lifestyle behaviours, risk perceptions may not even be necessary. Some individuals will take healthy levels of physical activity without ever understanding the risks of remaining sedentary; they may exercise for pleasure or for success. Other individuals will refuse to drink alcohol on religious grounds without ever considering their personal health. It could be argued that the costs and benefits of lifestyle choices need to be articulated to the young who may not yet understand the relationship between lifestyle and health but reiterating the same health messages to adults already aware of the risks and benefits of their lifestyle is unlikely to change their behaviour.

Self-efficacy

Although risk and benefit components of social cognitive models have been disappointing in their ability to predict or generate behavioural change useful factors have emerged from social cognitive research. The one consistent factor that is positively related to behavioural change in all lifestyle behaviours is self-efficacy (French et al. 1996; Plotnikoff and Higginbotham 1998; Marshall and Biddle 2001; Hagger et al. 2002; Rovniak et al. 2002; Cox et al. 2003; Kuther and Timoshin 2003; Siahpush et al. 2006; Epstein et al. 2007; Murgraff et al. 2007; Williams et al. 2007). Self-efficacy is the belief that one can carry out specific behaviours in specified situations (Bandura 1997). In other words, an individual who believes they can make a positive change is more likely to succeed in that attempt than another individual, who may be equally motivated but have less self-efficacy. This immediately begs the question: how can we increase individual self-efficacy? Self-efficacy has been argued to be enhanced by personal accomplishment or mastery, vicarious experience or verbal persuasion (Walker 2001). In the context of lifestyle change personal accomplishment is considered a more effective way of increasing self-efficacy than vicarious experience or persuasion (Walker 2001).

Ajzen (1988, 1998) has consistently argued that behaviour-specific constructs fare better than generalised dispositions in predicting behaviour, so specific experience of success in attempting to change behaviour is likely to increase the likelihood of continued positive change in that behaviour. Attempting to generalise successful change across behaviours is unlikely to be as effective as working within one behavioural context. However, the principles that underpin the promotion of self-efficacy will be the same across all lifestyle behaviours. Walker (2001) has argued that self-efficacy should be central to the design of interventions to help people adopt new behaviours. Kahn et al. (2002), Hillsdon et al. (2005) and NICE (2006b) report that interventions to teach behavioural change strategies that are focused on the importance of developing self-efficacy and perceived behavioural control are more likely to result in sustained behavioural change. Rovniak et al. (2002) have postulated that the positive impact of self-efficacy on lifestyle behaviours is mediated by the use of self-regulatory strategies. People with high self-efficacy are more likely to utilise self-regulatory strategies which in turn were found to exert a large total effect on physical activity in their study. Self-regulatory strategies include: goal setting, self-monitoring, planning and problem solving. Improving self-efficacy involves careful self-regulatory goal-setting that challenges but does not overwhelm the individual so that self-efficacy is developed not damaged. Such tailored interventions could be costly in terms of expert time and require a specialist who has both the physiological and psychological skills-base on which to base their recommendations and supportive strategies. Nevertheless, it is plausible that doctors, practice nurses, health visitors and other health professionals based in primary care could be taught appropriate psychological skills. Such generic skills would enable them to initiate and sustain preventative lifestyle change through improving self-efficacy in people with moderately deleterious lifestyles and no medical counter-indications. Individuals who are identified as dependent drinkers or who may have eating disorders can then be referred for specialist support. Self-efficacy focused primary care interventions for problem drinking are already well established and have had some degree of success (Moyer et al. 2002). Consequently, a clear framework for similar interventions with other deleterious behaviours is already in place.

Implementation intentions

It has been stated in previous chapters that intention to behave does not always lead to action. Even strong intentions can fail to materialise into behaviour. Gollwitzer (1999) has argued that implementation intentions can support goal intentions by specifying the when, where and how of responses leading goal attainment. Gollwitzer and Sheeran (2006: 70) have described implementation intentions as 'if-then' plans. For instance, if your goal is to lose weight you need to identify when you are likely to eat high-fat food and how you will respond to the external situation when your usual response has been to eat high-fat food. So if you usually have a biscuit with a cup of tea you need to formulate an alternative response, such as eating a low-fat cracker. The notion of planning how to implement an intention is not new. In the 1960s when the ineffectiveness of fear appeals was first recognised, Leventhal et al. (1967) argued that accompanying a fear appeal with a plan of action increased the likelihood of preventative action. Implementation intentions are hypothesised to create a mental representation of the anticipated situation. In this way, implementation intentions can initiate an automatic response to an external situation. Automatic responses can contribute to the development of positive lifestyle habits.

Social norms

Social norms are a key component of the theory of planned behaviour (TPB). Social norms have been consistently reported to be the least predictive component of the TPB (Godin and Kok 1996). However, many authors continue to argue that social normative behaviour is key in understanding and promoting positive lifestyle choices (Jones et al. 2007). Godin and Kok (1996) have argued that perhaps social norms are poorly conceptualised within the TPB framework. Similarly, McMillan and Conner (2003) conclude that the way that social norms are traditionally conceptualised with the TPB does not account for the various ways in which social influence is exerted. Traditionally, social norms are conceptualised and measured within the TPB framework by asking about the social approval or disapproval of others and are described as injunctive social norms by McMillan and Conner (2003). However, studies that report strong relationships between social norms and drinking behaviour ask about descriptive social norms. That is to say they ask individuals how much they think their peers are drinking (Kuther and Timoshin 2003). Using descriptive social norms as opposed to injunctive social norms with other lifestyle behaviours may well produce some useful evidence about the role of perceptions of other people's behaviour in lifestyle choices.

A related concept to social norms is unrealistic optimism. It is well reported that individuals tend to underestimate their personal risk for a number of health conditions and to underestimate their own deleterious behavioural practices. Social norms theory postulates that overestimation of the negative health behaviours of peers encourages individual deleterious behaviour. Providing people with evidence of actual peer behaviour can improve behaviour (Paglia and Room 1999; Ramos and Perkins 2006). While most of the evidence for the effectiveness of challenging social norms comes from studies of drinking behaviour, similar strategies may be effective in other behavioural contexts.

TTM and motivational interviewing

The transtheoretical model is a complex and comprehensive model of behavioural change which incorporates a number of potential mechanisms of behavioural change. However, it is the stages of change component of the model which has generated the most interest and frequently only that component of the model is utilised. The TTM conceptualises behavioural change as a process and identifies pre-contemplators, contemplators, preparers, people in action and people in maintenance. The evidence for the predictive power of this model is mixed and for all the behaviours research that supports (Marshall and Biddle 2001; Prochaska et al. 2004) or challenges the model (Riemsma et al. 2003; Michie and Abraham 2004; Williams et al. 2007) exists. The main tenet of the TTM is that different strategies will be required to help people move through the process of behavioural change. Often stage-based interventions report effective behavioural change but a careful analysis of what is effective often indicates that while a particular strategy may be effective the evidence for stage matching improving the efficacy of the intervention is not robust. A systematic review exploring the value of staged-based interventions has been completed by Riemsma et al. (2003), who concluded that 'Despite the widespread and uncritical use of stage based interventions in smoking cessation, we found only limited evidence for their effectiveness' (Riemsma et al. 2003: 5). Michie and Abraham (2004: 34) report that 'despite the popularity of this model, the psychological processes described by TTM are not well supported by available data'. Despite little concrete evidence about what will be most effective at any one stage and some evidence that strategies can be equally effective, particularly self-efficacy strategies, at any stage (Williams et al. 2007) stage-based interventions remain popular. Effective strategies that have been explored within the TTM framework include motivational interviewing (initially developed in order to move people from pre-contemplation and contemplation towards preparation and action) and interventions to increase self-efficacy which have been evaluated earlier.

Motivational interviewing

Motivational interviewing (MI) derives from the TTM and in particular from the notion that the motivation that individuals have for change will influence their success. Miller and Rollnick (2002) concluded that motivation is fundamental to change and they suggest motivational interviewing is the appropriate approach. Motivational interviewing can be defined as 'a client-centred, directive method for enhancing intrinsic motivation to change by exploring and resolving ambivalence' (Miller and Rollnick 2002: 25).

Motivational interviewing has as its goal the simple expectation that increasing an individual's motivation to consider change rather than showing them how to change should be the key step. If a person is not motivated to change, then it is irrelevant if they know how to do it or not. However, if a person is motivated to change then the interventions aimed at changing behaviour can begin. So in terms of stages of change motivational interviewing is focused at the pre-contemplative and contemplative.

Motivational interviewing is a technique based on cognitive-behavioural therapy which aims to enhance an individual's motivation to change health behaviour. The whole process aims to help the patient understand their thought processes and to identify how their thought processes help produce the inappropriate behaviour and how their thought processes can be changed to develop alternative, health-promoting behaviours.

Motivational strategies include eight components that are designed to increase the level of motivation the person has towards changing a specific behaviour. It is important to note that, similarly to self-efficacy, the motivation is specific to one behaviour, so being motivated to quit smoking does not simply transfer to being motivated to reduce alcohol consumption. The eight components are:

- giving advice (about specific behaviours to be changed)
- removing barriers (often about access to particular help)
- providing choice (making it clear that if they choose not to change that is their right and it is their choice; the therapist is there to encourage change but not insist on change)
- decreasing desirability (of the ambivalence towards change or the status quo)
- practising empathy
- providing feedback (from a variety of perspectives – family, friends, health professionals – in order to give the patient a full picture of their current situation)
- clarifying goals (feedback should be compared with a standard (an ideal), and clarification of the ideal can provide the pathway to the goal)
- active helping (such as expressing caring or facilitating a referral, all of which convey a real interest in helping the person to change).

Motivational interviewing has been found to be effective in increasing fruit and vegetable intake in smokers from the deprived socio-economic backgrounds (Ahluwalia et al. 2007), and in reducing the drinking of alcohol (Burke et al. 2003). Similarly, Dunn et al. (2001: 1725) report that there was 'substantial evidence that MI is an effective substance abuse intervention method'. Furthermore, other meta-analyses and systematic reviews have attested to the value and effectiveness of motivational interviewing in both specialist clinics (Burke et al. 2003) and in general practice (Rubak et al. 2005) and according to specific lifestyle behaviours (e.g. drinking: Vasilaki et al. 2006; smoking: Cofta-Woerpel et al. 2007; illicit drug use: Dunn et al. 2001; improving diet: Richards et al. 2006).

The effectiveness of motivational interviewing is encouraging but it does not indicate that the whole TTM model is valid. It would seem that motivational interviewing may be the first stage in a process that should move on to develop self-efficacy through effective goal setting once the motivation for change has been established. However, the TTM may not be a realistic representation of the process of behavioural change.

Enjoyment

People frequently, although not always, choose to do things that they enjoy. One of the negative aspects of the social cognitive approach to health behaviour is that the role of affect is marginalised. Pleasure can be argued to be the main motivation for lifestyle choices, particularly among the young (Orford 2001). Presumably most academics and health professionals know and understand this at a personal level yet their focus remains on cognitive decision making. Pleasure can be experienced either as a physiological sensation, such as a palatable food in the mouth or as a positive mood response or frequently as both. Ingesting food and drinking alcohol both have clear physiological effects that people can describe as enjoyable (Berridge 1996). Liking of sweet food is an innate response (Berridge 1996). Other pleasures are learnt and not initially enjoyable. Alcohol is not naturally palatable and people have to learn to enjoy it. Alcopops combine alcohol with sugar to increase its palatability to enable people to enjoy the taste and therefore experience the physiological effects of the drug. Such sweetened alcohol beverages are popular among young drinkers (Plant and Plant 2006).

Alcohol, tobacco and illicit drugs are powerful mood modifiers and a biological mechanism of how these substances influence mood is well understood (Chapters 5, 6 and 8). It is arguable that exercise, eating and sex can also be powerful means of emotional regulation. The biological mechanisms underpinning the mood-enhancing effects of food, exercise and sex are less well understood (Biddle and Mutrie 1991) and for these behaviours psychological mechanisms are postulated to be more important (Biddle and Mutrie 1991).

The mood-enhancing effects of lifestyle behaviours will be moderated to a greater or lesser degree by both biological and psychological processes and they will all sit somewhere along a continuum in terms of the involvement of the two processes in generating mood change (Figure 9.1). Exercise is different from other lifestyle behaviours in that health professionals wish to encourage people to be physically active when many people profess to not enjoy exercise whereas in the other behaviours health professionals aim to curtail activities experienced as enjoyable.

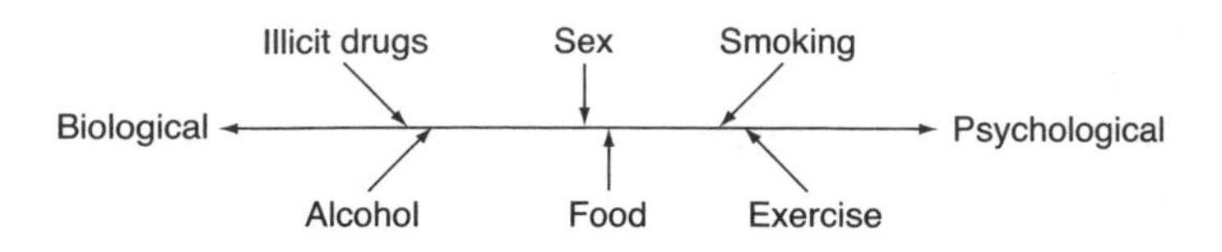

Figure 9.1 Control of mood-enhancing effects of lifestyle behaviours

Mood-enhancing effects of lifestyle behaviours can be straightforward in that they make people happy. However, the same mood-enhancing effects can also be used as an effective antidote to anxiety or tension. These dual effects are reported in a range of lifestyle behaviours (Orford 2001). Some authors are in favour of a deprivation reversal model of lifestyle and mood where a behaviour, such as smoking a cigarette, is conceptualised as necessary to restore normal mood. Other authors favour a resource model where nicotine, alcohol or whatever is a tool for providing pleasurable mood states (Orford 2001). It is not difficult to envisage that both strategies may be true and function in the same individual in different contexts.

If affect is considered at all within the social cognitive framework it is usually evaluated in terms of how it influences cognitive processes. For instance it has been argued that self-efficacy is increased when people are in a positive mood (Aarts et al. 1997). Alternatively, the relationship between affect and cognition can be conceptualised using a dual-processing framework where both a rational choice decision-making process and a heuristic alternative, such as affect or indeed some other sort of cognition-minimising shortcut are potential decision-making strategies. Finucane et al. (2003) neatly refer to the balance between affective and analytical thinking as 'the dance of affect and reason' and have argued that the emphasis in the dance will be mediated by a wide range of factors including both environmental conditions and individual characteristics. However, it has been argued that, as affective responses are immediate and cognitive decision making strategies are slower, often the affective response dominates (Loewenstein et al. 2001).

One approach to encouraging healthy lifestyle habits would be to try to elicit pleasurable responses to healthy behaviours. If healthy foods are not innately palatable then psychological mechanisms of initiating pleasurable responses could be explored. A similar exploration of what can make other lifestyle behaviours pleasurable may produce useful intervention strategies.

Establishing healthy habits and breaking bad habits

Past behaviour is a powerful predictor of future behaviour (Hagger et al. 2002; Conner and Norman 2007). In social cognitive models past behaviour is argued to influence the cognitive process of decision making by providing positive feedback which improves attitudes and perceived behavioural control. In terms of the TTM when people are in the maintenance stage of behavioural change their behaviour is considered established and as past behaviour is an excellent predictor of future behaviour the continuation of their newly established behaviour should be assured. Consistent patterns of past behaviours are often referred to as habits. Habits can be conceptualised as established patterns of behaviour that may once have been initiated by rational choice but which are now under the control of specific situational cues that trigger the behaviour without cognitive effort. Aarts et al. (1997) defined habitual behaviours as behaviours controlled by mental schemas that elicit specific behavioural patterns whenever specific external stimuli are experienced. Habits are therefore under the direct control of external stimuli rather than cognitive processes. Reasoned action as represented in social cognition models and habit can be considered as two extremes of a conscious decision-making continuum. In between may lie a number of heuristic decision-making strategies that involve varying degrees of cognition.

Many lifestyle behaviours have the potential to be habitual and in extreme cases addictive. Social cognition models may tell us something about the decision to initiate a behaviour. Research now needs to focus on the formation of habits. It is likely that positive feedback is necessary to reproduce a behaviour and develop a habit. Consequently, enjoyment and pleasure may play a central role in the development of habits (Aarts et al. 1997). If established lifestyle behaviours are fundamentally habitual, then health professionals are faced with the related problems of changing negative habits and initiating positive habits. Gollwitzer and Sheeran (2006: 70) have argued that forming 'if-then' plans can diminish the power of negative habits and support the development of the desired positive habitual behaviours.

Persuasion

The central tenet of health promotion in Britain has been one of informed consent and rational choice. Indeed one of the eight tenets of motivational interviewing is to establish that the decision to change is that of the interviewee and that the therapist will not persuade people to make a change. In 1986 WHO argued: 'The essence of health promotion is choice . . . people must be free to refuse' (WHO 1986: 123). UK government policy since the 1980s has followed the lead of WHO by emphasising individual choice. In 2002 the government stated: 'their role is to provide information so that individuals can decide how best to control their own exposure to risk' (Cabinet Office Strategy Unit 2002: 75).

Despite a clear message that lifestyle is one of individual choice, the UK government nevertheless sets itself and its health professionals clear targets to reduce lifestyle disease through the context of lifestyle behaviours (DoH 1999b; www.dh.gov.uk). Health professionals are then faced with a conundrum, providing people with information so that they can make informed choices is having little impact on lifestyle choices, but trying to persuade people through other means is out of line with the implied ethos of choice.

Risk information is often presented in persuasive contexts (Thirlaway and Heggs 2005). Dual process models of persuasion suggest that people can either carefully analyse the message content and arrive at a rational, systematic decision about its validity or they can use other characteristics of the message and its source to arrive at a decision (O'Keefe 2002). Rational systematic decision making is in line with modern concerns of informed consent and with the World Health Organisation's concern that people must be free to choose (WHO 1986). Social cognitive theories that emphasise the role of cognition in decision making also correspond with the rational choice arm of a dual process model of decision making. However, lay analyses of risk messages, health or otherwise, do not usually follow the analytical processes valued by experts (Thirlaway and Heggs 2005). Furthermore, there is evidence from clinical practice that patients who do think systematically about treatment options are more likely to be unsatisfied with the decision they arrive at and are more likely to report depression and/or anxiety during and after treatment (Pierce 1993).

Fear-inducing public health messages are examples of attempts to influence decisions by non-systematic processes, in this instance by inducing affective responses. While fear is often generated the response, as discussed earlier, is seldom behavioural change (Thirlaway and Heggs 2005). While negative, fear-focused, health messages have been less than successful, positive attempts to influence behavioural change via non-systematic processes are less common. It is possible that people may decide to concur with a message because it is delivered by a person they like, trust or find attractive. Some health behavioural messages are now aimed at utilising more positive heuristic strategies to persuade people to alter their behaviour. Images of Bob Monkhouse have been used posthumously to encourage men to be checked for prostate cancer. However, the use of celebrities to endorse healthy eating and moderate drinking is not a common strategy as yet (although some people may recall the use of Daley Thompson by the Milk Marketing Board to promote milk).

For some professionals a less informational more persuasive approach to lifestyle change is an anathema whereas others feel that the cost of adverse lifestyles for society require a more radical approach to behavioural change than has been adopted until now. The companies that promote unhealthy lifestyle choices have no such scruples and utilise many methods of persuasion to market their products vigorously with scant regard for the social consequences. The concept of social marketing has developed in an attempt to compete more effectively with those marketing components of adverse lifestyles.

Social marketing

Social marketing is becoming popular in the promotion of behavioural change. It takes lessons from commercial marketing about techniques that successfully influence consumer behaviour and applies them to health behaviour (Stead et al. 2006). Social marketing does not imply any particular intervention but rather a way of thinking strategically about change. The strategic approach is guided by the stages shown in Figure 9.2.

Defining the problem involves considering all the cultural, economic, societal and other forces that may be causing a particular problem such as binge drinking. Clear objectives ensure there is consensus between all about what is the goal of any planned intervention. Good objectives are measurable and realistic (Hastings et al. 2005). Understanding the consumer is the stage at which social marketing may challenge the current expert-led orthodoxy in which an expert decision is made about the appropriate behavioural goal. For example: 30 minutes of moderate activity on five or more days a week, or five portions of fruit

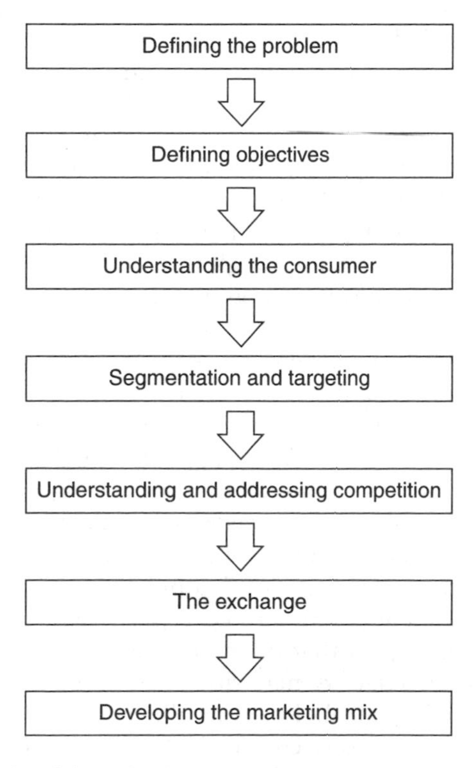

Figure 9.2 Stages of social marketing

and vegetables a day. Traditionally experts set such behavioural targets and health professionals try to promote them (MacFadyen et al. 2003). In Chapter 1 it was argued that lifestyle behaviours have non-health outcomes that may hold more resonance for individuals making choices about their behaviour. By attempting to understand the consumer, the importance of non-health outcomes can be recognised and incorporated into the aims and methods of any intervention.

Segmentation and targeting is a compromise between the ideal situation where every individual would be treated differently and a situation where everyone is treated exactly the same. By grouping people according to the similarity of their needs economic but tailored marketing strategies can be employed. The evidence discussed earlier in this chapter about sporting young men might indicate a potential segment that could be strategically targeted. Stead et al. (2006) argue that a target group should be substantial, accessible and actionable in order to have a realistic chance of meeting the objective of the intervention.

Understanding and addressing the competition can be complex for lifestyle interventions as competition can come from many sources as diverse as fast food outlets, the beverage industry, workplace ethos and the habitual nature of current behaviour which generates inertia for change. However, directly addressing the key 'competition' for any behaviour is postulated to increase the likelihood of success.

The exchange is easy to recognise in terms of products. Consumers exchange money for goods that they want. What respondents to a health intervention get is more difficult to conceptualise. One way of viewing it is to consider that the recipient gets a solution to a problem in exchange for their altered behaviour. However, this requires a number of assumptions. First, that individuals perceive themselves to have a problem, second that they are future orientated enough to wish to change, and third that they have confidence in the efficacy both of the solution and of their ability to perform it.

Finally, in developing a marketing mix the aim is to find a combination of variables that come closest to satisfying the needs of the consumer. This mix needs constant monitoring and review. So for instance initially consumers may not realise they have a problem with unsafe sex. Motivational interviewing and promotional campaigns may establish the recognition of the problem which then needs to be followed up with providing easy access to condoms and developing self-efficacy in condom use. In this way social marketing recognises that behavioural change is a process that will need constant adaptation to keep participants engaged.

Stead et al. (2006) report that interventions based on social marketing principles can be effective. A majority of interventions that sought to prevent youth smoking, alcohol use and illicit drug use were effective in the short term and several tobacco and alçohol interventions still displayed positive effects on behaviour after two years. There was also strong evidence that social marketing can increase fruit and vegetable consumption, rather limited evidence of its effect on fat intake and modest effects for physical activity. Stead et al. (2006: 57) recommend that public health promotion should adopt a target group approach and 'get to know' the problem from their perspective. Furthermore, public health strategies need to recognise the competition to behavioural change in order to make change as easy as possible.

Socio-environmental factors

Adverse environmental conditions are postulated to contribute to deleterious lifestyle choices. The term obesogenic environment is widely used to refer to the physical, economic, social and cultural aspects of the environment that lead to calorific intake being greater than calorific output (Swinburn et al. 1999). Aspects of the environment identified as being obesogenic are factors such as the easy availability of high fat food and the environmental obstacles to active commuting. However, perception of the environment appears to be more important than the environment per se (Jones et al. 2007). Consequently, environmental adaptations will need to be supported by behavioural interventions if positive changes in physical activity are to be acheived. For example, Mutrie et al. (2002) have argued that a significant shift to cycling is unlikely to happen by the provision of cycle routes alone. People may need support to believe that they can use cycle routes, to use the theory of planned behaviour's conceptualisation, improved perceptions of behavioural control will need to be developed by both providing good facilities and demonstrating how they can be utilised. Jones et al. (2007) raised the concern that the current focus on improving the environment to promote active travel may succeed only in encouraging those already cycling or walking regularly. While improving the experience of established walkers and cyclists is a good thing the primary goal is to encourage those who do not walk and cycle to do so. The government is also trying to dismantle the obesogenic nature of the environment from the other side of the energy balance coin. The government has promised to introduce a single, simple food labelling scheme – the traffic light system for food – but this was thwarted by different supermarkets backing different schemes. However, in January 2008 the Food Standards Agency (FSA 2008) commissioned a review of labelling with a hope of persuading the supermarkets to abide by the guidance.

For drinking, the key postulated environmental factors in the uptake and establishment of drinking are access to alcohol and societal acceptance of excess drinking. Despite repeated calls from alcohol addiction specialists (Plant and Plant 2006) for the government to reduce access to alcohol and to increase the price of alcohol, the UK government remains committed to a policy of changing the drinking culture in Britain away from acceptance of drunkenness and towards sensible drinking through non-legislative measures. This failure to act on alcohol has, of course, an impact on other lifestyle behaviours. For example it is well recognised that one of the key risk factors for having unprotected sex is a high level of alcohol (e.g. Celentano et al. 2005).

It is interesting to note that after many years of arguments the UK government has finally been persuaded to introduce smoking bans in public places (see Chapter 6). This has not led to mass riots, nor general discontent with the present government and was viewed as a sensible measure by the majority (ONS 2006a). The question is whether there will be the bravery, the political will and the ideological appreciation to implement any other such 'draconian' environmental measures, although it can be argued that they are ethically justified (Nuffield Council on Bioethics 2007).

Life course issues

Proceeding through the life course has a significant impact on all lifestyle choices. Drinking, smoking and exercising are all less common in older people (DoH 2003; Welsh Assembly Government 2007; Scottish Executive 2005; Department of Health, Social Services and Public Safety 2001). A poor diet is also more common in elderly people (Blaxter 1990). Some of the changes in lifestyle choices over the life course will be in response to physiological changes associated with chronological ageing. However, research has highlighted considerable variability in physiological response to ageing (Lawton 2002). Consequently, a functional age perspective rather than a chronological age perspective is indicated for future research into ageing and lifestyle choices. It is plausible that changing roles and responsibilities are influential in the different choices seen in younger and older people. Chronological age is a rather crude indicator of the roles that people are currently engaged in. People become parents or carers or retire over a wide range of chronological ages. It is possible that certain role changes may be particularly influential on lifestyle choices. The period of change from one role to another may be a particularly pertinent point at which to attempt interventions for lifestyle change. As highlighted earlier, dismantling established habitual behaviours is a challenge for health professionals which may be easier when a new role is starting and fewer external cues for deleterious behaviours are firmly established.

Progressing through the life course is associated with physiological ageing that may be experienced through ill health in oneself or in friends or family. Such reminders of mortality may change the emphasis of lifestyle choice towards health outcomes rather than the non-health outcomes that may have been more pertinent before (Lawton 2002). Health outcomes may be expected to take a more central role for individuals as they move through the life course. Consequently, it might be expected that social cognitive based interventions that focus on health outcomes may be more effective in older people. There is some evidence of this from the Scottish Health Survey where interventions to increase physical activity have been most effective in older people (Scottish Executive 2005). Consequently, it is argued that life course should take a central place in any comprehensive model of lifestyle change.

Ecological models of lifestyle change

Ecological models of health behaviour are argued to both focus attention on environmental causes of behaviour and also highlight the multiple levels of influence on health behaviour (Sallis and Owen 2002). Ecological models specify that intrapersonal, sociocultural factors, policies and physical environments can all influence lifestyle behaviours. Across all lifestyle behaviours the value of multilevel interventions has been demonstrated (Kahn et al. 2002; Prochaska et al. 2004). Well developed models will specify not only what variables are important for behavioural change but also how they interact to promote or impede behavioural change. For instance, it has been articulated that it is perception of the environment, rather than the objective environment that best predicts physical activity (Jones et al. 2007) (Figure 9.3). Although ecological models are postulated to be the best way forward for all aspects of lifestyle change, behaviour-specific ecological models are likely to be warranted. Although psychological aspects of behavioural change are consistent across many lifestyle behaviours environmental variables are often behaviour specific, with the accessibility of condoms having no relevance for the promotion of physical activity. Jones et al. (2007) present an ecological model of the determinants of physical activity which is particularly interesting because of the importance it gives to the lifecourse (Figure 9.3). Broad concepts may be identified in general lifestyle ecological models but specific concepts will require identification for specific behaviours. It is easy see how the broad framework adopted by Jones et al. (2007) for physical activity could be utilised with other lifestyle behaviours. General socio-economic conditions and the lifecourse are key axes within which the specific determinants of each lifestyle behaviour must operate.

Conclusion

The challenge now for lifestyle psychology is first, to develop behaviour-specific ecological models of lifestyle change, and second, to identify the generic psychological skills that are relevant to all lifestyles and the appropriate ways to apply these differentially for individuals at different stages in their lives within different socio-economic and environmental contexts.

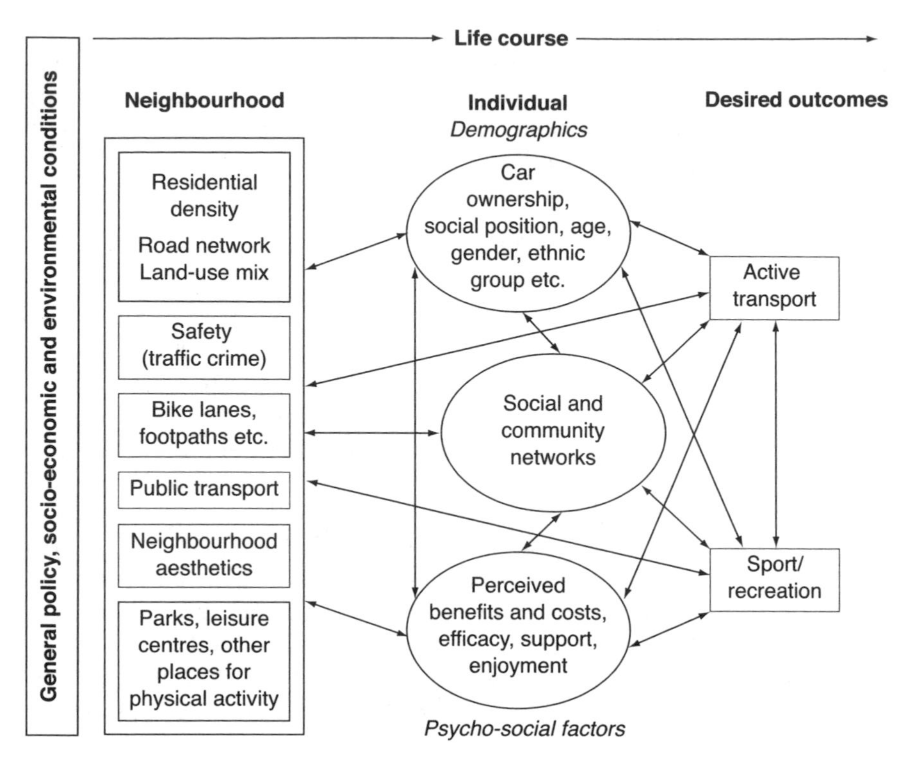

Figure 9.3 Evidence-informed model of the potential determinants of sport and physical activity
(Adapted from Jones et al. 2007)

Summary points

- Health promotion has successfully communicated the basis of a healthy lifestyle. The majority of people in the UK understand what constitutes a healthy lifestyle.
- Further education and risk communication is unlikely to promote major population lifestyle change
- Self-efficacy and perceived behavioural control are key psychological constructs that can enable positive lifestyle change.
- Motivational interviewing has been successful in supporting behavioural change.
- Many lifestyle behaviours are habitual and the mechanisms that underpin the development and maintenance of habitual behaviours need further exploration.
- Goal setting, self-regulation and implementation intentions are key psychological strategies that can empower behavioural change.

- Enjoyment is a key factor in the development and maintenance of lifestyle behaviours.
- Less cognitively based persuasive messages may be more effective in promoting behavioural change than more traditional information-based campaigns.
- Lifestyle behaviours have both health and non-health outcomes and the relative importance of these outcomes to individuals may change during the lifecourse.
- The wider social, cultural and physical environment may be influential in lifestyle choice but this effect will be mediated by perceptual processes and will not be a direct effect of the objective reality.

10 Strategies for the twenty-first century

At the end of this chapter you will:

- appreciate the arguments between libertarians and interventionists
- understand the current policy arguments and the developments that have occurred in this area
- appreciate the demands of the delivery of policy and the personnel most involved in behaviour change
- understand the role of the individual in changing their own behaviour
- explore the role of research and areas for further investigation.

Health professionals promoting evidence-based strategies for lifestyle change face fierce criticism and fierce competition from many sources, many of whom base their critiques and alternative solutions on personal experience. Dominic Lawson in the *Independent* (19 October 2007) has argued that the humiliation of being unable to purchase 42-inch waist trousers in Peter Jones drove him to lose weight and that stigmatising obesity is the way to get people to lose weight. Janet Street-Porter in the *Independent on Sunday* (27 January 2008) claimed that obesity is 'a result of wilful self-abuse'.

Both Dominic Lawson and Janet Street-Porter were opposed to any strategy that limits personal choice and both refer to the dangers of a 'nanny state'. However, Street-Porter had changed her mind a month later and was proposing rationing of sugar, chocolate, fats and salt (*Independent on Sunday*, 24 February 2008). Street-Porter also feels qualified to comment on drinking. She confidently stated, in direct contradiction to the research evidence (Room 2004), that 'there is absolutely no evidence that making drink more expensive will have any effect on the number of people getting slaughtered night after night' (Street-Porter, *Independent on Sunday*, 24 February 2008).

It is the job of columnists like Janet Street-Porter and Dominic Lawson to write controversial text. They are paid to generate controversy. On the one hand it is encouraging that lifestyle diseases and lifestyle behaviours are finally getting media coverage and that the health problems that arise from unsafe sex, binge drinking and so on are front page news. It was not long ago that Harrabin et al. (2003) were voicing concern at the media's lack of interest in lifestyle diseases. However, everybody is an expert on lifestyle, and alongside the columnists creating controversy are a plethora of lay persons offering health and lifestyle advice that ranges from the ill advised to the positively dangerous. It is impressive that key government health messages are so well understood in the population given the multitudes of health messages, both appropriate and inappropriate, that are reported through the media each day (Thirlaway and Heggs 2005).

Policy

Prevention of lifestyle diseases through promoting healthy lifestyle choices has been a central tenet of health policy in the UK since 1999 (DoH 1999b). The government faces two interrelated challenges. First, it needs to change the established lifestyle habits of the current generation of adults, and second, it needs to prevent the next generation of adults establishing similar or worse lifestyle habits. Lifestyle policy in the UK addresses these two issues by attempting to modify cultural norms: 'we need to work together to shape an environment that actively promotes sensible drinking' (HM Government 2007: 5).

> cultures exist where being active or eating 'healthy' foods are not top priorities. No matter how good the availability of high-quality food outlets and leisure facilities may be in the vicinity, certain individuals may never use them. The behaviour of these individuals may be the most difficult to modify due to both the difficulties in reaching them and overcoming their norms.
>
> (Jones et al. 2007: 38)

Changing cultural norms could both establish healthy lifestyle habits from the outset and make it easier for individuals to change established unhealthy lifestyles. Lifestyle policy clearly aims to direct cultural trends (DoH 1999b; HM Government 2007; Jones et al. 2007) but is itself a product of our history and culture. Every level of intervention proposed by the Nuffield Council on Bioethics (2007) has been utilised in the attempt to encourage positive lifestyle change (see Table 10.1) but the rationale for the levels of interventions utilised are not objectively or theoretically derived but instead reflect our historical and contemporary cultural and political climate. For example, illicit drugs are banned substances and include drugs such as cannabis and cocaine. Nicotine and alcohol are equally deleterious for health, and alcohol has behavioural consequences on a par with many illicit drugs but neither is illegal. The social acceptability of alcohol and the social unacceptability of illicit drugs have little to do with the properties of the

Table 10.1 The intervention ladder

Level	*Description*
Eliminate choice	Introduce laws that entirely eliminate choice
Restrict choice	Introduce laws that restrict the options available to people
Guide through disincentives	Introduce financial or other disincentives to influence behaviour
Guide through incentives	Introduce financial or other incentives to influence people's behaviour
Guide choices	Changing the default policy
Enable choice	Help individuals to change their behaviour

(Adapted from Nuffield Council on Bioethics 2007)

drugs in question and more to do with our long history of alcohol consumption and the value of alcohol as a commodity (Babor et al. 2003). The opening statement of *Safe. Sensible. Social.* (HM Government 2007) makes it clear that alcohol is seen as a primarily positive aspect of society despite the severe behavioural and health consequences the same document goes on to report: 'Alcohol can play an important and positive role in British culture' (HM Government 2007: 5).

Banning adverse lifestyle substances such as alcohol, nicotine or high-fat foods is not proposed here as a serious or sensible solution to excess drinking, smoking or poor diets. The banning of illicit drugs may have reduced the incidence of drug use in the population, compared to alcohol or nicotine use, but introduces other problems that arise from making a substance illegal, such as quality control, unsafe consumption practices, increased likelihood and extent of smuggling and other associated criminal activities.

For various reasons policy-driven interventions to support healthy lifestyles are not consistent across the lifestyle behaviours discussed in this book. The level of individual choice permitted varies considerably. People who use illicit drugs are breaking the law and run the risk of imprisonment. Nicotine is the next most strictly controlled substance in the UK: the recent legislation in England, Wales, Scotland and Northern Ireland has banned smoking in public places. Conversely, laws about drinking in public places have recently been eased. The Licensing Act 2005 removed blanket pub closing times in an attempt to encourage a more relaxed southern European-style drinking culture and reduce alcohol-related social disorder. According to a Home Office Review (Hough et al. 2007) there are no clear signs that the abolition of a standard closing time has significantly reduced alcohol-related crime and disorder. However, the chaos feared by those opposed to the new legislation has also not materialised. The net result of legislation, that both those in favour and those against believed would significantly impact on British drinking culture,

appears to be minimal. It is possible that in the longe
changes may occur, as cultural shifts can take time t

Laws that eliminate or restrict lifestyle choices are
protect others from harm not the individuals them
people can no longer smoke in a public place to prot
under the influence of alcohol is illegal. Other than
underage sex, the government does not interver
choices in order to protect individuals from self-h
commentators, health and non-health professionals,
UK government should restrict access to, and increase the cost of, harmful substances such as alcohol and fast food. There is considerable evidence that decreasing the availability and increasing the cost of alcohol would deter young people from drinking it (Room 2004; Plant and Plant 2006). Similar arguments can be made for unhealthy food (Jones et al. 2007). Until recently, the UK government has resisted calls for higher taxes on high fat foods and alcohol, preferring to cooperate with the beverage and food industry (HM Government 2007). However, growing concerns about 'Britain's binge-drinking culture' (*Daily Mail* 2008) have driven the UK government to consider raising the price of alcohol (*Independent*, 7 June 2008). While political parties are considering raising the price of alcohol, at the time of publication no additional taxes have been imposed on alcoholic beverages.

Critics of such interventionist policies (including Janet Street-Porter and Dominic Lawson) have argued that such measures are 'nanny statist' and an unnecessary intrusion into people's personal lives. The current UK government, and the official Opposition, distance themselves from such interventionist attitudes. However, this debate about the limits to state freedom and public health is not new. Libertarians have long argued that minimal state intervention is the way to protect individual freedom. For example, a commentator suggested that the original Public Health Act 1848 was 'paternalistic' and 'despotic' and 'a little dirt and freedom' was 'more desirable than no dirt at all and slavery' (Porter 1985).

It also appears as if there are some differences between the four UK countries in their approach to individual freedom. For example, the Welsh Assembly voted for smoke-free public places in 2003 but was unable to implement it, the Scottish Parliament passed legislation in 2005 but it was not until 2006 that England followed suit with considerable debate and lack of consensus among the two main political parties. Given the agonising over restricting a practice that is proven to be dangerous to other people, it seems unlikely the government will intervene with restrictive bans in other lifestyle behaviours where the danger to other people cannot be conclusively proven. However, as mentioned previously, the increasing concern about excessive heavy drinking means that increasing the cost of alcohol to curb drinking is being seriously debated for the first time in recent history (*Daily Mail* 2008; *Independent* 2008).

ne other end of the intervention ladder (Table 10.1) the govern-
emains committed to a policy of guiding choice despite the irrefu-
e evidence across all lifestyle behaviours that educational and risk
ommunication messages do not have any significant effect on lifestyle choices (Floyd et al. 2000; Milne et al. 2000; Ruiter 2004; Taubman Ben-Ari et al. 2005; Blue 2007). Nevertheless, in 2007 the government stated that it was committed to: 'Better education and communication' (HM Government 2007: 5).

The exasperation of many academics with policies that continue to ignore evidenced-based recommendations has been well articulated by Room (2004):

> where preventative measures are ranked roughly on the evidence of their effectiveness, there is an almost total correspondence between the measures proposed in the strategy recommendations and the measures that are ranked in the listing as 'ineffective'.
>
> (Room 2004: 1084)

A generous interpretation of this policy position is that the government is committed to individual choice as articulated by the World Health Organisation:

> The essence of health promotion is choice. If, in the process of promoting lifestyles conducive to health one tyranny, i.e. undue emphasis on health, is substituted for another, then the whole process will have failed. People must be free to refuse.
>
> (WHO 1986: 123)

A more cynical explanation of the government's refusal to legislate either by banning, restricting or taxing dangerous lifestyle substances such as smoking or alcohol is that it is unduly influenced by the hospitality industries (Babor et al. 2003; Room 2004; Plant and Plant 2006). This opinion is endorsed by Alcohol Concern who stated that legislation was: 'dangerously tilted towards the needs of the drinks industry' (Soodeen and Shenker 2008).

A similar argument can be made for the promotion of active transport. It has been focused on enabling individuals to be active rather than stopping them driving. The positive interpretation is that they are supporting individual choice; the more negative explanation is that they are unduly influenced by the car industry.

Enabling choice through developing life skills is an intervention where both the government and health professionals are agreed that progress can be made (McPearson 1992; Ashton and Seymour 1988, cited in Hansen and Easthope 2007), although appropriate funding for such interventions is limited (Room 2004).

In conclusion, it is clear that UK government lifestyle policies are many and varied and influenced by both health and non-health considerations. While totally banning substances can cause as many problems as it solves, there is considerable evidence that restricting the availability and increasing the cost of deleterious beverages and food would improve health. At the moment the government is not considering such tactics. However, it is important to continue to press for such interventions. It did not seem likely a decade before it happened that smoking in public places would be banned.

Policy documents have a clear focus on changing our lifestyle culture. Attempts to develop a culture of sensible drinking have been a dismal failure and young women are actually drinking more than ever. Cultural norms can be modified; drink-driving is no longer considered an acceptable behaviour and drink-related road accidents have been reduced. Smoking in public places is no longer acceptable and the move to this position was not nearly as contentious as was feared (ONS 2006a). However, all these cultural shifts have been supported by clear legislation; it is unlikely that health promotion alone will change lifestyle culture.

Heath professionals and policy makers now recognise that individuals cannot be left to take sole responsibility for their lifestyle choices and considerable interest has been shown in the concept of an obesogenic environment and methods of tackling it. It is encouraging to see that health and transport are working together to encourage active transport but it is clear that modifications to the environment must be supported by psychological interventions that provide people with the motivation and self-efficacy to utilise improved environments. Jones et al. (2007) argue that to increase activity it is necessary to 'create cultures of participation'. They conclude:

> It is certainly the case that changes to the environment alone are unlikely to solve the problems of increasing obesity and declining physical activity levels. Successfully tackling these issues will undoubtedly require a range of approaches, and complementary strategies addressing the individual, social and environmental determinants of activities may be a solution.
>
> (Jones et al. 2007: 39)

In summary, future policy should consider:

- increasing the price and reducing the availability of unhealthy food and alcoholic beverages
- supporting positive changes to the environment with psychological interventions which give people the confidence to use new facilities
- providing funding for theoretically based behavioural change interventions that focus on motivation and self-efficacy

- reducing the focus on educational and public information campaigns
- funding long-term evaluation of intervention strategies to inform future strategy
- adopting a policy of providing financial support only for evidence-based interventions
- whenever possible utilising multilevel interventions that address the individual, social and environmental determinants of lifestyle simultaneously.

Delivery of policy

The UK government has set many targets around reducing the incidence of lifestyle diseases and its main strategy to achieve these goals is to increase healthy and decrease unhealthy lifestyle choices. However, it is not entirely clear who is responsible for delivering these choices. In the alcohol policy document *Safe. Sensible. Social.* (HM Government 2007) virtually all public servants – the police, local authorities, the NHS, schools and voluntary organisations – are tasked with delivering the government's strategy. Furthermore, the government also identifies the alcohol industry and the wider business industry, the media and local communities as having a role to play in delivering its strategy. However, who is to deliver the behavioural change component of this strategy, which receives scant attention in the document but has the clearest evidence base as to its efficacy, is not addressed (Poikolainen 1999; Moyer et al. 2002; Mulvihill et al. 2005; Williams et al. 2007). Similarly, various public servants and businesses are involved in the promotion of healthy eating and physical activity but the central question of who should deliver the essential behavioural change component of the strategy remains unclear.

The principal candidates for the delivery of behavioural change interventions are primary care practitioners: general practitioners, practice nurses, health visitors and other associated health care professionals (Ashenden et al. 1997). Primary care has been central in the delivery of individual lifestyle advice for some time, and there is conflicting evidence about whether merely advising individuals to change their lifestyle can lead to lifestyle change (Ashenden et al. 1997; Moyer et al. 2002). However, it is clear that a psychologically based intervention is more likely to be successful (Biddle et al. 1997; Moyer et al. 2002). Biddle et al. (1997) reported that general practitioners were more involved in promoting physical activity than previously, primarily through exercise referral schemes. However, NICE (2006b) has concluded that there is no evidence that exercise referral schemes increased physical activity in participants. This is no great surprise; Biddle et al. (1997) nearly a decade earlier had argued that practice-managed physical activity schemes were more likely to be more successful than exercise referral schemes. Regardless of this warning exercise referral schemes have received the most support.

If primary care practitioners are to deliver psychologically based lifestyle interventions, they will need training and additional resources. However, the evidence presented in this book suggests that a single set of generic psychological techniques will be appropriate to encourage change in a range of lifestyle behaviours. Therefore, health professionals with training in delivering brief interventions for drinking may already have the skills to deliver brief interventions in other lifestyle behaviours.

In England, a new initiative to promote lifestyle change has been launched. Health trainers with a specific remit of promoting healthy lifestyles in the community are being trained in psychological behavioural techniques and employed to work in the community. These health trainers are being taught the key psychological techniques identified in this text to enable them to support individuals in the community to adopt healthy lifestyle habits. In essence, accredited health trainers will be trained to help people:

> Learn how to watch for things around them that can trigger or reinforce the behaviour they want to change;
>
> Set goals and plan how to achieve them;
>
> Build confidence to make the changes that they want to.
>
> (Michie et al. 2006: 4)

In this way, the training for health trainers will focus on recognising habitual behaviours, building motivation, encouraging self-regulation and increasing self-efficacy, which are the key aspects of lifestyle change identified in this text. The involvement of health psychologists in the development of the key competencies associated with this role has been a positive step forward in establishing the importance of psychology for effective health promotion and lifestyle change, but many other health professionals will still need to address lifestyle change with their patients. In order to deliver effect preventative lifestyle interventions, health practitioners will need a range of resources and skills. First, they will need to be able to measure current lifestyle behaviours quickly and reliably and to recognise individuals who have severe problems that need referral to a specialist. For example, they need to be able to distinguish between heavy and dependent drinkers and refer the dependent drinkers to an addiction specialist. They need to be able to recognise when individuals are in such poor health initially that an exercise programme could be introduced only under expert supervision. Similarly, they need to be able to recognise individuals who may have eating disorders. Many questionnaires are available to measure the various lifestyle behaviours. A consensus as to which should be utilised to inform preventative interventions needs to be reached as a matter of urgency. Measurement tools will need to be brief, reliable and valid if they are to be effective tools for primary care settings. Some progress in this area has been made in alcohol consumption. The UK government recommends the use of either the Alcohol Use Disorders Identification Test (AUDIT) or the briefer version of the AUDIT, the Fast Alcohol Screening Test (FAST) (HM Government 2007).

Health professionals who wish to enable the patients they work with to change their lifestyle need to take cognisance of the fact that providing people with information about the risks of unhealthy lifestyles will not result in lifestyle change. If health professionals wish to encourage lifestyle change they should be looking to increase self-motivation, increase self-regulatory skills, set achievable goals and increase self-efficacy in their clients. The template for brief interventions in drinking may well provide a useful template for interventions in other behaviours. Many health professionals may require training in order to support lifestyle change. There are training courses available in various appropriate psychological techniques but limited training tailored to lifestyle behavioural change. Spanou (2008) is currently evaluating the effectiveness of behavioural change counselling (BCC), which is specifically designed to encourage lifestyle change based on the principles of readiness, confidence and importance. The key psychological principles that underpin this approach are motivation and self-efficacy. This study is called 'Preventing disease through opportunistic, rapid, engagement by primary care teams using behavioural change counselling' (PRE-EMPT) and aims to evaluate whether exposing practitioners to blended learning of BCC will result in patients making more positive lifestyle changes. The results of this study will make an important contribution to the decision of how to encourage lifestyle change and the training required.

Individuals

There are many individuals who would like to change their lifestyle and have no idea where to find appropriate advice and support. Individuals who wish to change their lifestyle would be advised to find a professional to support them who is trained in behavioural change. However, for many individuals access to such professionals is difficult and in that case they may try to change their behaviour without professional support.

The key factors involved in successful behavioural change are the following:

- *Self-motivation:* it is important to want to change your behaviour. Trying to change your behaviour because you believe you should or someone else wants you to is unlikely to succeed.

- *Belief:* people who believe they can change their behaviour are the most likely to do so. Linked to the issue of self-belief is that of goal setting.
- *Goal-setting:* many people fail to change their behaviour because they set unrealistic goals. Even if you are determined to make a large change you should spilt it up into a number of smaller steps and focus on each step at a time.
- *Implementation:* most behavioural change goals involve replacing one habit with a healthier one. Habits are automatic responses to external stimuli. For instance; if you always have a biscuit with a coffee you will need to have a well-rehearsed alternative strategy to prevent this habit persisting. You need an implementation plan such as: 'When I have a cup of tea I will eat a low-fat cracker rather than a digestive biscuit'.

Research

We are at a turning point in health promotion. The ineffectiveness of the previous decades of educational interventions is irrefutable and policy makers and health professionals are both starting to recognise the importance of psychological processes in lifestyle change. Fortunately, psychology is a discipline with a strong record of high quality research and we are already in a position to provide evidenced-based advice about appropriate psychological interventions. Lifestyle behaviours are extremely varied but nevertheless the same psychological constructs are relevant to promoting change in them all. The potential opportunity to develop training and protocols for interventions that can be applied across all lifestyle behaviours should not be ignored. A recognition of a subdiscipline of lifestyle psychology could support a unified approach to lifestyle change. Future research in the area of lifestyle change will need to work within the key axes of the social, cultural and physical environment and the lifecourse (Figure 9.3). Very different psychological factors may be relevant for individuals at different points between these axes. Research will need to be multidisciplinary. Disciplines as wide ranging as urban policy makers and dieticians will need to work with lifestyle psychologists to ensure that the changes they make or the advice they give are utilised by individuals.

Social cognitive models of behavioural change have been central in identifying key factors involved in successful initiation of behavioural change. However, they are less useful for understanding habitual behaviour. The deleterious health outcomes associated with lifestyle behaviours are primarily chronic. They arise from persistent unhealthy choices over a long time period. Consequently, habitual lifestyle choices are the primary concern for public health. Research now needs to consider the mechanisms behind the establishment of habitual behaviours. Self-regulation and implementation intentions are both promising avenues in the pursuit of interventions that can support long-term lifestyle change. Behaviours need to be repeated frequently and regularly if they are to become habitual. Behaviours that are enjoyed are more likely to be repeated. Pleasure and enjoyment are key aspects of lifestyle choices. While some pleasures are innate, such as sweet food, there is a learnt element to enjoyment that is worth exploring.

Lifestyle choices vary over the lifecourse. Many studies attest to the reduction of unhealthy choices as people age. What makes people alter their choices as they age is not clear. Some changes may be a response to chronological ageing, others may be a response to a change of role. Lawson (2002) has argued that people change their behaviour reactively as their health deteriorates and the potential risks of unhealthy lifestyle choices become reality. The impact of progressing through the lifecourse on the role of psychological factors in lifestyle choice may well be key in identifying tailored strategies for lifestyle change.

Key areas for future research in lifestyle psychology include the following issues:

- We need to establish a range of reliable and valid measures of lifestyle activity so that practitioners can readily identify people who are in need of help. Consistent measurement criteria across interventions would make for easier evaluation of interventions.
- A reliable and valid tool for establishing levels of self-efficacy in lifestyle change is required.
- Research needs to identify the best mechanisms for increasing self-efficacy and to establish whether generic techniques to increase self-efficacy are equally effective across all lifestyle behaviours.
- The role of implementation intentions in behavioural change needs to be established.
- The effectiveness of implementation intentions in establishing habitual behaviours needs investigation.
- The role of descriptive norms in eating, smoking, physical activity, safe sex and drug taking needs to be established.
- The impact of progressing through the lifecourse on the relevance of health outcomes for individuals needs to be established.
- The role of family-based interventions for all lifestyle behaviours needs investigations.
- The relationship between actual environment and perceived environment on lifestyle choices needs to be evaluated.
- Multilevel interventions with a comprehensive scheme of evaluation need funding.
- Long-term evaluation of all interventions is required.

Conclusion

This final chapter recognises the key role of public policy in the promotion of healthy lifestyle. It stresses that there is a tension between the libertarian perspective currently predominant in our society and the evidence that a more interventionist approach to public health policy can have a significant impact on health and well-being. The focus of health policy, as many have stressed, should now be on the protection of health rather than the treatment of illness. Preventative policies need to be put into practice which requires health care professionals and individuals to make a commitment to lifestyle change. Motivation and self-efficacy have been established as key cognitive factors in successful lifestyle change. We need to explore further the role of non-cognitive factors such as habitual responses and enjoyment in the establishment of lifestyle choices. We need to develop research protocols, evidence-based interventions and strategies that can extend our understanding and implementation of successful lifestyle change. People do not usually make initial lifestyle choices based on future health implications and by the time they wish to protect their health need to overcome well established bad habits. Ultimately, it would be better if people established healthy lifestyles at the outset but if they wish to change we need to give them the resources to do so and help them believe that they can.

Summary points

- There are a wide range of views on lifestyle; everyone is an expert.
- There is a tension between libertarian and interventionist approaches to public health.
- Restricting lifestyle choices can play an important role in promoting health and reducing the long-term consequences on health.
- Health care professionals have a key role in promoting behaviour change.
- Lifestyle psychology can play a central role in the development of a healthy society.

References

Aarts, H., Paulussen, T. and Schaalma, H. (1997) Physical exercise habit: on the conceptualization and formation of habitual health behaviours. *Health Education Research* 21, 363–374.

Abraham, C.S. and Sheeran, P. (2005) The health belief model. In: M. Conner and P. Norman (eds) *Predicting Health Behaviour*. Berkshire: Open University Press.

Abraham, C.S., Sheeran, P., Abrams, D. and Spears, R. (1994) Exploring teenagers adaptive and maladaptive thinking in relation to the threat of HIW infection. *Psychology and Health* 9, 253–272.

Abraham, C., Krahé, B., Dominic, R. and Fritsche, I. (2002) Does research into the social cognitive antecedents of action contribute to health promotion? A content analysis of safer-sex promotion leaflets. *British Journal of Health Psychology, 7,* 227–246.

Abrahamsson, A., Springett, J., Karlsson, L. and Ottosson, T. (2005) Making sense of the challenge of smoking cessation during pregnancy: a phenomenographic approach. *Health Education Research* 20(3), 367–378.

Academy of Medical Sciences (2004) *Calling Time: The Nation's Drinking as a Health Issue.* London: Academy of Medical Sciences.

Acheson, D. (1998) *Independent Inquiry into Inequalities in Health.* London: Stationery Office.

Adams, K.F., Schatzkin, A., Harris, T.B., Kipnis, V., Mouw, T., Ballard-Barbash, R. et al. (2006) Overweight, obesity and mortality in a large prospective cohort of persons 50–71 years old. *New England Journal of Medicine* 355, 763–778.

Addley, K., McQuillan, P. and Ruddle, M. (2001) Creating healthy workplaces in Northern Ireland: evaluation of a lifestyle and physical activity programme. *Occupational Medicine*, 51, 439–449.

Adimora, A.A. and Schoenbach, V.J. (2005) Social context, sexual networks, and racial disparities in rates of sexually transmitted infections. *Journal Infectious Diseases* 191 (suppl 1), S115–122.

Agronick, G., O'Donnell, L., Stueve, A., San Doval, A., Duran, R. and Vargo, S. (2004) Sexual behaviours and risks among bisexually and gay-identified young Latino men. *AIDS and Behaviour*, 8(2), 185–197.

Ahluwalia, J.S., Nollen, N., Kaur, H., James, A.S. and Mayo, M.S. (2007) Pathways to health: Cluster-randomized trial to increase fruit and vegetable consumption among smokers in public housing. *Health Psychology* 26, 214–221.

Ajzen, I. (1985) From intention to actions: a theory of planned behaviour. In: J. Kuhl and J. Beckman (eds), *Action-Control: From Cognition to Behaviour.* Retrieved 20 December 2007 from http://www.people.umass.edu/aizen/publications.html.

Ajzen, I. (1988) *Attitudes, Personality and Behaviour*. Chicago: Dorsey Press

Ajzen, I. (1991) The theory of planned behavior. *Organizational Behavior and Human Decision Processes*, 50, 179–211.

Ajzen, I. (1998) Models of human social behaviour and their application to health psychology. *Psychology and Health* 13, 735–739.

Ajzen, I. (2001) Nature and operation of attitudes. *Annual Review of Psychology* 5, 27–58.

Ajzen, I., Timko, C. and White, J.B. (1982) Self-monitoring and the attitude–behavior relationship. *Journal of Personality and Social Psychology*, 42, 426–435.

Akers, R.L. (1977) *Deviant Behaviour: A Social Learning Approach*, 2nd edn, Belmont, California: Wadsworth Publishing Company.

Albanes, D., Jones, Y., Micozzi, M. and Mattson, M. (1987) Associations between smoking and body weight in the US population. *American Journal of Public Health* 77, 439–444.

Albarracin, D., Johnson, B.T., Fishbein, M. and Muellerleile, P. (2001) Theories of reasoned action and planned behavior as models of condom use: a meta-analysis. *Psychological Bulletin* 127, 142–161.

Alcohol Concern (2007) Factsheet: Young people's drinking. London: Alcohol Concern. Accessed 18 December 2007 at: http://www.alcoholconcern.org.uk/files/20070809_ 170143_Young%20people%20summary%20%20July%202007.pdf.

Alderson, T. and Ogden, J. (1999) What do mothers feed their children and why? *Health Education Research* 14(6), 717–727.

Ali, N.A. (2002) Prediction of coronary heart disease preventative behaviours in women: a test of the health belief model. *Women and Health* 35, 83–96.

American College of Sports Medicine (2005) *ACSM's Guidelines for exercise testing and prescription*. Philadelphia, PA: Lippincott, Williams & Wilkins.

American College of Sports Medicine (2007) Updated Physical Activity Guidelines. www.acsm.org accessed September 2007.

American Psychiatric Association (APA) (1987) *Diagnostic and Statistical Manual of Mental Disorders (DSM-IIIR)* 3rd edn, revised. Washington DC: American Psychiatric Association.

American Psychiatric Association (APA) (1994) *Diagnostic and Statistical Manual of Mental Disorders (DSM-IV)* 4th edn. Washington, DC: American Psychiatric Association.

Ames, G.M. and Grube, J.W. (2000) Social control and workplace drinking norms: a comparison of two organisational cultures. *Journal of Studies in Alcohol* 61, 203–219.

Amirkhanian, Y.A., Kelly, J.A. and McAuliffe, T.L. (2005) Identifying, recruiting, and assessing social networks at high risk for HIV AIDS: methodology, practice, and a case study in St Petersburg, Russia. *AIDS Care* 17, 58–75.

Anderson, A. (2002) Lifestyle interventions – how joined up are we? *Journal of Human Nutrition and Dietetics* 15, 241–242.

Anderson, J., Santelli, J. and Morrow, B. (2003) Trends in adolescent contraceptive use, unprotected and poorly protected sex, 1991–2003, *Journal of Adolescent Health* 38 (6), 734–739.

Anderson, J.V., Bybee, D.I., Brown, R.M., McLean, D.F., Garcia, E.M., Breer, M.L. and Schillo, B.A. (2001) 5 a day fruit and vegetable intervention improves consumption in a low income population. *Journal of the American Dietetic Association* 101, 195–202.

Anderson, P. (1993) Effectiveness of general practice interventions for patients with harmful alcohol consumption. *British Journal of General Practice* 43(374), 386–389.

Anderson, P., Cremona, A., Paton, A., Turner, C. and Wallace, P. (1993) The risk of alcohol. *Addiction* 88, 1493–1508.

Anderson, A.S., Cox, D.N., Mckellar, S., Reynolds, J., Lean, M.E.J. and Mela, D.J. (1998) Take Five, a nutrition education intervention to increase fruit and vegetable intakes: impact on attitudes towards dietary change. *British Journal of Nutrition* 80(2), 133–140.

Andreasen, A.R. (2002) Marketing social marketing in the social change marketplace. *Journal of Public Policy and Marketing* 21(1), 3–13.

Andreasen, A. R. (2006) *Social Marketing in the 21st Century*. Thousand Oaks, CA: Sage.

Anliker, J.A., Bartoshuk, L., Ferris, A.M. and Hooks, L.D. (1991) Children's food preferences and genetic sensitivity to the bitter taste of 6-n-propylthioouracil (prop) *American Journal of Clinical Nutrition* 54, 316–320.

Annandale, E. and Hunt, K. (2000) *Gender Inequalities in Health*. Buckingham: Open University Press.

Anthonisen, N. R., Skeans, M. A., Wise, R. A., Manfreda, J., Kanner, R. E. and Connett, J.E. (2005) The effects of a smoking cessation programme on survival in smokers with mild lung disease. *Annals of Internal Medicine* 142, 233–239.

Arent, S.M., Landers, D.M. and Etrier, J.L. (2000) The effects of exercise on mood in older adults: a meta-analysis review. *Journal of Aging and Physical Activity* 8, 407–430.

Armitage, C.J. and Conner, M. (2001) Efficacy of the Theory of Planned Behaviour: A meta-analytic review. *British Journal of Social Psychology* 40(4), 471–499.

Armitage, C.J., Conner, M., Loach, J. and Willets, D. (1999) Different perceptions of control: applying an extended theory of planned behaviour to legal and illegal drug use. *Basic and Applied Social Psychology* 21, 301–316.

Armstrong, C., Sallis, J., Hovell, M. and Hofstetter, C.R. (1993) Stages of change, self-efficacy and the adoption of vigorous exercise: a prospective analysis. *Journal of Sport and Exercise Psychology* 15, 390–402.

Armstrong, D. (1983) *The Political Anatomy of the Body: Medical Knowledge in the Twentieth Century*. Cambridge: Cambridge University Press.

Arnett, J.J. (2000) Optimistic bias in adolescent and adult smokers and nonsmokers. *Addictive Behaviors* 25(4), 625–632.

Ary, D., Tildseley, E., Hops, H. and Andrews, J. (1993) The influences of parents, siblings and peer modelling and attitudes on adolescent use of alcohol. *International Journal of Addictions* 28, 853–880.

ASH (2008) *Essential Information: Who Smokes and How Much*. London: ASH.

Ashenden, R., Silagy, C. and Weller, D. (1997) A systematic review of the effectiveness of promoting lifestyle change in general practice. *Family Practice* 14, 160–174.

Ashton, J. and Seymour, H. (1988) *The New Public Health: The Liverpool Experience*. Milton Keynes: Open University Press.

Astrom, A.N. and Okullo, I. (2004) Temporal stability of the Theory of Planned Behaviour: a prospective analysis of sugar consumption among Ugandan adolescents. *Community Dentistry and Oral Epidemiology* 32 (6), 426–434. Retrieved 20 December 2007 from Academic Search Premier.

Aveyard, P. and West, R. (2007) Managing smoking cessation. *British Medical Journal* 335, 37–41.

Axelson, M.L., Federline, T.L. and Brinberg, D. (1985) A meta-analysis of food and nutrition related research. *Journal of Nutrition Education* 17, 51–54.

Babor, T., Caetano, R., Casswell, S., Edwards, G., Giesbrecht, N., Graham, K. et al. (2003) *Alcohol: No Ordinary Commodity*. Oxford: Oxford University Press.

Bachanas, P.J., Morris, M.K., Lewis-Gess, J.K. et al. (2002) Predictors of risky sexual behavior in African American adolescent girls: implications for prevention interventions. *Journal of Pediatric Psychology* 27(6), 519–530.

Bajekal, M., Primatesta, P. and Prior, G. (2003) *Health Survey for England 2001*. London: The Stationery Office.

Baker, A. H. and Wardle, J. (2003) Sex differences in fruit and vegetable intake in older adults. *Appetite* 40(3), 269–275.

Bakker, F. and Vanwesenbeeck, I. (2002) *Veilig vrijen en condoomgebruik bij jongeren en jongvolwassenen* [Safe sex and condom use among adolescents and young adults]. Utrecht, The Netherlands: Rutgers Nisso Group.

Balbach, E.D., Smith, E.A. and Malone, R.E. (2006) How the Health Belief Model helps the tobacco industry: individual choice, and "information". *Tobacco Control* 15 (suppl IV), iv37–iv43.

Ballesteros, J., Gonzalez-Pinto, A., Querejeta, I. and Arino, J. (2004) Brief interventions for hazardous drinkers delivered in primary care are equally effective in men and women. *Addiction* 99 103–108.

Bandura, A. (1977) *Social Learning Theory*. Englewood Cliffs, NJ: Prentice-Hall.

Bandura, A. (1986) *Social Foundations of Thought and Action: A Social Cognitive Theory*. Upper Saddle River, NJ: Prentice Hall.

Bandura, A. (1997) *Self-efficacy. The Exercise of Control*. New York: WH Freeman.

Bandura, A. (1998) Health promotion from the perspective of social cognitive theory. *Psychology and Health* 13, 623–649.

Bansal, M.A., Cummings, K.M., Hyland, A. and Giovino, G.A. (2004) Stop-smoking medications: who uses them, who misuses them, and who is misinformed about them? *Nicotine and Tobacco Research* 6(S3), S303–S310.

Barnett, T., Parkhurst, J. (2005) HIV/AIDS: sex, abstinence, and behaviour change. *Lancet Infectious Diseases* 5, 590–593.

Barrett, A. (2004) Oral sex and teenagers: a sexual health educator's perspective. *Canadian Journal of Human Sexuality* 13, 197–200.

Barrientos-Gutierrez, T., Gimeno, D., Mangiane, T.W., Harrist, R.B. and Amick, B.C. (2007) Drinking social norms and drinking behaviours. *Occupational and Environmental Medicine* 64, 602–608.

Barry, P.M. and Klausner, J.D. (2006) The impact of STIs. *Clinical Issues*, Accessed 17 December 2007 at www.mioonline.com.

Bauld, L., Mackinnon, J. and Judge, K. (2002) *Community Health Initiatives: Recent Policy Developments and the Emerging Evidence Base*. Glasgow: Health Promotion Policy Unit, University of Glasgow.

Bauld, L., Chesterman, J., Judge, K., Pound, E. and Coleman, T. (2003) Impact of UK National Health Service smoking cessation services: variations in outcomes in England. *Tobacco Control* 12, 296–301.

Bauman, K.E., Foshee, V.A., Linzer, M.A. and Koch, G.G. (1990) Effect of parental smoking classification on the association between parental and adolescent smoking. *Addictive Behaviours* 15(5), 413–422.

BBC News (2006) Blair calls for lifestyle change. Accessed 29 September 2008 at: http://news.bbc.co.uk/1/hi/uk_politics/5215548.stm.

BBC News (2007) Exercise 'must be tough to work'. To be healthy, you really do need to break into a sweat when you exercise, say experts. Accessed 29 September 2008 at: http://news.bbc.co.uk/1/hi/health/6950856.stm.

Beck, U. (1990) *Risk Society: Towards a New Modernity*. London: Sage.

Becker, M.H. and Rosenstock, I.M. (1984) Compliance with medical advice. In: A. Steptoe and A. Mathews (eds), *Health Care and Human Behaviour*. London: Academic Press Inc.

Becker, M. H. and Rosenstock, I. M. (1987) Comparing social learning theory and the health belief model. *Advances in Health Education and Promotion* 2, 245–249.

Becker, M. H., Haefner, D. P., Kasl, S.V., Kirscht, J.P., Maiman, L.A. and Rosenstock, I.M. (1977) Selected psychosocial models and correlates of individual health-related behaviours. *Medical Care* 15 (supplement), 27–46.

Belcher, H.M. and Shinitzky, H.E. (1998) Substance abuse in children: prediction, protection and prevention. *Archives of Pediatrics and Adolescent Medicine 152,* 952–959.

Bell, D.W. and Esse, V.M. (2002) Ambivalence and response amplification: a motivational perspective. *Personality and Social Psychology Bulletin* 28, 1143–1152.

Bem, D. J. (1972) Self perception theory. In: L. Berkowitz (ed.) *Advances in Experimental Psychology*. New York: Academic Press.

Bengel, J. (1993) *Gesundheit, Risikowahrnehmung und Vorsorgeverhalten*. Göttingen: Hogrefe.

Bengel, J., Belz-Merk, M. and Farin, E. (1996) The role of risk perception and efficacy cognitions in the prediction of HIV-related preventive behavior and condom use. *Psychology and Health* 11, 505–525.

Bennett, G.G., Wolin, K.Y., Viswanath, K., Askew, S., Puleo, E. and Emmons, K.M. (2006) Television viewing and pedometer-determined physical activity amoung multi-ethnic residents of low income housing. *American Journal of Public Health* 96, 1681–1685.

Bennett, P. and Bozionelos, G. (2000) The theory of planned behaviour as predictor of condom use: a narrative review. *Psychology, Health, and Medicine* 5, 307–326.

Benton, D. (2004) Role of parents in the determination of the food preferences of children and the development of obesity. *International Journal of Obesity* 28, 858–869.

Berridge, K. (1996) Food reward: brain substrates of wanting and liking. *Neuroscience and Biobehavioral Reviews* 20, 1–25.

Berridge, V. (ed.) (2002) The Black report and the health divide. *Contemporary British History* 16, 131–171.

Bertrand, J.T., O'Reilly, K., Denison, J., Anhang, R. and Sweat, M. (2006) Systematic review of the effectiveness of mass communication programs to change HIV/AIDS-related behaviours in developing countries. *Health Education Research* 21, 567–597.

Biddle, S.J.H. and Mutrie, N. (1991) *Psychology of Physical Activity and Exercise*. London: Springer-Verlag.

Biddle, S., Edmunds, L., Bowler, I. and Killoran, A. (1997) Physical activity promotion through primary health care in England. *British Journal of General Practice* 47(419), 367–369.

Biener, L., Reimer, R., Wakefield, M., Szczypka, G., Rigotti, N. and Connolly, G. (2006) Impact of smoking cessation aids and mass media among recent quitters. *American Journal of Preventive Medicine* 30(3), 217–224.

Bimbi, D.S., Nanin, J.E., Parsons, J.T., Vicioso, K.J., Missildine, W. and Frost, D.M. (2006) Assessing gay and bisexual men's outcome expectancies for sexual risk under the influence of alcohol and drugs. *Substance Use & Misuse* 41, 643–652.

Birch, L.L. (1980) Effects of peer models' food choices and eating behaviours on preschoolers' food preferences. *Child development* 51, 489–496.

Birch, L.L. (1999) Development of food preferences. *Annual Review of Nutrition* 19, 41–62.

Birch, L.L. and Marlin, D.W. (1982) I don't like it; I never tried it: effects of exposure on two-year-old children's food preferences. *Appetite* 23, 353–360.

Birch, L.L., Zimmerman, S. and Hind, H. (1980) The influence of social-affective context on the development of children's food preferences. *Child Development* 55, 856–861.

Birch, L.L., Marlin, D.W. and Rotter, J. (1984) Eating as the 'means' activity in a contingency: effects on young children's food preference. *Child Development* 55, 431–439.

Birch, L.L., Birch, D., Marlin, D.W. and Kramer, L. (1982) Effects of instrumental consumption on children's food preference. *Appetite* 3, 125–134.

Birch, L.L., McPhee, L., Shoba, B.C., Pirok, E. and Steinberg, L. (1987) What kind of exposure reduces children's food neophobia? *Appetite* 9, 171–178.

Blaxter, M. (1990) *Health and Lifestyles*. London: Sage.

Blenkinsop, S., Bradshaw, S., Cade, J., Chan, D., Greenwood, D., Ransley, J. et al. (2007) Further evaluation of the school fruit and vegetable scheme. Retrieved 7 December 2007 from www.dh.gov.uk/prod_consum_dh/idcplg?IdcService=GET_FILEanddID=147851andRendition=Web.

Block, G., Patterson, B. and Subar, A. (1992) Fruit, vegetables, and cancer prevention: a review of the epidemiological evidence. *Nutrition and Cancer* 18(1), 1–29.

Blue, C.L. (2007) Does the theory of planned behaviour identify diabetes-related cognitions for intention to be physically active and eat a healthy diet? *Public Health Nursing* 24(2), 141–150.

Blume, A.W., Lostutter, B.S., Schaling, K.B. and Marlatt, G.A. (2003) Beliefs about drinking behaviour predict drinking consequences. *Journal of Psychoactive Drugs* 35, 395–399.

Blundell, J.E., Hill, A.J. and Lawton, C.L. (1989) Neurochemical factors involved in normal and abnormal eating in humans. In: R. Shepherd (ed.) *Handbook of the Psychophysiology of Human Eating*. London: Wiley.

Boer, A. and Seydel, E. (1996) Protection motivation theory. In: M. Conner and P. Norman (eds) *Predicting Health Behaviour*. Buckingham: Open University Press.

Bottorff, J. L., Johnson, J. L., Irwin, L. G. and Ratner, P. A. (2000) Narratives of smoking relapse: the stories of postpartum women. *Research in Nursing & Health 23*(2), 126–134.

Botvin, G. J. (1998) Preventing adolescent drug abuse through life skills training: theory, methods and effectiveness. In: J. Crane (ed.) *Social Programmes That Really Work*. New York: Russell Sage Foundation.

Bouchard, C., Shephard, R.J., Stephens, T. and Sutton, J.R. (1990) (eds) *Exercise, Fitness and Health: A Consensus of Current Knowledge*. Champaign, IL: Human Kinetics.

Bouchard, C. and Pérusse, L. (1993) Genetic aspects of obesity. *Annals of the New York Academy of Sciences* 699(1), 26–35.

Bourdieu, P. (1974) Der Habitus als Vermittlung zwischen Struktur und Praxis. In: P. Bourdieu (ed.) *Zur Soziologie der symbolischen Formen*. Frankfurt a.M: Suhrkamp.

Bourdieu, P. (1997) *Die feinen Unterschiede. Kritik der gesellschaftlichen Urteilskraft* (9th edn). Frankfurt a.M: Suhrkamp.

Bourn, J. (2001) *Tackling Obesity in England. Report by the Controller and Auditor General*. London: National Audit Office.

Boyce, T. (2007) The media and obesity. *Obesity Reviews* 8,(1), 201–205.

Brandon, T. H. and Brandon, K. O. (2005) Brother, can you spare a smoke? sibling transmission of tobacco use. *Addiction* 100(4), 439–440.

Brewer, N.T., Chapman, G.B., Gibbons, F.X., Gerrard, M., McCaul, K.D. and Weinstein, N.D. (2007) Meta-analysis of the relationship between risk perception and health behaviour: the example of vaccination. *Health Psychology* 26, 136–145.

Bricker, J.B., Rajan, K.B., Andersen, M.R., and Peterson, A.V. Jr (2005) Does parental smoking cessation encourage their young adult children to quit smoking? A prospective study. *Addiction* 100(3), 379–386.

British Crime Survey (2007) *Drug Misuse Declared: Findings from the 2006/07 British Crime Survey, England and Wales*. HMSO: London.

Britton, J (2004) Smoking cessation services: use them or lose them. *Thorax* 59 548–549.

Brown, S.L. and Morley, A.M. (2007) Risk perception, fuzzy representations and comparative optimism. *British Journal of Psychology* 98, 575–587.

Brown, W.J., Mummery, K., Eakin, E. and Schofield, G. (2006) 10,000 steps Rockhampton: evaluation of a whole community approach to improving population levels of physical activity. *Journal of Physical Activity & Health* 3, 1–14.

Brown, A., Yung, A., Cosgrave, E., Killackey E., Buckley, J., Stanford, C. et al. (2006) Depressed mood as a risk factor for unprotected sex in young people. *Australasian Psychiatry* 14(3), 310–312.

Browning, J. R., Hatfield, E., Kessler, D. and Levine, T. (2000) Sexual motives, gender, and sexual behavior. *Archives of Sexual Behavior* 29, 135–153.

Bruce, N. (1991) Epidemiology and the new public health: implications for training. *Social Science and Medicine* 32(1), 103–106.

Bruckner, H. and Bearman, P. (2005) After the compromise: the STD consequences of adolescent virginity pledges. *Journal of Adolescent Health* 56, 271–278.

Brug, J., De Vet, E., De Nooijer, J. and Verplanken, B. (2006) Predicting fruit consumption: cognitions, intention and habit. *Journal of Nutrition Education and Behaviour* 38, 73–81.

Brunnhuber, K., Cummings, K. M., Feit, S., Sherman, S. and Woodcock, J. (2007) *Putting Evidence into Practice: Smoking Cessation*. London: BMJ Publishing Group Limited.

Bryan, A.D., Aiken, L.S. and West, S.G. (1996) Increasing condom use: evaluation of a theory-based intervention to decrease sexually transmitted disease in women. *Health Psychology* 15, 371–382.

Bryan, A.D., Aiken, L.S. and West, S.G. (1997) Young women's condom use: the influence of responsibility for sexuality, control over the sexual encounter, and perceived susceptibility to common STDs. *Health Psychology* 16, 468–479.

Buckworth, J. and Dishman, R. (2002) *Exercise Psychology*. London: Human Kinetics.

Budd, T. (2003) Alcohol–related assault: findings from the British Crime Survey. Online Report 35/03. London: Home Office.

Budney, A. J. and Higgins, S.T. (2006) *A Community Reinforcement Plus Vouchers Approach: Treating Cocaine Addiction*. Rockville, MD: National Institute on Drug Abuse.

Bugel, S. (2003) Can human micronutrients status be improved by supplementing domestic animals? *Proceedings of the Nutrition Society* 62, 399–402.

Buhi, E.R. and Goodson, P. (2007) Predictors of adolescent sexual behavior and intention: a theory-guided systematic review. *Journal of Adolescent Health* 40(1), 4–21.

Bunton, R., Baldwin, S., Flynn, D. and Whitelaw, S. (2000) The 'Stages of Change' model in health promotion: science and ideology. *Critical Public Health* 10(1), 55–70.

Burke, B. L., Arkowitz, H. and Menchola, M. (2003) The efficacy of motivational interviewing: a meta-analysis of controlled clinical trials. *Journal of Consulting and Clinical Psychology* 71, 843–861.

Burke, V., Milligan, R.A., Beilin, L.J., Dunbar, D., Spencer, M., Balde, E. and Gracey, M.P. (1997) Clustering of health-related behaviours among 18 year old Australians. *Preventive Medicine* 26, 724–733.

Burr, V. (1998) *Gender and Psychology*. London: Routledge.

Butland, B., Jebb, S., Kopelman, P., McPherson, K., Thomas, S., Mardell, J. and Parry, V. (2007) *Foresight Tackling Obesities: Future Choices Project Report*. UK: Department of Innovation Universities and Skills.

Butler, C.C., Pill, R. and Stott, N.C.H. (1998) Qualitative study of patients' perceptions of doctors' advice to quit smoking: implications for opportunistic health promotion. *British Medical Journal* 316, 1878–1881.

Buunk, B.P., Bakker, A.B., Siero, F.W., van den Eijinden, R.J. and Yzer, M.C. (1998) Predictors of AIDS-preventive behavioral intentions among adult heterosexuals at risk for HIV-infection: extending current models and measures. *AIDS Education and Prevention* 10, 149–172.

Buysse A. (1996) Adolescents, young adults and AIDS: a study of actual knowledge vs. perceived need for additional information. *Journal of Youth and Adolescence* 25, 259–271.

Cabinet Office Strategy Unit (2002) *Risk: Improving Government Capability to Handle Risk and Uncertainty*. London: Cabinet Office.

Cacioppo, J.T. and Hawkley, L.C. (2003) Social isolation and health, with an emphasis on underlying mechanisms. *Perspectives in Biology and Medicine* 46, S39–S52.

Cade, J.E., Burley, V.J. and Greenwood, D.C. (2007) Dietary fibre and risk of breast cancer in the UK Women's Cohort Study. *International Journal of Epidemiology* 36 (2), 431–438.

Calabresa, R. L. and Adams, J. (1990) Alienation: a cause of juvenile delinquency. *Adolescence* 25, 435–440.

Campos, P., Saguy, A., Ernsberger, P., Oliver, E. and Gaesser, G. (2006a) The epidemiology of overweight and obesity: public health crisis or moral panic? *International Journal of Epidemiology* 35, 55–60.

Campos, P., Saguy, A., Ernsberger, P., Oliver, E. and Gaesser, G. (2006b) Lifestyle, not weight, should be the primary target. *International Journal of Epidemiology* 35, 81–82.

Cancer Research UK (2002) Alcohol, smoking and breast cancer: the definitive answer. Available at: www.cancerresearchuk.org.

Canoy, D. and Buchan, I. (2007) Challenges in obesity epidemiology. *Obesity Reviews* 8 (1), 1–11.

Caraher, M., Dixon, P., Lang, T. and Carr-Hill, R. (1998) Access to healthy foods: part I. Barriers to accessing healthy foods: differentials by gender, social class, income and mode of transport. *Health Education Journal* 57, 191–201.

Carey, R.F., Herman, W.A., Retta, S.M., Rinaldi, J.E., German, B.A., and Athey, T.W. (1992) Effectiveness of latex condoms as a barrier to human immunodeficiency virus-sized particles under conditions of simulated use. *Sexually Transmitted Diseases* 19, 230–234.

Carroll, K.M. and Onken, L.S. (2005) Behavioural therapies for drug abuse. *American Journal of Psychiatry* 162, 1–9.

Cartwright, M., Wardle, J., Steggles, N., Simon, A.E., Croker, H. and Jarvis, M.J. (2003) Stress and dietary practices in adolescents. *Health Psychology* 22, (4), 362–369.

Carvajal, S.C., Parcel, G.S. and Basen-Engquist, K., (1999) Psychosocial predictors of delay of first sexual intercourse by adolescents. *Health Psychology* 18(5), 443–452.

Case, S. and Haines, K. (2003) Promoting prevention: preventing youth drug use in Swansea, UK, by targeting risk and protective factors. *Journal of Substance Use* 8, 243–251.

Caspersen, C.J., Powell, K.E. and Christenson, G.M. (1985) Physical activity, exercise and physical fitness. Definitions and distinctions for health-related research. *Public Health Reports* 100, 126–131.

Celentano, D.D., Valleroy, L.A., Sifakis, F., Mackellar, D.A., Hylton, J., Thiede, H. et al. (2005) Associations between substance use and sexual risk among very young men who have sex with men. *Sexually Transmitted Diseases* 33, 1–7.

Centers for Disease Control (CDC) (2004b) Cigarette smoking among adults – United States, 2002. *Morbidity and Mortality Weekly Report* 53, 427–431.

Centers for Disease Control (CDC) (2006a) Can I get HIV from Oral Sex? Accessed 29 December 2007 at: www.cdc.gov.hiv/resources/qa/qa19.htm.

Centers for Disease Control (CDC) (2006b) Young people at risk: HIV/AIDS among America's youth. Retrieved from http://www.cdc.gov/hiv/pubs/facts/youth.pdf.

Centers for Disease Control (CDC) (2006c) Sexually Transmitted Disease Treatment Guidelines 2006. Accessed 20 December 2007 at: www.cdc.gov/std/treatment/2006/urethritis-and-cervicities.htm.

Centers for Disease Control (CDC) (2006d) Hepatitis A STD Treatment Guidelines. http://www.cdc.gov/std/treatment/2006/hepatitis-a.htm.

Centers for Disease Control (CDC) (2006e) Epidemiology of HIV/AIDS – United States, 1981–2005. MMRW Weekly, 55(21), 589–592. Accessed 17 December 2007 at: http://www.cdc.gov/mmwr/preview/mmwrhtml/mm5521a2.htm.

Centers for Disease Control (CDC) (2007a) HIV/AIDS and Men who have Sex with Men (MSM) Accessed 20 December 2007: http://www.cdc.gov/hiv/topics/msm/index.htm.

Centers for Disease Control and Prevention (CDC) (2007b) Healthy Youth! Sexual Risk Behaviours. Accessed 18 December 2007 at: http://www.cdc.gov/HealthyYouth/sexualbehaviors/index.htm.

Centers for Disease Control (CDC) (2007c) Chlamyda – CDC fact sheet. Accessed 18 December 2007 at: http://www.cdc.gov/std/chlamydia/STDFact-Chlamydia.htm.

Centers for Disease Control and Prevention (CDC) (2004a) Syphilis – CDC fact sheet. Accessed 18 December 2007 at: http://www.cdc.gov/std/syphilis/STDFact-Syphilis.htm#spread.

Challier, B., Chau, N., Predine, R., Choquet, M. and Legras, B. (2000) Associations of family environment and individual factors with tobacco, alcohol and illicit drug use in adolescents. *European Journal of Epidemiology* 16(1), 33–42.

Chambers, W.C. (2007) Oral sex: varied behaviours and perceptions in a college population. *Journal of Sex Research* 44(1), 28–42.

Chang, C.J., Wu, C.H. and Chang, C.S. (2003) Low body mass index but high percent body fat in Taiwanese subjects: implications of obesity cutoffs. *International Journal of Obesity and Related Metabolic Disorders* 27, 253–259.

Chapman, S. (2004) Evaluating social marketing interventions. In: M. Thorogood and Y. Coombes (eds) *Evaluating Health Promotion: Practice and Methods*, 2nd edn. Oxford: Oxford University Press.

Chavarria, F. (1989) Civilisation, diseases, time and space. In: R. Krieps (ed.) *Environment and Health a Holistic Approach*. Aldershot: Avebury.

Chen, K., Kandel, D.B. and Davies, M. (1997) Relationships between frequency and quantity of marijuana use and last year proxy dependence among adolescents and adults in the United States. *Drug and Alcohol Dependency* 46, 53–67.

Cherpes, T.L., Meyn, L.A. and Hiller, S.L. (2005) Cunnilingus and vaginal intercourse are risk factors for herpes simplex virus type 1 acquisition in women. *Sexually Transmitted Diseases* 32, 84–89.

Chesterman, J., Judge, K., Bauld, L, and Ferguson, J. (2005) How effective are the English smoking treatment services in reaching disadvantaged smokers? *Addiction* 100(s2), 36–45.

Childs, A. (2007) *Health Needs Assessment: Substance Misuse*. Cardiff: National Public Health Service for Wales.

Chiolero, A., Peytremann-Bridevaux, I. and Paccaud, F. (2007) Associations between obesity and health conditions may be overestimated if self-report body mass index is used. *Obesity Reviews* 8, 373–374.

Choi, K.H. and Catania, J.A. (1996) Changes in multiple sexual partnerships, HIV testing and condom use among US heterosexuals 18 to 49 years of age, 1990 and 1992. *American Journal of Public Health* 86, 554–556.

Chopra, M., Galbraith, S. and Darnton-Hill, I. (2002)A global response to a global problem: the epidemic of overnutrition. *Bulletin of the World Health Organisation* 80, 952–958.

Church, I.S., Earnest, C.P., Skinner, J.S. and Blair, S.N. (2007) Effects of different doses of physical activity on cardiorespiratory fitness among sedentary overweight or obese post menopausal women with elevated blood pressure: a randomised controlled trial. *Journal of American Medical Association* 297, 2081–2091.

Cinciripini, P.M., Lapitsky, L.G., Seay, S., Wallfisch, A., Kitchens, K. and van Vunakis, H. (1995) The effects of smoking schedules on cessation outcome: can we improve on common methods of gradual and abrupt nicotine withdrawal? *Journal of Consulting and Clinical Psychology* 63, 388–399.

Clark, D. (2004) The natural history of adolescent alcohol use disorders. *Addiction* 99(S2), 5–22.

Clark S. (2004) Early marriage and HIV risks in sub-Saharan Africa. *Studies in Family Planning* 35(3), 149–160.

Cobb, N.K., Graham, A.L., Bock, B.C., Papandonatos, G. and Abrams, D.B. (2005) Initial evaluation of a real-world Internet smoking cessation system. *Nicotine and Tobacco Research* 7(2), 207–216.

Cofta-Woerpel, L., Wright, K.L. and Wetter, D.W. (2006) Smoking cessation 1: pharmacological treatments. *Behavioral Medicine* 32(2), 47–56.

Cofta-Woerpel, L., Wright, K.L., Wetter, D.W. (2007) Smoking cessation 3: multicomponent interventions. *Behavioural Medicine*, 32, 135–149.

Cohen , J. (1992) A power primer. *Psychological Bulletin* 112, 155–159.

Cohen, S. (1972) Drug use: religion and secularization. *American Journal of Psychiatry* 129, 97.

Cole, T.J., Bellizzi, M.C., Flegal, K.M. and Dietz, W.H. (2000) Establishing a standard definition for child overweight and obesity worldwide: International Survey. *British Medical Journal* 320, 1240–1246.

Cole, J.C., Michailidou, K., Jerome, L. and Sumnall, H.R. (2006) The effects of stereotype threat on cognitive function in ecstasy users. *Journal of Psychopharmacology* 20, 518–525.

Coleman, L. and Cater, S. (2005) Underage 'binge' drinking: a qualitative study into motivations and outcomes. *Drugs: Education, Prevention and Policy* 12(2), 125–136.

Coleman, T. (2004) Use of simple advice and behavioural support. *British Medical Journal* 328(7436), 397–399.

Colfax, G.N., Vittinghoff, E., Husnik, M., McKirnan, D., Buchbinder, S., Koblin, B. et al. (2004) Substance use and sexual risk: a participant and episode-level analysis among a cohort of men who have sex with men. *American Journal of Epidemiology* 159, 1002–1012.

Collazo, A.A. (2004) Theory-based predictors of intention to engage in precautionary sexual behavior among Puerto Rican high school adolescents. *Journal of HIV/AIDS Prevention in Children and Youth* 6(1), 1–120.

Collins, F.S., Green, E.D., Guttmacher, A.E. and Guyer, M.S. (2003) A vision of the future for genomics research. *Nature* 422, 835–847.

Collins, G. (1985) Impact of AIDS: patterns of homosexual life changing. *New York Times*, 22 July, p. B4.

Condon, J. and Smith, N. (2003) *Prevalence of Drug Use: Key Findings from the 2002/2003 British Crime Survey*. London: Home Office Findings 229.

Conner, M. (1993) Pros and cons of social cognition models in health behaviour. *Health Psychology Update* 14, 24–31.

Conner, M. and Norman, P. (2005) *Predicting Health Behaviour*, 2nd edn. Berkshire: Open University Press.

Conner, M. and Sparks, P. (2005) Theory of planned behaviour and health behaviour. In: M. Conner and P. Norman *Predicting Health Behaviour*, 2nd edn. Berkshire: Open University Press.

Conner, M., Sherlock, K. and Orbell, S. (1998) Psychosocial determinants of ecstacy use in young people in the UK. *British Journal of Health Psychology* 3, 295–317.

Conner, M., Bell, R. and Norman, P. (2002) The Theory of Planned Behaviour and healthy eating. *Health Psychology* 21(2), 194–201.

Conner, M., Warren, R., Close, S. and Sparks, P. (1999) Alcohol consumption and the theory of planned behaviour: an examination of the cognitive mediation of past behaviour. *Journal of Applied Social Psychology* 29(8), 1676–1704.

Conner, M., Sandberg, T., McMillan, B. and Higgins, A. (2006) Role of anticipated regret in adolescent smoking initiation. *British Journal of Health Psychology* 11, 85–101.

Connolly, T., Arkes, H.R. and Hammond, K.R. (2000) *Judgement and Decision Making: An Interdisciplinary Reader*. Cambridge: Cambridge University Press.

Connor-Gorber, S., Tremblay, M., Moher, D. and Gorber, B. (2007) A comparison of direct vs. self-report measures for assessing height, weight and body mass index: a systematic review. *Obesity Reviews* 8(4), 307–326.

Consumer Council and Department of Health (2005) *National Social Marketing Strategy for Health*. Retrieved 16 July 2008 from http://www.nsms.org.uk/images/Corefiles/NSMSwebleaflet.pdf.

Contento, I.R., Basch, C., Shea, S., Gutin, B., Zybert, P., Michela, J.L. and Rips, J. (1993) Relationship of mothers' food choice criteria to food intake of pre-school children: identification of family subgroups. *Health Education Quarterly* 20, 243–259.

Coon, K.A. and Tucker, K. (2002) Television and children's consumption patterns: a review of the literature. *Minerva Pediatrica* 54, 423–436.

Cottew, G. and Oyefeso, A. (2005) Illicit drug use among bangladeshi women living in the United Kingdom: an exploratory qualitative study of a hidden population in East London. *Drugs: Education, Prevention and Policy* 12(3), 171–188.

Counterweight Project Team (2005) Empowering primary care to tackle the obesity epidemic: The Counterweight Programme. *European Journal of Clinical Nutrition* 59, 93–101.

Courtenay, W.H. (2000) Constructions of masculinity and their influence on men's well-being: a theory of gender and health. *Social Science and Medicine* 50(10), 1385–1401.

Cox, K.L., Gorely, T.J., Puddey, I.B., Beiline, L.J. (2003) Exercise behaviour change in 40 to 65-year-old women: the SWEAT Study (Sedentary Women Exercise Adherence Trial) *British Journal of Health Psychology* 8, 477–495.

Craig, J. (1985) A 1981 socio-economic classification of local and health authorities of Great Britain. *Studies on Medical and Population Subjects* 48, Office on Population Censuses and Surveys. London: HMSO.

Crowley, T.J. (1999) Research on contingency management treatment of drug dependence: clinical implications and future directions. In: S.T. Higgins and K. Silverman (eds) *Motivating Behaviour Change Among Illicit Drug Abusers*. Washington DC: American Psychological Association.

Cummings, K.M. and Hyland, A. (2005) Impact of nicotine replacement therapy on smoking behaviour. *Annual Review of Public Health* 26, 583–599.

Cummins, S. and Macintyre, S. (2006) Food environments and obesity – neighbourhood or nation? *International Journal of Epidemiology* 35, 100–104.

Cummins, S., Peticrew, M., Higgins, C., Findlay, A. and Sparks, L. (2005) Large-scale food retailing as health intervention: quasi-experimental evaluation of a natural experiment. *Journal of Epidemiology and Community Health* 59, 1035–1040.

Daily Mail (2008) We'll put up tax on alcopops and super-strength lager, say Tories. Daily Mail, Thursday 6 March.

Danaher, B. G. (1977) Rapid smoking and self-control in the modification of smoking behavior. *Journal of Consulting and Clinical Psychology* 45(6), 1068–1074.

Dandona, R., Dandona, L. and Gutierrez, J.P. (2005) High risk of HIV in non-brothel based female sex workers in India. *BMC Public Health* 5, 87.

Davis, A. (2007) Government to put graphic warning on tobacco products. *British Medical Journal* 335, 468

Davis, A.M., Giles, A. and Rona, R. (2000) *Tackling Obesity: A Toolbox for Local Partnership Action*. London: Faculty of Public Health Medicine.

Davis, C., Sloan, M., MacMaster, S. and Kilbourne, B.(2007) HIV/AIDS knowledge and sexual activity: an examination of racial differences in a college sample. *Health and Social Work* 32(3), 2–218.

De Bourdeaudhuij, I. and Van Oost, P. (1999) A cluster-analytical approach toward physical activity and other health related behaviours. *Medicine and Science in Sports and Exercise* 31(4), 605–612.

de la Cuesta, C. (2001) Taking love seriously: the context of adolescent pregnancy in Columbia. *Journal of Transcultural Nursing* 12, 180–192.

de Visser, R. and Smith, A. (2004) Which intention? Whose intention? Condom use and theories of individual decision making. *Psychology, Health and Medicine* 9, 193–204.

De Vries, H., Backbier, E., Kok, G. and Dijkstra, M. (1995) The impact of social influences in the context of attitude, self-efficacy, intention and previous behaviour as predictors of smoking onset. *Journal of Applied Social Psychology* 25, 237–257.

Dean, K. and Colomer, C. and Perez-Hoyos, S. (1995) Research on lifestyles and health: searching for meaning. *Social Science in Medicine* 41(6), 845–855.

Deas, D. and Thomas, S.E. (2001) An overview of controlled studies of adolescent substance abuse treatment. *American Journal of Addiction* 10(2), 178–189.

Delaney, W.P. and Ames, G. (1995) Work team attitudes, drinking norms and workplace drinking. *Journal of Drug Issues* 25, 275.

Dennis, K.E., Goldberg, A.P. (1996) Weight control self-efficacy types and transitions affect weight-loss outcomes in obese women. *Addictive Behaviour* 21, 103–116.

Denny-Smith, T., Bairan, A. and Page, M.C. (2006) A survey of female nursing students knowledge, health beliefs, perceptions of risk and risk behaviours regarding human paillomavirus and cervical cancer. *Journal of the American Academy of Nurse Practitioners* 18, 62–69.

Department of Health (DoH) (1999a) *Health Survey for England: The Health of Minority Ethnic Groups*. London: The Stationery Office.

Department of Health (DoH) (1999b) *Saving Lives: Our Healthier Nation*. London: The Stationery Office.

Department of Health (DoH) (2000a) *The NHS Plan*. London: The Stationery Office.

Department of Health (DoH) (2000b) *The NHS Cancer Plan*. London: The Stationery Office.

Department of Health (DoH) (2001) *Statistics on Smoking Cessation Services in Health Authorities: England, April 2001 to March 2002*. London: The Stationery Office.

Department of Health (DoH) (2002a) *National Alcohol Harm Reduction Strategy*. London: Cabinet Office.

Department of Health (DoH) (2002b) *Priorities and Planning Framework 2003–2006: Improvement, Expansion and Reform*. Department of Health: London.

Department of Health (DoH) (2003) *Health Survey for England*. London: The Stationery Office.

Department of Health (DoH) (2004a) *At Least 5 a Week: Evidence on the Impact of Physical Activity and its Relationship to Health*. London: Department of Health.

Department of Health (DoH) (2004b) New Drive to Tackle Rise in Sexual Diseases. Accessed 7 November 2007 at: http://www.dh.gov.uk/en/Publicationsandstatistics/Pressreleases/DH_4071087.

Department of Health (DoH) (2004c) *Improving Health: Changing Behaviour*. NHS Health Trainer Handbook.

Department of Health (DoH) (2005) *Choosing a Better Diet: A Food and Health Action Plan*. Retrieved 20 December 2007 from: http://www.dh.gov.uk/prod_consum_dh/groups/dh_digitalassets/@dh/@en/documents/digitalasset/dh_4105709.pdf.

Department of Health and Department for Education and Skills (2007) 'Condomessentialwear'. Accessed 19 December 2007 at: www.condomessentialwear.co.uk.

Department of Health, Physical Activity, Health Improvement and Prevention (2004) *At Least Five a Day*. London: Department of Health.

Department of Health and Social Security (1980) *Inequalities in Health: Report of a Research Working Group* (The Black Report). London: Department of Health and Society Security.

Department of Health, Social Services and Public Safety (2001) *Northern Ireland Health and Social Wellbeing Survey*. Belfast: Northern Ireland Statistical Research Agency.

Department of Health/Food Standards Agency (2002) *The National Diet and Nutrition Survey: Adults Aged 19 to 64 Years*. London: HMSO.

Department of Health, Social Services and Public Safety (DHSSPNI) (2007) *Statistics and Research*. Retrieved 01/12/07 from: http://www.dhsspsni.gov.uk/index/stats_research/public_health/statistics_and_research-drugs_alcohol-2.htm.

DePue, J.D., Clark, M.M., Ruggiero, L., Medeiros, M.L. and Pera, V. Jr. (1995) Maintenance of weight loss: a needs assessment. *Obesity Research* 3, 241–248.

Derby, C.A., Laster, T.M., Vass, K., Gonzalez, S. and Carleton, R.A. (1994) Characteristics of smokers who attempt to quit and of those who recently succeeded. *American Journal of Preventive Medicine* 10, 327–334.

Dicken-Kano, R. and Bell, M.M. (2006) Pedometers as a means to increase walking and achieve weight loss. *Journal of the American Board of Family Medicine* 19, 524–525.

DiClemente, C. C. (2005) A premature obituary for the transtheoretical model: a response to West (2005). *Addiction* 100(8), 1046–1104.

DiClemente, R. J. (1991) Predictors of HIV-preventive sexual behavior in a high-risk adolescent population: the influence of perceived peer norms and sexual communication on incarcerated adolescents' consistent use of condoms. *Journal of Adolescent Health* 12, 385–390.

Dietz, W. Jr. and Gortmaker, S.L. (1985) Do we fatten our children at the television set? Obesity and television viewing in children and adolescents. *Pediatrics* 75(5), 807–812.

Dijkstra, A., Sweeney, L. and Gebhardt, W. (2001) Social cognitive determinants of drinking in young adults: beyond the alcohol expectancies paradigm. *Addictive Behaviours* 26, 689–706.

Dillard, A., McCaul, K. and Klein, W. (2006) Unrealistic optimism in smokers: implications for smoking myth endorsement and self-protective motivation. *Journal of Health Communication* 11(S1), 93–102.

Dillon, L., Chivite-Matthews, N., Grewal, I., Brown, R., Webster, S. and Weddell, E. et al. (2007) *Risk, Protective Factors and Resilience to Drug Use: Identifying Resilient Young People and Learning From Their Experiences*. London: Home Office.

Dilorio, C., Dudley, W.N., Kelly, M., Soet, J., Mbwara, J. and Sharpe Potter, J. (2001) Social cognitive correlates of sexual experience and condom use among 13 through 15 year old adolescents. *Journal of Adolescent Health* 29, 208–216.

Dodge, B. and Sandfort, T.G.M. (2007) A review of mental health research on bisexual individuals when compared to homosexual and heterosexual individuals. In: B.A. Firestein (ed.) *Becoming Visible: Counseling Bisexuals Across the Lifespan*. New York: Columbia University Press.

Doll, R. and Hill, A.B. (1952) A study of the aetiology of carcinoma of the lung. *British Medical Journal* ii, 1271–1286.

Doll, R. and Peto, R. (1981) *The Cause of Human Cancer*. Oxford: Oxford University Press.

Doll, R., Peto, R., Boreham, J. and Sutherland, I. (2004) Mortality in relation to smoking: 50 years' observations on male British doctors. *British Medical Journal* 328, 1519.

Donenberg, G.R. and Pao, M. (2005) Youths and HIV/AIDS: psychiatry's role in a changing epidemic. *Journal of the American Academy of Child and Adolescent Psychiatry* 44, 728–47.

Donenberg, G.R., Emerson, E., Bryant, F.B. and King, S. (2006) Does substance use moderate the effects of parents and peers on risky sexual behaviour? *AIDS Care* 18(3), 194–200.

Donovan, J.E., Jessor, R. and Costa, F.M. (1991) Adolescent health behaviour and conventionality- unconventionality: an extension of problem-behaviour theory. *Health Psychology* 10(1), 52–61.

Doyle, R. (2001) By the numbers: lifestyle blues. *Scientific American* April.

Droomers, M., Schrijvers, C.T.M. and Mackenbach, J.P. (2002) Why do lower educated people continue smoking? Explanations from the longitudinal GLOBE Study. *Health Psychology* 21(3), 263–272.

Duncker, K. (1938) Experimental modification of children's food preferences through social suggestion. *Journal of Abnormal Social Psychology* 33, 490–507.

Dunn, C., Deroo, L. and Rivara, F.P. (2001) The use of brief interventions adapted from motivational interviewing across behavioural domains: a systematic review. *Addiction* 96, 1725–1742.

Dunn, L., Ross, B., Caines, T. and Howorth, P. (1998) A school-based HIV/AIDS prevention education program: outcomes of peer-led versus community health nurse-led interventions. *Canadian Journal of Human Sexuality*, 7, 339–345.

Duryea, E.J. and Okwumabua, J.O. (1988) Effects of a preventive alcohol education programme after 3 years. *Journal of Drug Education* 18, 23–31.

Dye, C. and Upchurch, D.M. (2006) Moderating effects of gender on alcohol use: implications for condom use at first intercourse. *Journal of School Health* 76(3), 111–116.

Ebbeling, C., Pawlak, D. and Ludwig, D. (2002) Childhood obesity: public-health crisis, common sense cure. *Lancet* 360, 473–482.

Edwards, R. (2004) The problem of tobacco smoking. *British Medical Journal* 328 (7433), 217–219.

Ellickson, P.L. and Bell, R.M. (1990) Drug prevention in junior high: a multi-site longitudinal test. *Science* 247 (4948), 1299–1305.

Emslie, C., Hunt, K. and Macintyre, S. (2002) How similar are the smoking and drinking habits of men and women in non-manual jobs? *European Journal of Public Health* 12, 22–28.

Epstein, J. A. and Botvin, G. J. (2002) The moderating role of risk taking and refusal assertiveness on social influences in alcohol use among inner-city adolescents. *Journal of Studies on Alcohol* 63, 456–459.

Epstein, J. A., Bang, H. and Botvin, G. J. (2007) Which psychosocial factors moderate or directly affect substance use among inner-city adolescents? *Addictive Behaviours* 32, 700–713.

Erens, B. and Laiho, J. (2001) Alcohol consumption. In: B. Erens, P. Primatesta and G. Prior (eds) *Health Survey for England: the Health of Minority Ethnic Groups '99*. Vol 1. London: The Stationery Office.

Erens, B., Primatesta, P. and Prior, G. (eds) (2001) *Health Survey for England: the Health of Minority Ethnic Groups '99*. London: The Stationery Office.

Etter, J. (2005) Comparing the efficacy of two internet-based, computer-tailored smoking cessation programs: a randomized trial. *Journal of Medical Internet Research* 7(1), e2.

Etter, J. and Perneger, T. V. (1999) A comparison of two measures of stage of change for smoking cessation. *Addiction* 94(12), 1881–1889.

Etter, J. and Sutton, S. (2002) Assessing 'stage of change' in current and former smokers. *Addiction* 97(9), 1171–1182.

EUROHIV (2006) HIV/*AIDS Surveillance in Europe. End-year Report 2006. No. 75*. Accessed 18 December at: www.eurohiv.org.

European Heart Network (2002) Food, nutrition and cardiovascular disease prevention in the European region: challenges for the new millennium. Retrieved 3 December 2007 from http://www.ehnheart.org/files/millenium-143851A.pdf.

Evans, D.G.R., Greenhalgh, R., Hopwood, P. and Howell, A. (1994) The impact of genetic counselling on risk perception in women with a family history of breast cancer. *British Journal of Cancer* 70, 934–938.

Faculty of Family Planning & Reproductive Health Care (2007) *FFPRHC Guidance (January 2007) Male and Female Condoms*. Accessed 17 December 2007 at: http://www.ffprhc.org.uk/admin/uploads/CEUguidanceMaleFemaleCondomsJan07.pdf.

Faryna, E. and Morales, E. (2000) Self-efficacy and HIV-related risk behaviors among multiethnic adolescents. *Cultural Diversity and Ethnic Minority Psychology* 6(1), 42–56.

Fergusson, D.M. and Horwood, L.J. (2000) Does cannabis use encourage other forms of illicit drug use? *Addiction* 95, 505–520.

Fergusson, D.M., Boden, J.M. and Horwood, L.J. (2006a) Cannabis use and other illicit drug use: testing the cannabis gateway hypothesis. *Addiction* 101, 556–569.

Fergusson, D.M., Poulton, R., Smith, P.F. and Boden, J.M. (2006b) Cannabis and psychosis. *British Medical Journal* 332, 172–175.

Finch, E. and Welch, S. (2006) Classification of alcohol and drug problems. *Psychiatry* 5(12), 423–426.

Finucane, M.L., Peters, E. and Slovic, P. (2003) Judgment and decision making: the dance of affect and reason. In: S.L. Schneider and J. Shanteau (eds) *Emerging Perspectives on Judgement and Decision Research*. Cambridge: Cambridge University Press.

Fiore, M.C., Jaén, C.R., Baker, T.B. and Bailey, W.C. (2008) *Treating Tobacco Use and Dependence: 2008 Update*. Rockville, MD: US Department of Health and Human Services, Public Health Service.

Fiore, M.C., Bailey, W.C., Cohen, S.J., et al. (2000) *Treating Tobacco Use and Dependence: Clinical Practice Guideline*. Rockville, MD: US Department of Health and Human Services, Public Health Service.

Fischer, M. and Barkley, R.A. (2003) Childhood stimulant treatment and risk for later substance abuse. *Journal of Learning Disabilities* 15, 280–289.

Fischoff, B., Bostrom, A. and Quadrel, M. (2000a) Risk perception and communication. In: T. Connolly, H. Arkes and K. Hammond (eds) *Judgement and Decision Making*. Cambridge: Cambridge University Press.

Fischoff, B., Slovic, P., Lichtenstein, S., Read, S. and Combs, B. (2000b) How safe is safe enough? A psychometric study of attitudes toward technological risks and benefits. In: P. Slovic (ed) *The perception of risk*. London. Earthscan Publications Ltd.

Fishbein, M. and Ajzen, I. (1975) *Belief, Attitude, Intention and Behaviour. An Introduction to Theory and Research*. Retrieved 20 December 2007 from http://www.people.umass.edu/aizen/publications.html.

Fishbein, M., Trafimow, D., Middlestadt, S., Helquist, M., Francis, C. and Eustace, M.A. (1995) Using an AIDS KABP survey to identify determinants of condom use among sexually active adults from St. Vincent and The Grenadines. *Journal of Applied Social Psychology* 25, 1–20.

Fisher, J.D. and Fisher, W.A. (1992) Changing AIDS-risk behavior. *Psychological Bulletin* 111(3), 455–474.

Fisher, J.D., Fisher, W.A., Williams, S.S. and Malloy, T.E. (1994) Empirical tests of the information motivation-behavioral skills model of AIDS preventive behavior with gay men and heterosexual university students. *Health Psychology* 13, 238–250.

Flegal, K.M. (2006) The epidemic of obesity – what's in a name? *International Journal of Epidemiology* 35, 72–74.

Flegal, K.M., Carroll, M.D., Kuczmarski, R.J. and Johnson, C.L. (1998) Overweight and obesity in the United States: prevalence and trends, 1960–1994. *International Journal of Obesity* 22, 39–47.

Flegal, K.M., Graubard, B.I., Williamson, D.F. and Gail, M.H. (2005) Excess deaths associated with underweight, overweight and obesity. *Journal of the American Medical Association* 293, 1861–1867.

Flegal, K.M., Graubard, B.I., Williamson, D.F. and Gail, M.H. (2007) Cause-specific excess deaths associated with underweight, overweight and obesity. *Journal of the American Medical Association* 298(17), 2028–2037.

Floyd, D.L., Prentice-Dunn, S. and Rogers, R.W. (2000) A meta-analyses of protection motivation theory. *Journal of Applied Social Psychology* 30, 407–429.

Flynn, B.S., Worden, J.K., Secker-Walker, R.H., Pirie, P.L. Badger, G.J., Carpenter, J.H., and Geller, B.M. (1994) Mass-media and school interventions for cigarette smoking prevention: effects 2 years after completion. *American Journal of Public Health* 84, 1148–1150.

Folkard, S., Lombardi, D.A. and Tucker, P.T. (2005) Shiftwork: safety, sleepiness and sleep. *Industrial Health* 43, 20–23.

Foltin, R.W., Fischman, M.W. and Byrne, M.F. (1988) Effects of smoked marijuana on food intake and body weight of humans living in a residential laboratory. *Appetite* 11(1), 1–14.

Food Dude Healthy Eating Programme (2006) *The Food Dude 1 page summary*. Retrieved 22 December 2007 from http://www.fooddudes.co.uk/documents/one_page_summary.pdf.

Food Standards Agency (FSA) (2001) The balance of good health: information for educators and communicators. Retrieved 18 December 2007 from: http://www.food.gov.uk/multimedia/pdfs/bghbooklet.pdf.

Food Standards Agency (FSA) (2004) Defusing the diet time bomb. Food and Beverage Conference, Queen Elizabeth Conference Centre. FSA: London.

Food Standards Agency (FSA) (2007) Agency's new traffic light TV add launched. Retrieved 4 December 2007 from: http://www.food.gov.uk/news/newsarchive/2007/mar/tvadsignpost.

Food Standards Agency (FSA) (2008) The eatwell plate. Retrieved 2 April 2008 from: http://www.eatwell.gov.uk/healthydiet/eighttipssection/8tips/.

Forney, M.A., Forney, P.D. and Ripley, W.K. (1989) Predictor variables of adolescent drinking. *Advances in Alcohol & Substance Abuse* 8(2), 97–117.

Foster, C., Hillsdon, M., Cavill, N., Bull, F., Buxton, K. and Crombie, H. (2006) *Interventions That Use the Environment to Encourage Physical Activity: Evidence Review*. London: National Institute for Health and Clinical Excellence.

Foster, P. (1995) *Women and the Health Care Industry: An Unhealthy Relationship?* Buckingham: Open University Press.

Fox, K.R. and Hillsdon, M. (2007) Physical activity and obesity. *Obesity Reviews* 8(s1), 115–121.

Foxcroft, D.R., Ireland, D., Lister-Sharp, D.J., Lowe, G. and Breen, R. (2003) Longer-term primary prevention for alcohol misuse in young people. *Addiction* 98, 397–411.

Foxcroft, R. (2003) *Alcohol Misuse Prevention for Young People: Psychosocial and Educational Interventions*. London: Alcohol Concern.

FPA (2007) Family Planning Association Information for Young People. Accessed 19 December 2007 at: http://www.fpa.org.uk/information/detail.cfm?contentid=120.

Frazäo, E. and Golan, E. (2005) Diets high in fruit and vegetables are more expensive than diets high in fats and sugars. *Evidence-Based Healthcare and Public Health* 9, 104–107.

French, M.T. and Zavala, S.K. (2007) The health benefits of moderate drinking revisited: alcohol use and self-reported health status. *American Journal of Health Promotion* 21, 484–491.

French, S.A., Perry, C.L., Leon, G.R., Fulkerson, J.A. (1996) Self-esteem and change in body mass index over 3 years in a cohort of adolescents. *Obesity Research* 4(1), 27–33.

Frieden, T.R., Mostashari, F., Kerker, B.D., Miller, N., Hajat, A. and Frankel, M. (2005) Adult tobacco use levels after intensive tobacco control measures: New York City, 2002–2003. *American Journal of Public Health* 95(6), 1016–1023.

Frischer, J., Crome, I., MacLeod, J., Bloor, R. and Hickman. (2007) Predictive factors for illicit drug use among young people: a literature review. Retrieved 23/07/07 from: http://www.homeoffice.gov.uk/rds/pdfs07/rdsolr0507.pdf.

Gallo, M.F., Steiner, M.J., Warner, L., Hylton-Kong, T., Figueroa, J.P., Hobbs, M.M. and Behets, F.M. (2007) Self-reported condom use is associated with reduced risk of chlamydia, gonorrhea, and trichomoniasis. *Sexually Transmitted Diseases* 34(10), 829–833.

Gard, M. and Wright, J. (2005) *The Obesity Epidemic*. London: Routledge.

Gebhardt, W.A., Kuyper, L. and Dusseldorp, E. (2006) Condom use at first intercourse with a new partner in female adolescents and young adults: the role of cognitive planning and motives for having sex. *Archives of Sexual Behavior* 35(2), 217–223.

Gee, C. (2006) Does alcohol stimulate appetite and energy intake? *British Journal of Community Nursing* 11(7), 298–302.

Gerrish, C.J. and Mennella, J.A. (2001) Flavour variety enhances food acceptance in formula fed infants. *American Journal of Clinical Nutrition* 73, 1080–1085.

Giddens, A. (1991) *Modernity and Self-Identity*. Oxford: Polity Press.

Giddens, A. (2006) *Sociology* (5th edn) London: Polity Press.

Godin, G. and Kok, G. (1996) The theory of planned behaviour: a review of its applications to health-related behaviours. *American Journal of Health Promotion* 11, 87–98.

Godin, G., Gagnon, H., Lambert, L.D. and Conner, M. (2005) Determinants of condom use among a random sample of single heterosexual adults. *British Journal of Health Psychology* 10, 85–100.

Godin, G., Fortin, C., Michaud, F., Bradet, R. and Gok, K. (1997) Use of condoms: intention and behaviour of adolescents living in juvenile rehabilitation centres. *Health Education Research* 12, 289–300.

Godin, G., Maticka-Tyndale, E., Adrien, A., Mason-Singer, S., Willms, D., Cappon, P. et al (1996) Cross-cultural testing of three social cognitive theories: an application to condom use. *Journal of Applied Social Psychology* 26, 1556–1586.

Goldberg, J.H., Halpern-Felsher, B.L. and Millstein, S.G. (2002) Beyond invulnerability: the importance of benefits in adolescents decision to drink alcohol. *Health Psychology* 21, 477–484.

Gollwitzer, P.M. (1999) Implementation intentions. *American Psychologist* 54, 493–503

Gollwitzer, P.M. and Sheeran, P. (2006) Implementation intentions and goal achievement: a meta-analysis of effects and processes. *Advances in Experimental Social Psychology* 38, 69–119.

Goode, E. (1974) Marijuana use and the progression to dangerous drugs. In L.L. Miller (ed.) *Marijuana: Effects on Human Behaviour* New York: Academic Press.

Goode, J., Beardsworth, A., Haslam, C., Keil, T. and Sherratt, E. (1995) Dietary dilemmas: nutritional concerns of 1995. *British Food Journal* 97(11), 3–12.

Gordon, R., McDermott, L., Stead, M., Angus, K. and Hastings, G. (2006a) *A Review of the Effectiveness of Social Marketing Physical Activity Interventions*. London: National Social Marketing Centre for Excellence.

Gordon, R., McDermott, L., Stead, M. and Angus, K. (2006b) The effectiveness of social marketing interventions for health improvement: what's the evidence? *Public Health* 120, 1133–1139.

Gourlay, S.G., Forbes, A., Marriner, T., Pethica, D. and McNeil, J.J. (1994) Prospective study of factors predicting outcome of transdermal nicotine treatment in smoking cessation. *British Medical Journal* 309, 842–846.

Graham, H. (1987) Women's smoking and family health. *Social Science and Medicine* 25(1), 47–56.

Gredig, D., Nideroest, S. and Parpan-Blaser, A. (2006) HIV-protection through condom use: testing the theory of planned behaviour in a community sample of heterosexual men in a high-income country. *Psychology and Health* 21, 541–555.

Greening, L., Stoppelbein, L. and Jackson, M. (2001) Health education programs to prevent teen pregnancy. *Journal of Adolescent Health* 28, 257–258.

Greeno, C.G. and Wing, R.R. (1994) Stress-induced eating. *Psychological Bulletin* 115, 444–464.

Gregg, E.W., Cheng, Y.J., Cadwell, B.L., Imperatore, G., Williams, D.E., Flegal, K.M., et al. (2005) *Journal of the American Medical Association* 293, 1868–1874.

Griep, M.I., Mets, T.F., Vercruysse, A., Cromphout, I., Ponjaert, I., Toft, J. and Massert, D.L. (1995) Food odour thresholds in relation with age, nutritional and health status. *Journal of Gerontology* 503, B407–B414.

Grier, S. and Bryant, C.A. (2005) Social marketing in public health. *Annual Review Public Health* 26, 319–339.

Grillo, C.M. and Pogue-Geile, M.F. (1991) The nature of environment influences on weight and obesity : a behaviour genetic analysis. *Psychological Bulletin* 110, 520–537.

Grube, J., Morgan, M. and McGree, S. (1986) Attitudes and normative beliefs as predictors of smoking intentions and behaviours: a test of three models. *British Journal of Social Psychology* 25, 81–93.

Grunseit, A., Richters, J., Crawford, J., Song, A. and Kippax, S. (2005) Stability and change in sexual practices among first-year Australian university students (1990–1999) *Archives of Sexual Behaviour* 34, 557–568.

Guiguet, M., Lepont, F., Retel, O. and Valleron, A.J. (1994) Changes in HIV behavior among French heterosexuals: patterns of sexual monogamy and condom use between 1988 and 1991. *Journal of Acquired Immune Deficiency Syndromes* 7, 1290–1291.

Gutschoven, K. and Van den Bulck, J. (2005) Television viewing and age at smoking initiation: does a relationship exist between higher levels of television viewing and earlier onset of smoking? *Nicotine and Tobacco Research* 7(3), 381–385.

Hagger, M.S., Chatzisarantis, N.L.D. and Biddle, S.J.H. (2002) A meta-analytic review of the theories of reasoned action and planned behaviour in physical activity: predictive validity and the contribution of additional variables. *Journal of Sport and Exercise Psychology* 24, 3–32.

Hahm, H.C., Lahiff, M. and Barreto, R.M. (2006) Asian American adolescents' first sexual intercourse: gender and acculturation differences. *Perspectives on Sexual and Reproductive Health* 38(1), 28–36.

Halford, J.C.G., Harrold, J.A., Boyland, E.J., Lawton, C.L. and Blundell, J.E. (2007) Serotonergic drugs: effects on appetite expression and use for the treatment of obesity. *Drugs* 67(1), 27–55.

Halkitis, P.N., Shrem, M.T. and Martin, F.W. (2005) Sexual behaviour patterns of methamphetamine-using gay and bisexual men. *Substance Use and Misuse* 40, 703–719.

Hall, W.D. (2006) Cannabis use and the mental health of young people. *Australian and New Zealand Journal of Psychiatry* 40, 105–113.

Halley, J.A., Valdez, A. and Kaplan, C.D. (2007) *Ecstasy Use and Sexual Behavior in the South Texas Club Scene: A Study of Mexican American Ecstasy Users*. University of Texas at San Antonio, Center for Drug and Social Policy Research, San Antonio, accessed 19 December 2007 at: http://www.drugtext.org/.

Hallfors, D. and Van, D. (2002) Strengthening the role of two key institutions in the prevention of adolescent substance abuse. *Journal of Adolescent Health* 30, 17–28.

Halperin, D.T., Steiner, M.J., Cassell, M.M., Green, E.C. and Hearst, N. (2004) The time has come for common ground on preventing sexual transmission of HIV. *Lancet* 364, 1913–15.

Hammond, D., Fong, G.T., McDonald, P.W., Brown, K.S. and Cameron, R. (2004) Graphic Canadian cigarette warning labels and adverse outcomes: evidence from Canadian smokers. *American Journal of Public Health* 94(8), 1442–1445.

Hammond, D., Fong, G., Borland, R., Cummings, K., McNeill, A. and Driezen, P. (2007) text and graphic warnings on cigarette packages: findings from the International Tobacco Control Four Country Study. *American Journal of Preventive Medicine* 32(3), 202–209.

Hancox, R.J. and Poulton, R. (2006) Watching television is associated with childhood obesity: but is it clinically important? *International Journal of Obesity* 30, 171–175.

Hansen, E. and Easthope, G. (2007) *Lifestyle in Medicine*. London: Routledge.

Harper, L.V. and Sanders, K.M. (1975) The effect of adults' eating on young children's acceptance of unfamiliar foods. *Journal of Experimental Child Psychology* 20, 206–214.

Harrabin, R., Coote, A. and Allen, J. (2003) Health in the news: risk, reporting and media influence. London: King's Fund.

Harrison, J.A., Mullen, P.D. and Green, L.W. (2002) A meta-analysis of studies of the health belief model with adults. *Health Education Research* 7, 107–116.

Haslam, D. (2007) Obesity: a medical history. *Obesity Reviews* 8(1), 31–36.

Haslam, D.W. and James, W.P. (2005) Obesity. *Lancet* 366, 1197–1209.

Hastings, G. and McLean, N. (2006) Social Marketing, smoking cessation and inequalities. *Addiction* 101(3), 303–304.

Hastings, G.B., Devlin, E. and MacFadyen, L. (2005) Social marketing. In: J. Kerr, R. Weitkunat and M. Morettie (eds) *ABC of Behavior Change: A Guide to Successful Disease Prevention and Health Promotion*. Oxford: Elsevier Churchill Livingstone.

Hatherall, B., Ingham, R., Stone, N. and McEachran, J. (2007) How, not just if, condoms are used: the timing of condom application and removal during vaginal sex among young people in England. *Sexually Transmitted Infections* 83, 68–70.

Hawkins, J.D., Catalano, R.F., and Miller, J.Y. (1992) Risk and protective factors for alcohol and other drug problems in adolescence and early adulthood: implications for substance abuse prevention. *Psychological Bulletin* 112(1), 64–105.

Hawkins, J.D., Graham, J.W., Maguin, E., Abbott, R., Hill, K.G. and Catalano, R.F. (1997) Exploring the effects of alcohol use initiation and psychosocial risk factors on subsequent alcohol misuse. *Journal of Studies on Alcohol* 58, 280–290.

He, F.J., Nowson, C.A. and Macgregor, G.A. (2006) Fruit and vegetable consumption and stroke: meta-analysis of cohort studies. *Lancet* 367, 320–326.

Health Protection Agency (HPA) (2005) *General Information – Syphilis*. Accessed 18 December 2007 at: http://www.hpa.org.uk/infections/topics_az/hiv_and_sti/sti-syphilis/general.htm.

Health Protection Agency (HPA) (2007a) HIV and Other STIs – 2.1 HIV. Accessed 18 December 2007 at: www.hpa.org.uk/infections/topics_az/hiv_and_sti/publications/AnnualReport/2007/chap2/hiv.htm.

Health Protection Agency (HPA) (2007b) Gonorrhoea. Accessed 18 December 2007 at: http://www.hpa.org.uk/infections/topics_az/hiv_and_sti/Stats/STIs/gonorrhoea/default.htm.

Health Protection Agency (HPA) (2007c) Statistics – Genital Herpes. Accessed 18 December 2007 at: http://www.hpa.org.uk/infections/topics_az/hiv_and_sti/Stats/STIs/herpes/statistics.htm.

Health Protection Agency (HPA) (2007d) Hepatitis B – General Information. Accessed 18 December 2007 at: http://www.hpa.org.uk/infections/topics_az/hepatitis_b/gen_info.htm.

Health Protection Agency (HPA) (2007e) Hepatitis C. Accessed 18 December 2007 at: http://www.hpa.org.uk/infections/topics_az/hepatitis_c/phlsgen_info.htm.

Health Protection Agency (HPA) (2007f) Human Papillomavirus (HPV) – cervival cancer and genital warts. Accessed 18 December 2007 at: http://www.hpa.org.uk/infections/topics_az/hiv_and_sti/Stats/STIs/warts/default.htm.

Healthcare Commission (2007) *No Ifs, No Buts: Improving Services for Tobacco Control*. London: The Stationery Office.

Henderson, L., Gregory, J. and Swan, G. (2002) *The National Diet and Nutrition Survey: Volume 1: Adults aged 19 to 64 years. Types and Quantities of Foods Consumed*. Retrieved 3 December 2007 from: http://www.food.gov.uk/multimedia/pdfs/ndnsprintedreport.pdf.

Hendry, L.B. and Kloep, M. (2002) *Life-span Development: Resources, Challenges and Risks*. London: Thomas Learning.

Herbert, A., Gerry, N.P., McQueen, M.B., Heid, I.M., Pfeufer, A., Illig, T., et al. (2006) A common genetic variant is associated with adult and childhood obesity. *Science* 312(5771), 279–283.

Herzog, T.A. (2007) Are the stages of change for smokers qualitatively distinct? Analysis using an adolescent sample. *Psychology of Addictive Behaviours* 21, 120–125.

Herzog, T.A. and Blagg, C.O. (2007) Are most precontemplators contemplating smoking cessation? Assessing the validity of the stages of change. *Health Psychology* 26, 222–231.

Hiddink, G.J., Hautvast, J.G., Van Woerkaum, C.M., Fieren, C.J. and Van't Hof, M.A. (1997) Consumer's expectations about nutrition guidance: the importance of primary care physicians. *American Journal of Clinical Nutrition* 65, (Supplement), 1974–1979.

Higgins, A. and Conner, M. (2003) Understanding adolescent smoking: the role of the Theory of Planned Behaviour and implementation intentions. *Psychology, Health and Medicine* 8(2), 173–186.

Hill, J., Melanson, E. and Wyatt, H. (2000) Dietary fat intake and regulation of energy balance: implications for obesity. *Journal of Nutrition* 130, 284S–88S.

Hillier, L., Dempsey, D. and Harrison, L. (1999) "I'd never share a needle" – [but I often have unsafe sex]: considering the paradox of young people's sex and drugs talk. *Culture, Health and Sexuality* 1, 347–361.

Hillsdon, M., Foster, C., Cavill, N., Crombie, H. and Naidoo, B. (2005) *The Effectiveness of Public Health Interventions for Increasing Physical Activity Among Adults: A Review of Reviews*, 2nd edn. London: Health Development Agency.

Hirshfield, S., Remien, R.H., Walavalker, I. and Chiasson, M.A. (2004) Crystal methamphetamine use predicts incident STD infection among men who have sex with men recruited online: a nested case-control study. *Journal of Medical Internet Research* 6(4), e41.

HM Government (2005) *Every Child Matters: Change for Young People and Drugs*. Retrieved 23/07/07 from: http://www.nelincs.gov.uk/NR/rdonlyres/B4E19F5F-1558-42A9-AAC9-D1F5BC6D46/22950/ECMchangeforyoungpeopleanddrug2005.pdf.

HM Government (2007) *Safe. Sensible. Social. The Next Steps in the National Alcohol Strategy*. London: Department of Health and The Home Office.

Hoare, J., Henderson, L., Bates, C.J., Prentice, A., Birch, M., Swan, G. and Farron, M. (2004) *National Diet and Nutrition Survey: Volume 5: Adults aged 19 to 64 years, Summary Report*. Retrieved 6 November 2007 from: http://www.food.gov.uk/multimedia/pdfs/ndns5full.pdf.

Hobden, K. and Pilner, P. (1995) Effects of a model on food neophobia in humans. *Appetite* 25, 101–114.

Hoffmann, J.P. and Cerbone, F.G. (2002) Parental substance use disorder and the risk of adolescent drug abuse: an event history analysis. *Drug and Alcohol Dependence* 66(10), 255–264.

Hofler, M., Lieb, R. and Perkonigg, A. (1999) Covariates of cannabis use progression in a representative population sample of adolescents: a prospective examination of vulnerability and risk factors. *Addiction*, 94, 1679–1694.

Holland, J., Ramazanoglu, C., Scott, S., Sharpe, S. and Thomson, R. (1991) Between embarrassment and trust: young women and the diversity of condom use. In: P. Aggleton, G. Hart and P. Davies (eds). *AIDS: Responses, Interventions and Care*. London: Falmer Press.

Home Office (2005) *Drug Misuse Declared: Findings from the 2004/05 British Crime Survey*. London: The Stationery Office.

Home Office (2006) *Measuring the harm from illegal drugs using the Drug Harm Index – an update*. Retrieved 27/07/07 from: http://www.homeoffice.gov.uk/rds/pdfs06/rdsolr0806.pdf.

Home Office (2007) *FRANK: Brain warehouse Performance Summary*. Retrieved 3/12/07 from http://drugs.homeoffice.gov.uk/publication-search/frank/brainwarehousetrackingsummary?view=binary.

Honjo, K., Tsutsumi, A., Kawachi, I. and Kawakami, N. (2006) What accounts for the relationship between social class and smoking cessation? Results of a path analysis. *Social Science and Medicine* 62(2), 317–328.

Hopkins, R.H., Mauss, A.L., Kearney, K.A. and Weisheit, R.A. (1988) Comprehensive evaluation of a model alcohol education curriculum. *Journal of Studies on Alcohol* 49, 38–50.

Horne, P.J., Tapper, K., Lowe, C.F., Hardman, C.A., Jackson, M.C. and Woolner, J. (2004) Increasing children's fruit and vegetable consumption: a peer modelling and rewards-based intervention. *European Journal of Clinical Nutrition* 58, 1649–1660.

Hough, M., Hunter, G., Jacobson, J. and Cossalter S. (2007) *The Impact of the Licensing Act 2003 on Levels of Crime and Disorder: An Evaluation.* London: Home Office.

Howard, D.E. and Qi Wang, M. (2004) Multiple sexual-partner behavior among sexually active US adolescent girls. *American Journal of Health Behaviour* 28(1), 3–12.

Hughes, J. R., Goldstein, M. G., Hurt, R. D. and Shiffman, S. (1999) Recent advances in the pharmacotherapy of smoking. *Journal of the American Medical Association* 281, 72–76.

Hume-Hall, R. (1990) *Health and the Global Environment*. Cambridge: Polity Press.

Hursti, U.K.K. and Sjöden, P.O. (1997) Food and general neophobia and their relationship with self-reported food choice: familial resemblance in Swedish families with children of ages 7–17 years. *Appetite* 29, 89–103.

Husemoen, L.L.N., Osler, M., Godtfredsen, N.S. and Prescott, S. (2004) Smoking and subsequent risk of early retirement due to permanent disability. *The European Journal of Public Health* 14(1), 86–92.

Huver, R.M.E., Engels, R.C.M.E., and de Vries, H. (2006) Are anti-smoking parenting practices related to adolescent smoking cognitions and behaviour? *Health Education Research* 21(1), 66–77.

Hyland, A., Li, Q., Bauer, J.E., Giovino, G.A., Steger, C. and Cummings, K.M. (2004) Predictors of cessation in a cohort of current and former smokers followed over 13 years. *Nicotine and Tobacco Research* 6(S3), S363–S369.

Hymowitz, N., Cummings, K.M., Hyland, A., Lynn, W.R., Pechacek, T.F. and Hartwell, T. D. (1997) Predictors of smoking cessation in a cohort of adult smokers followed for five years. *Tobacco Control* 6(S2), S57–S62.

Iannotti, R.J., Schneider, S., Nansel, T.R., Haynie, D.L., Plotnick, L.P., Clark, L.M. et al. (2006) Self-efficacy, outcome expectations and diabetes self-management in adolescents with Type 1 diabetes. *Developmental and Behavioural Pediatrics* 27, 98–105.

Independent (2008) Budget set to increase duty on spirits. 7 March.

Information Centre (2006) *Statistics on Obesity, Physical Activity and Diet: England, 2006.* Retrieved 19 December 2007 from: http://www.ic.nhs.uk/webfiles/publications/opan06/OPAN%20bulletin%20finalv2.pdf.

Irvin, J.E., Bowers, C.A., Dunn, M.E., and Wang, M.C. (1999) Efficacy of relapse prevention: a meta-analytic review. *Journal of Consulting and Clinical Psychology* 67, 563–570.

Irwin, L., Johnson, J. and Bottorff, J. (2005) Mothers who smoke: confessions and justifications. *Health Care for Women International* 26(7), 577–590.

Jackson, A.S., Stanforth, P.R., Gagnon, J., Rankinen, T., Leon, A.S., Rao, D.C. et al. (2002) The effect of sex, age and race on estimating percentage body fat from body mass index: The Heritage Family Study. *International Journal of Obesity and Related Metabolic Disorders* 26, 789–796.

James, W.P., Nelson, M., Ralph, A. and Leather, S. (1997) Socio-economic determinants of health: the contribution of nutrition to inequalities in health. *British Medical Journal* 314, 1545–1555.

Janis, I.L. (1968) *The Contours of Fear*. London: John Wiley and Sons.

Janis, I.L. and Mann, L. (1977) *Decision Making: A Psychological Analysis of Conflict, Choice and Commitment.* New York: Free Press.

Jansen, A. and Tenney, N. (2001) Seeing mum drinking a 'light' product: is social learning a stronger determinant of taste preference acquisition than caloric conditioning? *European Journal of Clinical Nutrition* 55, 418–422.

Janz, N. and Becker, H.M. (1984) The health belief model: a decade later. *Health Education Quarterly* 11, 1–47.

Jarvis, M.J. (2004) Why people smoke. *British Medical Journal* 328, 277–279.

Jarvis, M.J. and Wardle, J. (1999) Social patterning of health behaviours: the case of cigarette smoking. In: M. Marmot and R. Wilkinson (eds) *Social Determinants of Health*. Oxford: Oxford University Press.

Jarvis, M.J., Wardle, J., Waller, J. and Owen, L. (2003) Prevalence of hardcore smoking in England, and associated attitudes and beliefs: cross sectional study. *British Medical Journal* 326, 1061.

Jefferis, B.J.M.H., Manor, O., Power, C. (2006) Social gradients in binge drinking and abstaining: trends in a cohort of British adults. *Journal of Epidemiological Community Health* 61, 150–153.

Jefferson, D.J., Breslau, K., Darman, J., Childress, S., Juarez, V. and Williams, K. (2005) *Newsweek* 145, 9.

Jeffery, R.W., Baxter, J.E., McGuire, M.T. and Linde, J.A. (2006) Are fast food restaurants an environmental risk factor for obesity? *International Journal of Behaviour, Nutrition and Physical Activity* 3, 2.

Jeffery, R.W., Bjornson-Benson, W.M., Rosenthal, B.S., Lindquist, R.A., Kurth, C.L. and Johnson, S.L. (1984) Correlates of weight loss and its maintenance over two years of follow-up among middle-aged men. *Preventive Medicine* 13, 155–168.

Jeffries, W.L. and Dodge, B. (2007) Male bisexuality and condom use at last sexual encounter: results from a national survey. *Journal of Sex Research* 44(3), 278–289.

Jemmott, L.S. and Jemmott, J.B. (1991) Applying the theory of reasoned action to AIDS risk behaviour: condom use among black women. *Nursing Research* 40, 228–234.

Jemmott, J.B., and Jemmott, L.S. (2000) HIV risk reduction behavioural interventions with heterosexual adolescents. *AIDS* 14(S2), S40–S52.

Jemmott, J.B., Jemmott, L.S. and Fong, G.T. (1998) Abstinence and safer sex HIV risk-reduction interventions for African American adolescents. *Journal of the American Medical Association* 279, 1529–1536.

Jemmott, J.B., Jemmott, L.S., Fong, G.T. and McCaffree, K. (1999) Reducing HIV risk-associated sexual behavior among African American adolescents: testing the generality of intervention effects. *American Journal of Community Psychology* 27, 161–187.

Jenkins, J.E. (1996) The influence of peer affiliation and student activities on adolescent drug involvement. *Adolescence* 31, 297–306.

Job, R.F.S. (1988) Effective and ineffective use of fear in health promotion campaigns. *American Journal of Public Health* 78(2), 163–167.

Jochelson, K. (2006) Nanny or steward? The role of government in public health. *Public Health* 120, 1149–1155.

Joffe, H. (2003) Risk: from perception to social representation. *British Journal of Social Psychology* 42, 55–73.

John, J.H. and Ziebland, S. (2004) Reported barriers to eating more fruit and vegetables before and after participation in a randomized controlled trial: a qualitative study. *Health Education Research* 19(2), 165–174.

Johnson, S.L. and Birch, L.L. (1991) Conditioned preferences: young children prefer flavours associated with high dietary fat. *Physiology and Behaviour* 50, 1245–1251.

Johnston, L.D., O'Malley, P.M. and Bachman, J.G. (2003) *Monitoring the Future: National Survey Results on Adolescent Drug Use: Overview and Key Findings*. Bethesda,

MD: National Institute on Drug Abuse, US Department of Health and Human Services.

Jones, A., Bentham, G., Foster, C., Hillsdon, M. and Panter, J. (2007) *Tackling Obesities: Future choices – Obesogenic Environments – Evidence Review*. London: Foresight.

Jotangia, D., Moody, A., Stamatakis, E. and Wardle, H. (2005) Obesity among children under 11. Retrieved 4 December 2007 from http://www.sepho.org.uk/Download/Public/9449/1/Obesity%20report_text_FINAL_v3.doc.

Kahn, E., Ramsey, L., Brownson, R., Heath, G., Howze, E., Powell, K., Stone E. et al., Task Force on Community Preventive Services (2002) The effectiveness of interventions to increase physical activity: a systematic review. *American Journal of Preventive Medicine* 22, 73–107.

Kalat, J.W. and Rozin, P. (1973) Learned safety as a mechanism in long delay taste aversion learning in rats. *Journal of Comparative and Physiological Psychology* 83, 198–207.

Kalichman, S.C., Simbayi, L.C., Jooste, S. and Cain, D. (2007) Frequency, quantity, and contextual use of alcohol among sexually transmitted infection clinic patients in Cape Town, South Africa. *American Journal of Drug and Alcohol Abuse* 33, 687–698.

Kandel, D.B. (2003) Does marijuana use cause use of other drugs? *Journal of the American Medical Association* 289, 482–483.

Kassem, N.O. and Lee, J.W. (2004) Understanding soft drink consumption among male adolescents using the Theory of Planned Behaviour. *Journal of Behavioural Medicine* 27(3), 273–296.

Kaur, G. and Kulkarni, S.K. (2002) Studies on modulation of feeding behaviour by atypical antipsychotics in female mice. *Progress in Neuro-Psychopharmacology and Biological Psychiatry* 26(2), 277–285. Retrieved 21 December 2007 from Science Direct.

Kearney, M., Bradbury, C., Ellahi, B., Hodgson, M. and Thurston, M. (2005) Mainstreaming prevention: prescribing fruit and vegetables as a brief intervention in primary care. *Journal of the Royal Institute of Public Health* 119, 981–986.

Kennedy, S.B., Nolen, S., Appleswhite, J., Waiters, E. and Vanderhoff, J. (2007a) Condom use behaviours among 18–24 year-old urban African American males: a qualitative study. *AIDS Care* 19(8), 1032–1038.

Kennedy, S.B., Nolen, S., Applewhite, J., Pan, Z., Shamblen, S. and Vanderhoff, K.J. (2007b) A quantitative study on the condom-use behaviors of eighteen- to twenty-four-year-old urban African American males. *AIDS Patient Care and STDs* 21, 5.

King, K. M. and Chassin, L. (2004) Mediating and moderated effects of adolescent behavioural undercontrol and parenting in the prediction of drug use disorders in emerging adulthood. *Psychology of Addictive Behaviors* 18, 239–249.

Kirby, D. (1980) The effects of school sex education programs: a review of the literature. *Journal of School Health* 50, 559–563.

Kirby, D., Laris, B.A. and Rolleri, L. (2006) *Impact of Sex and HIV Education Programs on Sexual Behaviours of Youth in Developing and Developed Countries: FHI Youth Research Working Paper No 2*. North Carolina: Family Health International (Youth Net Program)

Kirby, D., Korpi, M., Adivi, C. and Weissman, J. (1997) An impact evaluation of project SNAPP: an AIDS and pregnancy prevention middle school program. *AIDS Education and Prevention* 9(S4), S44–S61.

Kirkland, S., Greaves, L. and Devichand, P. (2004) Gender differences in smoking and self reported indicators of health. *BMC Women's Health* 4(S1), 7.

Kitchen, J.M.W. (1889) On the value to man of the so-called divinely beneficient gift, tobacco. *Medical Record* 35, 459–460.

Kiviniemi, M., Voss-Humke, A.M. and Seifert, A.L. (2007) How do I feel about the behavior? The interplay of affective associations with behaviour and cognitive beliefs as influences on physical activity behaviour. *Health Psychology* 26, 152–158.

Klepp, K.I., Schmid, L.A. and Murray, D.M. (1996) Effects of increased minimum drinking age law on drinking and driving behaviour among adolescents. *Addiction Research* 4, 237–244.

Koivisto, U.K. and Sjöden, P.O. (1996) Food and general neophobia in Swedish families: parent child comparisons and relationships with serving specific foods. *Appetite* 26, 107–118.

Kotz, D. (2007) Sex ed for Seniors: you still need those condoms. *US News and World Report* 143(5), 45–46.

Kouvonen, A., Kivimäki, M., Virtanen, M., Pentti, J. and Vahtera, J. (2005) Work stress, smoking status, and smoking intensity: an observational study of 46 190 employees. *Journal of Epidemiology and Community Health* 59, 63–69.

Kozlowski, L.T., Goldberg, M.E., Yost, B.A., White, E.L., Sweeney, C.T. and Pillitteri, J.L. (1998) Smokers' misperceptions of light and ultra-light cigarettes may keep them smoking. *American Journal of Preventive Medicine* 15(1), 9–16.

Krahé, B. and Reiss, C. (1995) Predicting intentions of AIDS-preventive behavior among adolescents. *Journal of Applied Social Psychology* 25, 2118–2140.

Kreitman, N. (1986) Alcohol consumption and the preventative paradox. *British Journal of Addiction* 81, 353–363.

Krista, A.M. and Caspersen, C.J. (1997) Introduction to a collection of physical activity questionnaires. *Medicine and Science in Sports and Exercise* 29(6) supplement, 5–9.

Kruglanski, A.W. and Webster, D.M. (1996) Motivated closing of the mind: 'Seizing' and 'Freezing'. *Psychological Review* 103, 263–283.

Kurz, M. (2003) Early interventions strategies in substance abuse. *Journal of Neural Transmission* 66, 85–96.

Kuther, T.L. and Timoshin, A. (2003) A comparision of social cognitive and psychosocial predictors of alcohol use by college students. *Journal of College Student Development* 44, 143–154.

Laflin, M.T., Moore-Hirschl, S., Weis, D.L. and Hayes, B.E. (1994) Use of the theory of reasoned action to predict drug and alcohol use. *International Journal of Addiction* 29, 927–940.

Lancaster, T., Hajek, P., Stead, L., West, R. and Jarvis, M.J. (2006) Prevention of relapse after quitting smoking. *Archives of Internal Medicine* 166, 828–835.

Lannotti, R.J., Schneider, S., Nansel, T.R., Haynie, D.L., Plotnick, L.P., Clark, L.M. et al. (2006) Self-efficacy, outcome expectations and diabetes self-management in adolescents with Type 1 diabetes. *Developmental and Behavioural Pediatrics* 27, 98–105.

Lapointe, M. (2008) *Adolescent Smoking and Health Research*. New York: Nova Scientific Publishing.

Lawlor, D.A., Frankel, S., Shaw, M., Ebrahim, S. and Davey Smith, G. (2003) Smoking and ill health: does lay epidemiology explain the failure of smoking cessation programs among deprived populations? *American Journal of Public Health* 93(2), 266–270.

Lawson, D. (2007) We can seek a cure for obesity. But it might be more effective to start stigmatising it. *The Independent*, 19 October.

Lawton, J. (2002) Colonising the future: temporal perceptions and health-relevant behaviors across the adult lifecourse. *Sociology of Health and Illness* 24, 714–733.

Lawton, R. and Conner, M. (2007) Beyond cognition: predicting health risk behaviours from instrumental and affective beliefs. *Health Psychology* 26, 259–267.

Leach, K. (2006) *The Overweight Patient: A Psychological Approach to Understanding and Working with Obesity*. London: Jessica Kingsley.

Lean, M.E., Han, T.S. and Morrison, C.E. (1995) Waist circumference as a measure for indicating need for weight management. *British Medical Journal* 311, 158–161.

Lear, D. (1995) Sexual communication in the age of AIDS: the construction of risk and trust among young adults. *Social Science and Medicine* 41, 1311–1323.

Lear, D. (1996) 'You're gonna be naked anyway': college students negotiating safer sex. *Qualitative Health Research* 6, 112–134.

Lee, I. (2007) Dose response relations between physical activity and fitness:even a little is good, more is better. *Journal of American Medical Association* 297, 2137–2138.

Lee, C. and Kahende, J. (2007) Factors associated with successful smoking cessation in the United States, 2000. *American Journal of Public Health* 97(8), 1503–1509.

Lepper, M.R. and Greene, D. (1978) *The Hidden Costs of Reward: New Perspectives on the Psychology of Human Motivation*. New Jersey: Lawrence Erlbaum.

Lescano, C.M., Vazquez, E.A., Brown, L.K., Litvin, E.B., Pugatch, D., Project SHIELD Study Group (2006) Condom use with "casual" and "main" partners: what's in a name? *Journal of Adolescent Health* 39(3), 443e.1–443e.7. 2007.

Lesch, E. and Kruger, L. (2005) Mothers, daughters and sexual agency in one low-income South African community. *Social Science and Medicine* 61, 1072–1082.

Leventhal, H., Kelly, K. and Leventhal, E.A. (1999) Population risk, actual risk, perceived risk and cancer control: a discussion. *Journal of the National Cancer Institute Monographs* 25, 81–85.

Leventhal, H., Watts, J. and Pagano, F. (1967) Effects of fear and instructions on how to cope with danger. *Journal of Personality and Social Psychology* 6(3), 313–321.

Levinson, R.A., Sadigursky, C. and Erchak, G.M. (2004) The impact of cultural context on brazilian adolescents sexual practices. *Adolescence* 39, 154, 203–227.

Levy, K.B., O'Grady, K., Wish, E.D. and Arria, A.M. (2005) An in-depth qualitative examination of the ecstasy experience: results of a focus group with ecstasy-using college students. *Substance Use and Misuse* 40, 1427–1441.

Li, C., Pentz, M.A. and Chou, C.-P. (2002) Parental substance use as a modifier of adolescent substance use risk. *Addiction* 97, 1537–1550.

Li, C., Unger, J.B., Schuster, D., Rohrbach, L.A., Howard-Pitney, B. and Norman, G. (2003) Youths' exposure to environmental tobacco smoke (ETS) associations with health beliefs and social pressure. *Addictive Behaviours* 28, 39–53.

Liddle, R. (2008) Laugh at lard butts – but just remember Fatty Fritz lives longer. *Sunday Times*, January 27.

Liddle, H.A., Dakof, G.A., Parker, K., Diamond, G.S., Barrett, K. and Tejeda, M. (2001) Multidimensional family therapy for adolescent drug abuse: results of a randomized clinical trial. *The American Journal of Drug and Alcohol Abuse* 27, 651–688.

Likeitis (2007) Love Bugs. Accessed on 19 December 2007 at: http://www.likeitis.org/love_bugs.html.

Lindsey, R. (1985) Bathhouse curbs called help in coast AIDS fight. *New York Times*, October 24, p. A19.

Littell, J.A. and Girvin, H. (2002) Stages of change: a critique. *Behavior Modification* 26, 223–273.

Ljubotina, D., Galic, J. and Jukic, V. (2004) Prevalence and risk factors of substance use among urban adolescents: questionnaire study. *Croatian Medical Journal* 45(1), 88–98.

Lloyd, C. (1998) Risk factors for problem drug use: identifying vulnerable groups. *Drug education* 5(3), 217–232.

Lloyd, P.J. and Foster, S.L. (2006) Creating healthy, high performance workplaces: strategies from health and sports psychology. *Consulting Psychology Journal: Practice and Research* 58, 23–39.

Lobb, E.A., Butow, P.N., Meiser, B., Barratt, A., Gaff, C., Young, M.A. et al. (2003) Women's preferences and consultants' communication of risk in consultations about familial breast cancer: impact on patient outcomes. *Journal of Medical Genetics* 40(e), 56–72.

Lobstein, T. and Dibb, S. (2005) Evidence of a possible link between obesogenic food advertising and child overweight. *Obesity Reviews* 6(3), 203–208.

Loewenstein, G.F., Weber, E.U., Hsee, C.K. and Welch, N. (2001) Risk as feelings. *Psychological Bulletin* 127, 267–286.

Logan, T., Cole, J. and Leukefeld, C. (2003) Gender differences in the context of sex exchange among crack users. *AIDS Education and Prevention* 15(5), 448–464.

Lowe, C.E., Dowey, A.J. and Horne, P.J. (1998) Changing what children eat. In: A. Murcott (ed.) *The Nation's Diet: The Social Science of Food Choice*. London: Longman.

Lowe, C.F., Horne, P.J., Bowdery, M.A., Egerton, C. and Tapper, K. (2001) Increasing children's consumption of fruit and vegetables. *Public Health Nutrition* 4(2a), 387.

Lowe, C.F., Horne, P.J., Tapper, K., Jackson, M., Hardman, C.A., Woolner, J. et al (2002) *Changing the Nation's Diet: A Programme to Increase Children's Consumption of Fruit and Vegetables*. End of project report. University of Wales, Bangor.

Lowe, F., Horne, P. and Hardman, C. (2007) *Changing the Nation's diet: A Programme to Increase Children's Consumption of Fruit and Vegetables: Working Paper No. 5*. Retrieved 11 December 2007 from: http://www.fooddudes.co.uk/documents/Working_paper_no5.pdf.

Lupton, D. (1995) *The Imperative of Health: Public Health and the Regulated Body*. London: Sage Publications.

Luszczynska, A. and Schwarzer, R. (2005) Social Cognitive Theory. In: M. Conner and P. Norman (eds) *Predicting Health Behaviour*. Berkshire: Open University Press.

Lynskey, M.T., Heath, A.C., Nelson, E.C., Bucholz, K.K., Madden, P.A.F., Slutske, W.S. et al. (2002) Genetic and environmental contributions to cannabis dependence. *Addiction* 97(12), 1508–1509.

MacDougall, D.B. (1987) Effects of pigmentation, light scatter and illumination on food appearance and acceptance. In J. Solms, D.A. Booth, R.M. Pangborn and O. Raunhardt (eds) *Food Acceptance and Nutrition*. London: Academic Press.

MacFadyen, L., Stead, M., Hasting, G.B. (2003) Social marketing. In: M.J. Baker (ed.) *The Marketing Book*, 5th edn. Oxford: Butterworth-Heinneman.

MacIntosh, H. and Coleman, T. (2006) Characteristics and prevalence of hardcore smokers attending UK general practitioners. *BMC Family Practice* 7, 24.

Macintyre, S. (2001) Understanding the social patterning of health: the role of the social sciences. *Journal of Public Health* 16(1), 53–59.

Macleod, Z. R., Charles, M. A., Arnaldi, V. C. and Adams, I. M. (2003) Telephone counselling as an adjunct to nicotine patches in smoking cessation: a randomised controlled trial. *Medical Journal of Australia* 179(7), 349–352.

Maes, S. and Gebhardt, W.A. (2000) Self regulation and health behaviour: the health behaviour goal model. In: M. Boekaerts, P.R. Pintrich and M. Zeidner (eds) *Handbook of Self Regulation: Theory, Research and Applications*. San Diego, CA: Academic Press.

Maio, G.R., Haddock, G. and Jarman, H.L. (2007) Social psychological factors in tackling obesity. *Obesity Reviews* 8(1), 123–125.

Manning, W.G., Blumberg, L. and Moulton, L.H. (1995) The demand for alcohol: the differential response to price. *Journal of Health Economics* 14, 123–148.

Manoff, R.K. (1985) *Social Marketing: New Imperative for Public Health*. New York: Praeger.

Manson, J.E., Willett, W.C., Stampfer, M.J., Colditz, G.A., Hunter, D.J., Hankinson, S.E. et al. (1995) Body weight and mortality among women. *New England Journal of Medicine* 333, 677–685.

Marcoux, B.C. and Shope, J.T. (1997) Application of the theory of planned behaviour to adolescent use and misuse of alcohol. *Health Education Research* 12, 323–331.

Marks, D.F. and Yardley, L. (2004) *Research Methods for Clinical and Health Psychology*. London: Sage.

Marks, D.F. (1998) Addiction, smoking and health: developing policy-based interventions. *Psychology, Health and Medicine* 3, 97–111.

Marks, D.F., Murray, M., Evans, B., Willig, C., Woodall, C. and Sykes, C.M. (2005) *Health Psychology: Theory Research and Practice*, 2nd edn. Thousand Oaks, CA: Sage.

Marlatt, G.A. and Gordon, J.R. (eds) (1985) *Relapse Prevention: Maintenance Strategies in Addictive Behavior Change*. New York: Guilford.

Marsh, A. and McKay, S. (1994) *Poor Smokers*. London: Policy Studies Institute.

Marshall, D. (1995). Eating at home: meals and food choice. In: D. Marshall (ed.) *Food Choice and the Consumer*. Glasgow: Blackie Academic and Professional.

Marshall, S.J. and Biddle, S.J.H. (2001) The transtheoretical model of behavior change: a meta-analysis of applications to physical activity and exercise. *Annals of Behavioral Medicine* 23, 229–246.

Marshall, S., Bower, J.A. and Schröder, M.J.A. (2007) Consumer understanding of UK salt intake advice. *British Food Journal* 109(3), 233–245.

Marshall, S.J., Biddle, S.J., Gorely, T., Cameron, N. and Murdey, I. (2004) Relationships between media use, body fatness and physical activity in children and youth: a meta-analysis. *International Journal of Obesity and Metabolic Disorders* 28, 1238–1246.

Marston, C. and King, E. (2006) Factors that shape young people's sexual behaviour: a systematic review. *Lancet* 368(9547), 1581–1586.

Marston, C., Meltzer, H. and Majeed, A. (2005) Impact on contraceptive practice of making emergency hormonal contraception available over the counter in Great Britain; repeated cross-sectional surveys. *British Medical Journal* 331(7511), 271–273.

Marteau, T.M. and Lerman, C. (2001) Genetic risk and behavioural change. *British Medical Journal* 322: 1056–1058.

Martinez, J. (2000) Obesity in young Europeans: genetic and environmental influences. *European Journal of Clinical Nutrition* 54(Suppl 1), S56–60.

Masalu, J.R. and Astrom A.N. (2001) Predicting intended and self-perceived sugar restriction among Tanzanian students using the Theory of Planned Behavior. *Journal of Health Psychology* 6(4), 435–445.

Mathews, S. and Richardson, A. (2005) *Findings from the 2004 Offending, Crime and Justice Survey: Alcohol Related Crime and Disorder*. London: Home Office Research Findings No 261.

Maynard, A. (2001) Sense and nonsense in British drug policy. *Eurohealth* 7, 6–7.

McAuley, E. (1992) The role of efficacy cognitions in the prediction of exercise behaviour in middle-aged adults. *Journal of Behavioural Medicine* 15, 65–88.

McCambridge, J. and Strang, J. (2004) Drug problems – what problems? Concurrent predictors of selected types of drug problems in a London community sample of young people who use drugs. *Addiction Research and Theory* 12, 55–66.

McClenahan, C.M., Shevlin, M., Adamson, G., Bennett, C. and O,Neill, B. (2007) Testicular self-examination: a test of the health belief model and the theory of planned behaviour. *Health Education Research* 22, 272–284.

McCrory, M.A., Fuss, P.J., Hays, N.P., Vinken, A.G., Greenberg, A.S. and Roberts, S.B. (1999) Overeating in America: association between restaurant food consumption and body fatness in healthy adult men and women aged 19 to 80. *Obesity Research* 7, 564–571.

McCullough, F.S.W., Yoo, S. and Ainsworth, P. (2004) 'Food choice, nutrition education and parental influence on British and Korean primary school children' *International Journal of Comsumer Studies* 28(3), 235–244.

McElrath, K. (2005) MDMA and sexual behaviour: ecstasy users perceptions about sexuality and sexual risk. *Substance Use and Misuse* 40, 1461–1477.

McEwen, A. and West, R. (2001) Smoking cessation activities by general practitioners and practice nurses. *Tobacco Control* 10, 27–32.

McEwen, A., Akotia, N. and West, R. (2001) General practitioners' views on the English national smoking cessation guidelines. *Addiction* 96(7), 997–1000.

McGrath, Y.T., Sumnall, H.R., McVeigh, J. and Bellis, M.A. (2006) *Drug Use Prevention Among Young People: A Review of Reviews*. Evidence Briefing Update. London: NICE.

McIntyre, J.A. (2005) Sex, pregnancy, hormones, and HIV. *Lancet* 366, 1141–1142.

McKeown, T. (1979) The direction of medical research. Lancet 2(8155), 1281–1284.

Mckinlay, J.B. (1994) Towards appropriate levels of analysis, research methods and health public policy. Paper presented at the *International Symposium on Quality of Life and Health: Theoretical and Methodological Considerations* 25–27 May, Berlin.

McKinley, J.B. (1993) The promotion of health through planned socio-political change: challenges for research and policy. *Social Science and Medicine* 60, 1099–1106.

McLean, G., Sutton, M. and Guthrie, B. (2006) Deprivation and quality of primary care services: evidence for persistence of the inverse care law from the UK Quality and Outcomes Framework. *Journal of Epidemiology and Community Health* 60, 917–922.

McMillan, B. and Conner, M. (2003) Applying an extended version of the theory of planned behaviour to illicit drug use among students. *Journal of Applied Social Psychology* 33, 1662–1683.

McMillan, B., Higgins, A. R. and Conner, M. (2005) Using an extended theory of planned behaviour to understand smoking amongst schoolchildren. *Addiction Research and Theory* 13(3), 293–306.

McPearson, P.D. (1992) Health for all Australians. In: H. Gardner (ed.) *Health Policy*. Melbourne: Churchill Livingstone.

McPherson, K., Marsh, T. and Brown, M. (2007) *Foresight Tackling Obesities: Future choices – Modelling Future Trends in Obesity and Their Impact on Health*. London: Department of Innovation Universities and Skills.

Mercer, C.H., Bailey, J.V., Johnson A.M., Erens, B., Wellings, K., Fention, K.A. and Copas, A.J. (2007) Women who report having sex with women: British national probability data on prevalence, sexual behaviors, and health outcomes. *American Journal of Public Health* 97(6), 1126–1133.

Merikangas, K.R. (2000) Genetic epidemiology of drug use disorders. *Trends in Neurosciences* 2, 55–62.

Merikangas, K.R. (2002) Genetic epidemiology of substance-use disorders. In: H. D'haenen, J. Den Boer and P. Willner (eds) *Textbook of Biological Psychiatry*. New York: John Wiley and Sons.

Merikangas, K. and Avenevoli, S. (2000) Implications of genetic epidemiology for the prevention of substance use disorders. *Addictive Behaviors* 25, 807–820.

Michaud, C.I., Kahn, J.P., Musse, N., Burlet, C., Nicholas, J.P. and Mejean, J. (1990) Relationships between critical life event and eating behaviour in high-school students. *Stress Medicine* 6, 57–64.

Michie, S. and Abraham, C. (2004) Interventions to change health behaviours: evidence-based or evidence-inspired? *Psychology and Health* 19(1), 29–49.

Michie, S., Lester, K., Pinto, J. and Marteau, T. (2005) Communicating risk information in generic counselling: an observational study. *Health Education and Behaviour* 32, 589–598.

Michie, S., Rumsey, N., Fussell, A., Hardman, W., Johnston, M., Newman, S. and Yardley, L. (2006) *Improving Health: Changing Behaviour. NHS Health Trainer Handbook*. London: Department of Health.

Miles, A., Rapoport, L., Wardle, J., Afuape, T. and Duman, M. (2001) Using the mass media to target obesity: an analysis of the characteristics and reported behaviour change of participants in the BBC's Fighting Fat, Fighting Fit campaign. *Health Education Research* 16, 357–372.

Miller, A.M. and Vance, C.S. (2004) Sexuality, human rights, and health. *Health and Human Rights* 7, 5–16.

Miller, M.A, Alberts, J.K., Hecht, M.L. and Krizek, R.L. (2000) *Adolescent Relationships and Drug Use*. Mahwah, NJ: Lawrence Erlbaum.

Miller, W.R. and Rollnick, S. (2002) *Motivational Interviewing: Preparing People for Change*, 2nd edn. New York: Guilford.

Miller, W.R., Yahne, C.E. and Tonigan, J.S. (2003) Motivational interviewing in drug abuse services: a randomized trial. *Journal of Consulting and Clinical Psychology* 71, 754–763.

Millett, G., Malebranche, D., Mason, B. and Spikes, P. (2005) Focusing down low: bisexual black men, HIV risk and heterosexual transmission. *Journal of the National Medical Association* 97(Suppl. 7), 52S–59S.

Milne, S., Sheeran, P. and Orbell, S. (2000) Prediction and intervention in health-related behaviour: a meta-review of protection motivation theory. *Journal of Applied Social Psychology* 30, 106–143.

Milner, D. and Bates, C. (2002) *Smoking Interventions in the New GP Contract*. Retrieved 14/06/08 from: http://www.ash.org.uk/index.php?navState=factsandgetpage=?.?html/cessation/gpcontract.html.

Minugh, A.P., Rice, C. and Young, L. (1998) Gender, health beliefs, health behaviours and alcohol consumption. *American Journal of Alcohol Abuse* 24, 483–497.

Mitchie, S. and Abraham, C. (2004) Interventions to change health behaviours: evidence-based or evidence-inspired? *Psychology and Health* 19, 29–49.

Moher, M., Hey, K. and Lancaster, T. (2005) Workplace interventions for smoking cessation. *Cochrane Database of Systematic Reviews* 2, Art. No. CD003440.

Moore, L., Campbell, R., Whelan, A., et al. (2002) Self-help smoking cessation in pregnancy: cluster randomised control trial. *British Medical Journal* 325, 1383–1387.

Morin, S.F., Charles, K.A. and Malyon, A.K. (1984) The psychological impact of AIDS on gay men. *American Psychologist* 39,1288–1293.

Morrison, D.M., Golder, S., Keller, T.E. and Gillmore, M.R. (2002) The theory of reasoned action as a model of marijuana use: tests of implicit assumptions and applicability to high-risk young women. *Psychology of Addictive Behaviours* 16(3), 212–224.

Moskowitz, J.M., Assunta Ritieni, A., Tholandi, M. and Xia, M. (2006) How do Californians define safe sex? *Californian Journal of Health Promotion* 4(1), 109–118.

Moyer, A., Finney, J.W., Swearingen, E. and Vergun, P. (2002) Brief interventions for alcohol problems a meta-analytic review of controlled investigations in treatment seeking and non-treatment seeking populations. *Addiction* 97, 279–292.

MTP Research Group (2004). Brief treatments for cannabis dependence: findings from a randomized multisite trial. *Journal of Consulting Clinical Psychology* 72, 455–466.

Mulvihill, C., Taylor, L., Waller, S., Naidoo, B. and Thom, B. (2005) *Prevention and Reduction of Alcohol Misuse: Evidence Briefing*, 2nd edition. London: Health Development Agency.

Muraven, M. and Baumeister, R.F. (2000) Self regulation and depletion of limited resources: does self control resemble a muscle? *Psychological Bulletin* 126, 247–259.

Murgraff, V., Abraham, C. and McDermott, M. (2007) Reducing Friday alcohol consumption among moderate women drinkers: evaluation of a brief evidence-based intervention. *Alcohol and Alcoholism* 42, 37–41.

Murgraff, V., White, D. and Phillips, K. (1999) An application of protection motivation theory to riskier single-occasion drinking. *Psychology and Health* 14, 339–350.

Murray, M. and Jarrett, L. (1985) Young people's perception of health, illness and smoking. *Health Education Journal* 44(1), 18–22.

Mutrie, N., Carney, C., Blamey, A., Crawford, F., Aitchison, T. and Whitelaw, A. (2002) 'Walk in to Work Out': a randomised controlled trial of a self help intervention to promote active commuting. *Journal of Epidemiology and Community Health* 56, 407– 412.

Myers, K.P. and Sclafani, A. (2006) Development of learned flavour preferences. *Developmental Psychobiology* 48, 380–388.

Myslobodsky, M. (2003) Gourmand savants and environmental determinants of obesity. *Obesity Reviews* 4, 121–128.

Nabi, R.L. (2002) Discrete emotions and persuasion. In: J.P. Dillard and M. Pfau (eds) *The Persuasion Handbook: Developments in Theory and Practice*. London: Sage.

Naidoo, B., Stephens, W. and McPherson, K. (2000) Modelling the short term consequences of smoking cessation in England on the hospitalisation rates for acute myocardial infarction and stroke. *Tobacco Control* 9, 397–400.

Najman, J.M. (1980) Theories of disease causation and the concept of general susceptibility: a review. *Social Science and Medicine, Medical Psychology and Medical Sociology* 14A(3), 231–237.

Nandwani, R., on behalf of the Clinical Effectiveness Group of the British Association for Sexual Health and HIV (BASHH) *2006 United Kingdom Guideline on the Sexual Health of People with HIV: Sexually Transmitted Infections*. Accessed 25 November 2007 at: http://www.bashh.org/guidelines/2006/sexual_health_hiv_0406. pdf.

National AIDS Trust (2006) Public Attitudes towards HIV. Accessed 18 December 2007 at: www.nat.org.uk/document/122.

National Center for Health Statistics (2004) *Health, United States, 2004 with Chartbook on Trends in the Health of Americans*. Hyattsville, MD: NCHS.

National Assembly for Wales (2000) *A Strategic Framework for Promoting Sexual Health in Wales*. Cardiff: National Assembly for Wales.

National Assembly for Wales (2006) *Welsh Health Survey: 2003/05 Local Authority Report*. Cardiff: National Assembly for Wales.

National Audit Office (2001) *Tackling Obesity in England*. London: The Stationery Office.

National Cancer Institute (2000) *Population Based Smoking Cessation: Proceedings of a Conference on What Works to Influence Cessation in the General Population*. Smoking and Tobacco Control Monograph no. 12, Bethesda, MD, USA. NIH publication no. 00–4892. Department of Health and Human Services, National Institutes of Health, National Cancer Institute.

National Consumer Council (2002) Running risks: summary research into consumers' view on risk. London: National Consumer Council.

National Institute for Health and Clinical Excellence (NICE) (2006a) *Obesity: Guidance on the Prevention, Identification, Assessment and Management of Overweight and Obesity in Adults and Children.* Retrieved 11 December 2007 from: http://www.nice.org.uk/nicemedia/pdf/word/CG43NICEGuideline.doc.

National Institute for Health and Clinical Excellence (NICE) (2006b) Public Health Intervention Guidance no. 2. Four commonly used methods to increase physical activity: brief interventions in primary care, exercise referral schemes, pedometers and community-based exercise programmes for walking and cycling. London: NICE.

National Public Health Service for Wales (2005) *Framework for Action: Physical Activity.* Cardiff: Welsh Assembly Government.

National Treatment Agency for Substance Misuse (2005) *A National Survey of Inpatient Services in England.* The Stationery Office: London.

Natsal (2000) *National Survey of Sexual Attitudes and Lifestyles II, 2000–2001 (NATSAL II; NATSAL 2000*) Accessed 20 December 2007 at: http://www.data-archive.ac.uk/findingData/snDescription.asp?sn=5223.

Ness, A.R. and Powles, J.W. (1997) Fruit and vegetables and cardiovascular disease: a review. *International Journal of Epidemiology* 26, 1–13.

Newman, J. and Taylor, A. (1992) Effect of a means-end contingency on young children's food preferences. *Journal of Experimental Child Psychology* 64, 200–216.

News (2007) Alcohol, breast and colorectal cancer. *European Journal of Cancer* 43, 1225–1229.

NHS Information Centre (2007) Statistics on Drug Use: England, 2007. ICS: London.

Nicholas, J., Wood, L. and Nelson, M. (2007) *Second annual survey of take-up of school meals in England.* Retrieved 9 December 2007 from: http://www.schoolfoodtrust.org.uk/UploadDocs/Library/Documents/second_annual_survey_of_take_up_final.pdf.

NIDA (National Institute on Drug Abuse) (1997) *Preventing drug use among children and adolescents: a research based guide.* National Institute of Health Publication No. 04–4212.

Nielsen, S.J. and Popkin, B.M. (2003) Patterns and Trends in Food Portion Sizes, 1977–1998 *Journal of the American Medical Association* 289, 450–453.

NISRA (2006) *Northern Ireland Health and Social Wellbeing Survey 2006.* NISRA: Belfast.

Norman, E. (1994) Personal factors related to substance misuse: risk abatement and/or resiliency enhancement. In: T.P. Gullotta, G.R. Adams and R. Montemayor (eds) *Substance Misuse in Adolescence.* Thousand Oaks, CA: Sage Publications.

Norman, P., Boer, H. and Seydel, E.R. (2005) Protection motivation theory. In: Conner and Norman (eds) *Predicting Health Behaviour,* 2nd edn. Berkshire: Open University Press.

Northern Ireland Executive (2000) *Investing for Health.* Belfast: NI Executive.

NSOS (2007) Omnibus Survey Report No. 33 Contraception and Sexual Health 2006/07: A report on research using the National Statistics Omnibus Survey produced on behalf of the Information Centre for health and social care. Accessed 7 Nov 2007 at http://www.statistics.gov.uk/downloads/theme_health/contraception2006-07.pdf.

Nuffield Council on Bioethics (2007) *Public Health Ethical Issues.* London: Nuffield Council.

Oakley, A., Fullerton, D., Holland, J., Arnold, S., France-Dawson, M., Kelley, P. and McGrellis, S. (1995) Sexual health education interventions for young people: a methodological review. *British Medical Journal* 310, 158–162.

Oatley, K. (2996) Emotions, rationality and informal reasoning. In: J. Oakhill and A. Garnham (eds) *Mental Models in Cognitive Science: Essays in Honour of Phil Johnson-Laird*. Hove: Psychology Press.

O'Connor, M.L. and Parker, E. (1995) *Health Promotion: Principles and Practice in the Australian Context.* St Leonards, NSW: Allen and Unwin.

Oesterle, S., Hill, K.G., Hawkins, J.D., Guo, J., Catalano, R.F. and Abbott, R.D. (2004) Adolescent heavy episodic drinking trajectories and health in young adulthood. *Journal of Studies on Alcohol* 65, 204–212.

Oetting, E.R. and Beauvais, F. (1986) Peer cluster theory: drugs and the adolescent. *Journal of Counselling and Development* 65, 17–22.

Oetting, E.R. and Beauvais, F. (1987) Common elements in youth drug abuse: peer clusters and other psychosocial factors. *Journal of Drug Issues* 17, 133–151.

Ofcom (2004) *Childhood Obesity: Food Advertising in Context.* Retrieved 20 December 2007 from: http://www.ofcom.or.uk/research/tv/reports/food_ads/report.pdf.

Ofcom (2006) Annex 7 – Impact Assessment Consultation on Television Advertising of Food and Drink to Children. Joint FSA/DoH Analysis; 2.

Office for National Statistics (ONS) (2003) *National Travel Survey: 2003 Final Results*. London: The Stationery Office.

Office for National Statistics (ONS) (2006b) *Sexual Health*. Accessed on 18 December 2007 at: http://www.statistics.gov.uk/CCI/nugget.asp?ID=1330andPos=andColRank=2andRank=224.

Office for National Statistics (ONS) (2006a) *General Household Survey, 2005*. London: Office for National Statistics.

Office for National Statistics (ONS) (2007) *Social Trends*. London: HMSO.

Office for National Statistics (ONS) (2008) *News Release: Alcohol-related Death Rates Continue to Rise*. London: Office for National Statistics.

Office of the Surgeon General (1964) *Smoking and Health*. Washington, DC: US Department of Health, Education and Welfare.

Official Journal of the European Union (2003) http://eur-lex.europa.eu/LexUriServ/site/en/oj/2003/l_226/l_22620030910en00240026.pdf.

Ogden, J. (2003a) *The Psychology of Eating: From Healthy to Disordered Behaviour*. Oxford: Blackwell.

Ogden, J. (2003b) Some problems with Social Cognition Models: a pragmatic and conceptual analysis. *Health Psychology* 22(4), 424–428.

Ogilvie, D., Egan, M., Hamilton, V. and Pettricrew, M. (2004) Promoting walking and cycling as an alternative to using cars: systematic review. *British Medical Journal Online*: BMJ,doi:10.1136/bmj.38216.714560.55.

O'Keefe, D.J. (2002) *Persuasion: Theory and Research*, 2nd edn. London: Sage.

Okuyemi, K.S., Nollen, N.L. and Ahluwalia, J.S. (2006) Interventions to facilitate smoking cessation. *American Family Physician* 74, 262–271.

Oliver, G. and Wardle, J. (1999) Perceived effects of stress on food choice. *Physiological Behaviour* 66, 511–515.

Olivera, S.A., Ellison, R.C., Moore, L.L., Gillman, M.W., Garrahie, E.J. and Singer, M.R. (1992) Parent–child relationships in nutrient intake: the Framingham children's study. *American Journal of Clinical Nutrition* 56, 593–598.

Olsson, C., Coffey, C., Bond, L., Toumbourou, J. and Patton, G. (2003) Family risk factors for cannabis use: a population based survey of Australian secondary school students. *Drug and Alcohol Review* 22, 143–152.

Onat, A., Avci, G.S., Barlan, M.M., Uyarel, H., Uzunlar, B. and Sansoy, V. (2004) Measures of abdominal obesity assessed for visceral adiposity and relation to coronary risk. *International Journal of Obesity and Related Metabolic Disorders* 28, 1018–1025.

Orbell, S., Blair, C., Sherlock, K. and Conner, M. (2001) The theory of planned behaviour and ecstacy use: role for habit and perceived control over taking versus obtaining substances. *Journal of Applied Social Psychology* 31, 31–47.

Orford, J. (2001) *Excessive Appetites: A Psychological View of Addictions*, 2nd edn. Chichester: John Wiley and Sons Ltd.

O'Sullivan, L.F., Udell, W. and Patel, V.L. (2006) Young urban adults' heterosexual risk encounters and perceived risk and safety: a structured diary study. *The Journal of Sex Research* 43(4), 343–351.

Owen, N., Leslie, E., Salmon, J. and Fotheringham, J. (2000) Environmental determinants of physical activity and sedentary behaviour. *Exercise and Sport Sciences Reviews* 28, 153–158.

Paglia, A. and Room, R. (1999) Preventing substance use problems among youth: a literature review and recommendations. *The Journal of Primary Prevention* 20, 3–50.

Paisley, C.M. and Sparks, P. (1998) Expectations of reducing fat intake: the role of perceived need within the Theory of Planned Behaviour. *Psychology and Health* 13, 341–353.

Palo Alto Medical Foundation (2005) *Safer Oral Sex*. Accessed 19 December 2007 from: http://www.pamf.org/teen/sex/std/oral/.

Parker, D., Manstead, A.M.R. and Stradling, S. (1995) Extending the theory of planned behaviour: the role of the personal norm. *British Journal of Social Psychology* 35, 127–137.

Parrott, S. and Godfrey, C. (2004) Economics of smoking cessation. *British Medical Journal* 328(7445), 947–949.

Parsons, J.T., Vicioso, K.J., Punzalan, J.C., Halkitis, P.N., Kutnick, A. and Velasquez, M.M. (2004) The impact of alcohol use on the sexual scripts of HIV-positive men. *Journal of Sex Research*, May.

Pate, R.R., Pratt, M., Blair, S.N., Haskell, W.L., Macera, C.A., Bouchard, C. et al. (1995) Physical activity and public health – a recommendation from the Centers for Disease Control and Prevention and the American College of Sports Medicine. *Journal of the American Medical Association* 273, 402–407.

Patel, V.L., Gutnik, L.A., Yoskowitz, N.A., O'Sullivant, L.F. and Kaufman, D.R. (2006) Patterns of reasoning and decision making about condom use by urban college students. *AIDS Care* 18(8), 918–930.

Peattie, S. and Peattie, K. (2003) Ready to fly solo? Reducing social marketing's dependence on commercial marketing theory. *Marketing Theory* III(3), 365–385.

Peretti-Watel, P., Constance, J., Guilbert, P., Gautier, A., Beck, F. and Moatti, J. (2007) Smoking too few cigarettes to be at risk? Smokers' perceptions of risk and risk denial, a French survey. *Tobacco Control* 16, 351–356.

Perkins, K.A. (1992) Effects of tobacco smoking on caloric intake. *British Journal of Addiction* 87, 193–205. Retrieved 20 December 2007 from Academic Search Premier.

Perkins, K.A., Conklin, C.A. and Levine, M.D. (2008) *Cognitive-Behavioural Therapy for Smoking Cessation*. New York: Routledge.

Peto, R. and Lopez, A.D. (1990) Worldwide mortality from current smoking pattern. In: B. Durston and K. Jamrozik (eds) *Tobacco and Health: The Global War*. Perth: Health Department of Western Australia.

Petraitis, J., Flay, B.R. and Miller, T.Q. (1995) Reviewing theories of adolescent substance use: organising piece in the puzzle. *Psychological Bulletin* 117, 67–86.

Phillips, R., Amos, A., Ritchie, D., Cunningham-Burley, S. and Martin, C. (2007) Smoking in the home after the smoke-free legislation in Scotland: qualitative study. *British Medical Journal* 335, 553.

Piasecki, T.M. (2006) Relapse to smoking. *Clinical Psychology Review* 26(2), 196–215.

Pierce, J.P. and Gilpin, E.A. (2002) Impact of over-the-counter sales on effectiveness of pharmaceutical aids for smoking cessation. *Journal of the American Medical Association* 288, 1260–1264.

Pierce, J.P., Stefanick, M.L., Flatt, S.W., Natarajan, L., Sternfeld, B., Madlensky, L. et al. (2007) Greater survival after breast cancer in physical active women with high vegetable-fruit intake regardless of obesity. *Journal of Clinical Onocology* 17, 2345–2351.

Pierce, P.F. (1993) Deciding on breast cancer treatment: a description of decision behaviour. *Nursing Research* 42, 22–28.

Plant, M. and Plant, M. (2006) *Binge Britain*. Oxford: Oxford University Press.

Plotnikoff, R.C. and Higginbotham, N. (1998) Protection motivation theory and the prediction of exercise and low-fat diet behaviours among Australian cardiac patients. *Psychology and Health* 13, 411–429.

Plotnikoff, R.C. and Higginbotham, N. (2002) Protection motivation theory and exercise behaviour change for the prevention of coronary heart disease in a high risk Australian representative community sample of adults. *Psychology, Health and Medicine* 7, 87–98.

Poikolainen, K. (1999) Effectiveness of brief interventions to reduce alcohol intake in primary care populations: a meta analysis. *Preventive Medicine* 28, 503–509.

Porter, R. (1985) The drinking man's disease: the prehistory of drinking in Georgian Britain. *British Journal of Addiction* 80, 385–396.

Portnoy, B. (1980) Effects of a controlled usage alcohol education program based on the health belief model. *Journal of Drug Education* 10, 181.

Poulton, R., Caspi, A., Milne, B.J. et al. (2002) Association between children's experience of socio-economic disadvantage and adult health: a life-course study. *Lancet* 360, 1640–1645.

Pound, E., Coleman, T., Adams, C., Bauld, L. and Ferguson, J. (2005) Targeting smokers in priority groups: the influence of government targets and policy statements. *Addiction* 100(S2), S28–S35.

Prentice-Dunn, S. and Rogers, R.W. (1986) Protection motivation theory and preventive health: beyond the Health Belief Model. *Health Education Research* 1, 153–161.

Primatesta, P. (2004) *Health Survey for England 2004 – Updating of Trend Tables to Include 2005 Data*. London. The Stationery Office.

Prime Minister's Strategy Unit (2004) *Alcohol Harm Reduction Strategy for London*. London: Strategy Unit.

Prochaska, J.O. (2005) Further commentaries on West (2005) *Addiction* 101, 768–778.

Prochaska, J.O. and DiClemente, C.C. (1983) Stages and processes of self-change smoking: towards an integrative model of change. *Journal of Consulting and Clinical Psychology* 51, 390–395.

Prochaska, J.O. and Goldstein M.G. (1991) Process of smoking cessation: implications for clinicians. *Clinics in Chest Medicine* 12(4), 727–735.

Prochaska, J.O. and Velicer, W.F. (1997) The transtheoretical model of health behavior change. *American Journal of Health Promotion* 12(1), 38–48.

Prochaska, J.O., DiClemente, C.C. and Norcross, J.C. (1992) In search of how people change: applications to addictive behaviours. *American Psychologist* 47, 1102–1114.

Prochaska, J.O., Velicer, W.F., Prochaska, J.M. and Johnston, J.L. (2004) Size consistency and stability of stage effects for smoking cessation. *Addictive Behaviours* 29, 207–13.

Prochaska, J.M., Prochaska, J.O., Cohen, F.C., Gomes, S.O., Laforge, R.G. and Eastwood, B.S. (2004) The transtheoretical model of change for multi-level interventions for alcohol abuse on campus. *Journal of Alcohol and Drug Education* 47, 34–50.

Puska, P. (2001) Commentary: physical activity promotion in primary care. *International Journal of Epidemiology* 30, 815–816.

Quetelet, L. (1869) *Physique sociale ou essai sur le développement des facultes de l'homme*. Bruxelles: C. Murquardt.

Quinlan, K.B. and McCaul, K.D. (2000) Matched and mismatched interventions with young adult smokers: testing a stage theory. *Health Psychology* 19, 165–171.

Radlo, S.J., Steinberg, G.M., Singer, R.M., Barba, D.A. and Melnikov, A. (2002) The influence of an attentional focus strategy on alpha brain wave activity, heart rate and dart throwing performance. *International Journal of Sport Psychology* 33, 205–217.

Ramisetty-Mikler, S., Caetano, R., Goebert, D. and Nishimura, S. (2004) Ethnic variation in drinking, drug use, and sexual behaviour among adolescents in Hawaii. *Journal of School Health* 74(1), 16–22.

Ramos, D. and Perkins, D.F. (2006) Goodness of fit assessment of an alcohol intervention program and the underlying theories of change. *Journal of American College Health* 55, 57–64.

Rana, R.K., Pimenta, J.M., Rosenberg, D.M., Warren, T., Sekhin, S., Cook, S.F., Robinson, N.J., Valociclovir HSV Transmission Study Group (2006) Sexual behaviour and condom use among individuals with a history of symptomatic genital herpes. *Sexually Transmitted Infections* 82(1), 69–74.

Raw, M., Anderson, P., Batra, A., Dubois, G., Harrington, P., Hirsch, A. et al. (2002) WHO Europe evidence based recommendations on the treatment of tobacco dependence. *Tobacco Control* 11, 44–46.

Rayner, M. (2007) Social marketing: how might this contribute to tackling obesity? Short Science Review. Foresight Tackling Obesities: Future Choices. *Obesity Reviews* 8(s1), 195–199.

Rayner, M. and Scarborough, P. (2005) The burden of food related ill health in the UK. *Journal of Epidemiology and Community Health* 59, 1054–1057.

Reaich, D. (1997) Odour perception in chronic renal disease. *Lancet* 350, (9086), 1191–1193. Retrieved 20 December 2007 from Academic Search Premier.

Rehm, J., Room, R., Monteiro, H., Gmel, G., Graham, K., Rehn, N., Sempos, C. and Jerrigan, D. (2003) Alcohol as a risk factor for global burden of disease. *European Addiction Research* 9, 157–164.

Reilly, J. and Dorosty, A. (1999) Epidemic of obesity in UK children. *Lancet* 354, 1874–1875.

Reinherz, H.Z., Giacconia, R.M., Carmola Hauf, A.M. et al. (2000) General and specific childhood risk factors for depression and drug disorders by early adulthood. *Journal of the American Academy of Child and Adolescent Psychiatry* 39, 223–231.

Remennick, L. (1998) Race, class and occupation as determinants of cancer risk and survival: trend report: the cancer problem in the context of modernity: sociology, demography, politics. *Current Sociology* 46(1), 25–39.

Reniscow, K., Davis-Hearn, M., Smith, M., Baranowski, T., Lin, L.S., Baraowski, J. et al. (1997) Social-cognitive predictors of fruit and vegetable intake in children. *Health Psychology* 16, 272–276.

Repetti, R.L., Taylor, S.E. and Seeman, T.E. (2002) Risky families: family social environments and the mental and physical health of offspring. *Psychological Bulletin* 128(2), 330–366.

Richards, A., Kattelmann, K. and Ren, C. (2006) Motivating 18- to 24-year-olds to increase their fruit and vegetable consumption. *Journal of the American Dietetic Association* 106, 1405–1411.

Richardson, K. and Crosier, A. (2002) *Smoking and Health Inequalities* London: ASH and the Health Development Agency.

Riemsma, R.P., Pattenden, J., Bridle, C., Sowden, A.J., Mather, L., Watt, I.S. and Walker, A. (2003) Systematic review of the effectiveness of stage based interventions to promote smoking cessation. *British Medical Journal* 326, 1175–1177.

Rigby, K., Brown, M., Anagnostou, P., Ross, M.W. and Rosser, B.R.S. (1989) Shock tactics to counter AIDS: the Australian experience. *Psychology and Health*, 3, 145–159.

Rimm, E.B., Stampfer, M.J., Giovannucci, E., Ascherio, A., Spiegelman, D., Colditz, G.A. and Willett, W. (1995) Body size and fat distribution as predictors of coronary heart disease among middle-aged and older US men. *American Journal of Epidemiology* 141(12), 1117–1127.

Robbins, T.W. and Fray, P.J. (1982) Stress induced eating: fact, fiction or misunderstanding. *Appetite* 1, 103–133.

Roberts, A.B., Oyun, C., Batnasan, E., Laing, L. (2005) Exploring the social and cultural context of sexual health for young people in Mongolia: implications for health promotion. *Social Science and Medicine* 60, 1487–1498.

Robinson, K.L., Price, J.H., Thompson, C.L. and Schmalzried, H.D. (1998) Rural junior high school students' risk factors for and perceptions of teenage parenthood. *Journal of School Health* 68(8), 334–338.

Robinson, K., Telljohann, S. and Price, J. (1999) Predictors of sixth graders engaging in sexual intercourse. *Journal of School Health* 69(9), 369–375.

Rodgers, W.M., Hall, C.R., Blanchard, C.M., McAuley, E. and Munroe, K.J. (2002) Task and scheduling self efficacy as predictors of exercise behaviour. *Psychology and Health* 27, 405–416.

Rodin, J., Elias, M., Silberstein, L.R. and Wagner, A. (1988) Combined behavioural and pharmacologic treatment for obesity: predictors of successful weight maintenance. *Journal of Consulting and Clinical Psychology* 56, 399–404.

Rogers, P.J. and Blundell, J.E. (1990) Umami and appetite: effects of mono-sodium glutamate on hunger and food intake in human subjects. *Physiology and Behaviour* 48, 801–804.

Rogers, R.W. (1975) A protection motivation theory of fear appeals and attitude change. *Journal of Psychology* 91, 93–114.

Rogers, R.W. (1983) Cognitive and physiological processes in fear appeals and attitude change: a revised theory of protection motivation. In: J.T. Cacioppo and R.E. Petty (eds) *Social Psychophysiology: A Source Book*. New York: Guildford Press.

Rogers, R.W. (1985) Attitude change and information integration in fear appeals. *Psychological Reports* 56, 179–182.

Rohsenow, D.J., Monti, P.M., Martin, R.A., Michalec, E. and Abrams, D.B. (2000) Brief coping skills treatment for cocaine abuse: 12-month substance use outcomes. *Journal of Consulting Clinical Psychology* 68, 515–520.

Rome Declaration on World Food Security and World Food Summit Plan of Action. (1996) World Food Summit 13–17 November. Rome.

Room, R. (2004) Disabling the public interest: alcohol strategies and policies for England. *Addiction* 99, 1083–1089.

Room, R., Babor, T. and Rehm, J. (2005) Alcohol and public health. *Lancet* 365, 519–530.

Rose, J.E. and Behm, F.M. (1995) There is more to smoking than the CNS effects of nicotine. In: P.B.S. Clark (ed.) *Effects of Nicotine on Biological Systems II*. Basel: Burkhauser Verlang.

Rose, J.E., Behm, F.M. and Levin, E.D. (1993) Role of nicotine dose and sensory cues in the regulation of smoke intake. *Pharmacology Biochemistry and Behaviour* 44(4), 891–900.

Rosen, C.S. (2000) Is the sequencing of change processes by stage consistent across health problems? A meta-analysis. *Health Psychology* 19, 593–604.

Rosenstein, D. and Oster, H. (1988) Differential facial responses to four basic tastes in newborns. *Child Development* 59, 1555–1568.

Rosenstock, I.M. (1974) Historical origins of the health belief model. *Health Education Monographs* 2, 1–8.

Rosenstock, I. (1990) The Health Belief Model: Explaining health behaviour through expectancies. In: K. Glanz, F.M. Lewis and B.K. Rimmer (eds) *Health Behaviour and Health Education: Theory, Research and Practice*. San Francisco: Jossey-Bass.

Rosenstock, I.M., Strecher, V.J. and Becker, M. H. (1988) Social learning theory and the health belief model. *Health Education and Quarterly* 15, 175–183.

Rothman, K.J. (1998) *Modern Epidemiology*. Philadelphia, PA: Lippincott, Williams and Wilkins.

Rovniak, L.S., Anderson, E.S., Winett, R.A. and Stephens, R.S. (2002) Social cognitive determinants of physical activity in young adults: a prospective structural equation analysis. *Annals of Behavioural Medicine* 24, 149–156.

Rubak, S., Sandbaek, A., Lauritzen, T. and Christensen, B. (2005) Motivational interviewing: a systematic review and meta-analysis. *British Journal of General Practice* 55(513), 305–312.

Ruiter R.A.C. (2004) *Effecten van angstaanjagende tv-spotjes [Effects of fear-arousing TV commercials]. Final report.* Maastricht, Netherlands: Maastricht University, Department of Experimental Psychology.

Ruiter, R.A.C. and Kok, G. (2005) Saying is not (always) doing: cigarette warning labels are useless. *European Journal of Public Health* 15(3), 329.

Ruiter, R.A.C. Abraham, C. and Kok, G. (2001) Scary warnings and rational precautions: a review of the psychology of fear appeals. Psychology and Health 16(6), 613–630.

Rusch, M., Lampinen, T., Schilder, A. and Hogg, R. (2004) Unprotected anal intercourse associated with recreational drug use among young men who have sex with men depends on partner type and intercourse role. *Sexually Transmitted Diseases* 31, 492–498.

RUThinking (2007) Safer Sex. Accessed 19 December 2007 at: http://www.ruthinking.co.uk/about_sex/contraception/safer_sex.aspx.

Saguy A.C. and Almeling, R. (2005) *Fat devils and moral panics: News reporting on obesity science.* Presented at the SOMAH workshop. UCLA Department of Sociology.

Salber, E.J. MacMahon B. and Harrison, S.V. (1963) The influence of siblings on student smoking patterns. *Pediatrics* 31(4), 569–572.

Sallis, J.F. and Owen, N. (2002) Ecological models of health behaviour, In: J.F. Sallis (ed.) *Health Behaviour and Health Education*, 3rd edn. San Francisco: Jossey Bass.

Sanderson, C.A. (2000) The effectiveness of a sexuality education newsletter in influencing teenagers' knowledge and attitudes about sexual involvement and drug use. *Journal of Adolescent Research* 15, 674–681.

Santelli, J.S., Kaiser, J., Hirsch, L. et al. (2004) Initiation of sexual intercourse among middle school adolescents: the influence of psychosocial factors. *Journal of Adolescent Health* 34, 200–208.

Sareen, J., Chartier, M., Paulus, M.P. and Stein, M.B. (2006) Illicit drug use and anxiety disorders: findings from two community surveys. *Psychiatry Research* 142(1), 11–17.

Scambler, G. (ed.) (2003) *Sociology as Applied to Medicine*, 5th edn. London: Elsevier.

Schaalma, H.P., Abraham, C., Gillmore, M.R. and Kok, G. (2004) Sex education as health promotion: what does it take? *Archives of Sexual Behavior* 33(3), 259–269.

Schachter, S., Silverstein, B., Kozlowski, L.T., Herman, C.P. and Liebling, B. (1977) Effects of stress on cigarette smoking and urinary pH. *Journal of Experimental Psychology: General* 106, 24–30.

Schagen, S., Blenkinsop, S., Schagen, I., Scott, E., Teeman, D., White, G. et al. (2005) *Evaluation of the School Fruit and Vegetable Scheme: Final Report.* Retrieved 7 December 2007 from: http://www.nfer.ac.uk/publications/pdfs/downloadable/NFSfinal.pdf.

Schar, E.H. and Gutierrez, K.K. (2001) *Smoking Cessation Media Campaigns From Around the World: Recommendations From Lessons Learned.* Copenhagen, Denmark: World Health Organization, Regional Office for Europe. Available at: http://www.euro.who.int/document/e74523.pdf.

Schluter, G. and Lee, C. (1999) Changing food consumption patterns: their effect on the US food system, 1972–1992. *Food Review* 22, 35–37.

Schoeller, D.A., Shay, K. and Kushner, R. (1997) How much physical activity is needed to minimize weight gain in previously obese women? *American Journal of Clinical Nutrition* 66: 551–556.

School Food Trust (2006) *'Eat better, do better'. Strategic plan 2006–2009.* Retrieved 5 December 2007 from: http://www.schoolfoodtrust.org.uk/UploadDocs/Contents/Documents/SFT%20Strategic%20Plan%2029032006.pdf.

Schubotz, D., Simpson, A. and Rolston, B. (2003) *Towards Better Sexual Health: A Survey of Sexual Attitudes and Lifestyles of Young People in Northern Ireland.* Research Report. Belfast: fpaNI in partnership with University of Ulster.

Schwarcz, S., Scheer, S., McFarland, W., Katz, K., Valleroy, L., Chen, S. and Catania, J. (2007) Prevalence of HIV infection and predictors of high-transmission sexual risk behaviors among men who have sex with men. *American Journal of Public Health* 97(6), 1067–1075.

Schwarzer, R. (1992) Self efficacy in the adoption and maintenance of health behaviours: theoretical approaches and a new model. In: R. Schwarzer (ed.) *Self Efficacy: Thought Control of Action.* Washington, DC: Hemisphere.

Scotland Public Health Observatory (2007) *Drug Misuse in Scotland.* National Information Services: Edinburgh.

Scottish Executive (2005) *The Scottish Health Survey 2003.* Edinburgh: Scottish Executive.

Segaar, D., Willemsen, M.C., Bolman, C. and De Vries, H. (2007) Nurse adherence to a minimal-contact smoking cessation intervention on cardiac wards. *Research in Nursing and Health* 30(4), 429–444.

Shafil, T., Stovel, K. and Holmes, K. (2007) Association between condom use at sexual debut and subsequent sexual trajectories: a longitudinal study using biomarkers. *American Journal of Public Health* 97(6), 1090–1095.

Shaw, J.M., Dzewaltowski, D.A. and McElroy, M. (1992) Self-efficacy and causal attributions as mediators of perceptions of psychological momentum. *Journal of Sport and Exercise Behaviour* 14, 134–147.

Shaw, M., Dorling, D., Gordon, D. and Davey Smith, G. (2005) Health inequalities and New Labour: how the promises compare with real progress. *British Medical Journal* 330, 1016–1021.

Shaw, M., Gordon, D., Dorling, D., Mitchell, R. and Davey Smith, G. (2000) Increasing mortality differentials by residential area level of poverty: Britain 1981–1997. *Social Science and Medicine* 51, 151–153.

Sheeran, P. and Orbell, S. (1998) Does intention predict condom use? A meta analysis and test of four moderators. *British Journal of Social Psychology* 37, 231–250.

Sheeran, P. and Taylor, S. (1999) Predicting intentions to use condoms: a meta-anaylsis and comparison of the theories of reasoned action and planned behaviour. *Journal of Applied Social Psychology* 29, 1624–1675.

Sheeran, P., Abraham, C. and Orbell, S. (1999) Psychosocial correlates of heterosexual condom use: a meta-analysis. *Psychological Bulletin* 125, 90–132.

Sheeran, P., Milne, S., Webb, T.L. and Gollwitzer, P.M. (2007) Implementation intentions and health behaviour. In: M. Conner, and P. Norman (eds) *Predicting Health Behaviour*. Berkshire: Open University Press.

Shepherd, R. and Farleigh, C.A. (1989) Sensory assessment of foods and the role of sensory attributes in determining food choice. In: R. Shepherd (ed.) *Handbook of the Psychophysiology of Human Eating*. London: Wiley.

Shiffman, S., Paty, J.A., Rohay, J.M., Di Marino, M.E. and Gitchell, J.G. (2001) The efficacy of computer-tailored smoking cessation material as a supplement to nicotine patch therapy. *Drug and Alcohol Dependence* 64(1), 35–46.

Shiloh, S. and Saxe, L. (1989) Perceptions of recurrence risk by genetic counselees. *Psychological Health* 3(1), 45–61.

Shrier, L.A., Ancheta, R., Goodman, E., Chiou, V.M., Lyden, M.R. and Emans, S.J. (2001) Randomized controlled trial of a safer sex intervention for high-risk adolescent girls. *Archives of Pediatrics and Adolescent Medicine* 155, 73–79.

Siahpush, M., McNeill, A., Borland, R. and Fong, G.T. (2006) Socioeconomic variations in nicotine dependence, self efficacy, and intention to quit across four countries: findings from the International Tobacco Control (ITC) Four Country Survey. *Tobacco Control* 15(Siii), iii71–iii75.

Sigal, R., Kenny, G.P., Wasserman, D.H., Castaneda-Sceppa, C. and White, R. (2006) Physical activity/exercise and Type 2 diabetes: a consensus statement from the American Diabetes Association. *Diabetes Care* 29, 1433–1438.

Silagy, C., Lancaster, T., Stead, L., Mant, D. and Fowler, G. (2002) Nicotine replacement therapy for smoking cessation. *Cochrane Database of Systematic Reviews* 4, CD000146.

Simon, S. and Paxton, S.J. (2004) Sexual risk attitudes and behaviours among young adult Indonesians: a focus group study. *Culture, Health and Sexuality* 6, 303–409.

Sionéan, C., DiClemente, R.J. and Wingood, G.M. (2002) Psychosocial and behavioral correlates of refusing unwanted sex among African-American adolescent females. *Journal of Adolescent Health* 30, 55– 63.

Skills for Health (2007) *Competencies for Health Trainers*. London: Skills for Health.

Skolbekken, J.A. (1995) The risk epidemic in medical journals. *Social Science and Medicine* 40, 291–305.

Slack, M.K. (2006) Interpreting current physical activity guidelines and incorporating them into practice for health promotion and disease prevention. *American Journal of Health System Pharmacy* 63, 1647–1653.

Slevin, A.P. and Marvin, C.L. (1987) Safe sex and pregnancy prevention: a guide for health practitioners working with adolescents. *Journal Community Health Nursing* 4, 235–241.

Slovic, P. (2000) Do adolescent smokers know the risks? In: *The Perception of Risk*. P. Slovic (ed.) London: Earthscan Publications Ltd.

Smoking and Health: Report of the Advisory Committee to the Surgeon General of the Public Health Service. Washington, DC: Public Health Service, Center for Disease Control (1964). PHS publication 103.

Sniehotta, F.F., Schols, U. and Schwarzer, R. (2004) Bridging the intention–behaviour gap: planning, self-efficacy, and action control in the adoption and maintenance of physical exercise. *Psychology and Health* 20(2), 143–160.

Snijder, M.B., Van Dam, R.M., Visser, M. and Seidell, J.C. (2006) What aspects of body fat are particularly hazardous and how do we measure them? *International Journal of Epidemiology* 35, 83–92.

Society of Sexual Health Advisers (SSHA) (2007) *Sexually Transmitted Infections*. Accessed 19 December 2007 at: www.ssha.info/public/infections/index.asp.

Soodeen, F. and Shenker, D. (2008) *Licensing Act 2003: A Lopsided Policy*. London: Alcohol Concern.

Sorensen, G., Emmons, K., Stoddard, A.M. et al. (2002) Do social influences contribute to occupational differences in quitting smoking and attitudes towards quitting? *American Journal of Heath Promotion* 16, 135–141.

Spanou, C. (2008) *Health Behaviour Change: Theory and Practice*. Conference presentation. Behaviour Change: Putting Theory into Action. Physical Activity Network Wales.

Sparks, P., Shepherd, R. and Frewer, L.J. (1995) Assessing and structuring attitudes toward the use of gene technology in food production: the role of perceived ethical obligation. *Basic and Applied Social Psychology* 16, 267–285.

Sparks, P., Connor, M., James, R., Shepherd, R. and Povey, R. (2001) Ambivalence about health-related behaviours: an exploration in the domain of food choice. *British Journal of Health Psychology* 6, 53–68.

Spooner, C. (1999) Causes and correlates of adolescent drug abuse and implications for treatment. *Drug and Alcohol Review* 18(4), 453–475.

Spoth, R.L., Redmond, C. and Shin, C. (2001) Randomised trial of brief family interventions for general populations: adolescent substance use outcomes 4 years following baseline. *Journal of Consulting and Clinical Psychology* 69, 627–642.

Springett, J., Owens, C. and Callaghan, J. (2007) The challenge of combining 'lay' knowledge with 'evidence-based' practice in health promotion: Fag Ends Smoking Cessation Service. *Critical Public Health* 17(3), 243–256.

Stacy, A.W., Newcombe, M.S. and Bentler, P.M. (1992) Interactive and high-order effects of social influences on drug use. *Journal of Health and Social Behaviour* 33, 226–241.

Stapleton, J. (1997) Cigarette smoking prevalence, cessation and relapse. *Statistical Methods in Medical Research* 7(2), 187–203.

Stead, M., Hastings, G. and McDermott, L. (2007b) The meaning, effectiveness and future of social marketing. *Obesity Reviews* 8(s1), 189–193.

Stead, M., McDermott, L., Angus, K. and Hastings, G. (2006) *Marketing Review: Final Report*. ISM Institute for Social Marketing. London: NICE.

Stead, M., Gordon, R., Angus, K. and McDermott, L. (2007a) A systematic review of social marketing effectiveness. *Health Education* 107(2), 126–191.

Stephens, R.S., Roffman, R. A. and Curtin, L. (2000) Comparison of extended versus brief treatments for marijuana use. *Journal of Consulting and Clinical Psychology* 68, 898–908.

Stevens, P.E. and Galvao, L. (2007) 'He Won't Use Condoms': HIV-infected women's struggles in primary relationships with serodiscordant partners. *American Journal of Public Health* 97(6), 1015–1022.

Stitzer, M.L., Iguchi, M.Y. and Felch, L.J. (1992) Contingent takehome incentive: effects on drug use of methadone maintenance patients. *Journal of Consulting and Clinical Psychology* 60, 927– 934.

Strategy Unit (2008) *Food: an analysis of the issues*. Retrieved 15/07/08 from: http://www.cabinetoffice.gov.uk/strategy/~/media/assets/www.cabinetoffice.gov.uk/strategy/food/food_analysis%20pdf.ashx.

Street-Porter, J. (2008a) Let adults fatties eat themselves to death. The kids we can save. *Independent on Sunday*, January.

Street-Porter, J. (2008b) A return to the ration book is the answer to obesity. *Independent on Sunday*, February.

Street-Porter, J. (2008c) Don't blame it on the young we're a nation of boozers. *Independent on Sunday*, February.

Stroebe, W. and Stroebe, M.S. (1995) *Social Psychology and Health*. Suffolk: Open University Press.

Sullivan, R. and Wilson, M.F. (1995) New directions for research in prevention and treatment of delinquency: a review and proposal. *Adolescence* 30, 1–17.

Sumnall, H.R. and Bellis, M.A. (2007) Can health campaigns make people ill? The iatrogenic potential of population-based cannabis prevention. *Journal of Epidemiology and Community Health* 61, 930–931.

Sutton, M. and Godfrey, C. (1995) A grouped data regression approach to estimating economic and social influences on individual drinking behaviour. *Health Economics* 4, 237–247.

Sutton, S. (1982) Fear-arousing communications: a critical examination of theory and research. In: J.R. Eiser (ed.) *Social Psychology and Behavioural Medicine*. London: Wiley.

Sutton, S. (1998) Predicting and explaining intentions and behaviour: how well are we doing? *Journal of Applied Social Psychology* 28, 1317–1338.

Sutton, S. (2001) Back to the drawing board? A review of applications of the transtheoretical model to substance use. *Addiction* 96(1), 175–186.

Sutton, S. (2005) Stage theories of behavioural change. In: M. Conner and P. Norman *Predicting Health Behaviour*, Berkshire: Open University Press.

Swinburn, B. and Egger, G. (2002) Preventive strategies against weight gain and obesity. *Obesity Reviews* 3, 289–301.

Swinburn, B.A., Egger, G.J. and Raza, F. (1999) Dissecting obesogenic environments: the development and application of a framework for identifying and prioritising environmental interventions for obesity. *Preventive Medicine* 29, 563–570.

Tang, J.L., Muir, J., Jones, L., Lancaster,, T. and Fowler, G. (1997) Health profiles of current and former smokers and lifelong abstainers. *Journal of Royal College of Physicians of London* 31(3), 304–309.

Taubman Ben-Ari, O. and Findler, L. (2005) Proximal and distal effects of mortality salience on willingness to engage in health promoting behavior along the life span. *Psychology and Health* 20, 303–318.

Taylor, T., Lader, D., Bryant, A., Keysee, L. and McDuff, T.J. (2006) Smoking-related behaviour and attitudes. London: ONS.

Taylor, A. et al. (1998) 'The Governments Ten-Year Strategy for Tackling Drug Misuse' Cm 3945. Retrieved 25/07/08 from http://www.archive.official-documents.co.uk/document/cm39/3945/strategy.htm.

Terence Higgins Trust (THT) (2007) Survey *Highlights Shocking Ignorance about HIV 25 Years After Death of Terry Higgins*. Accessed 18 December 2007: www.tht.org.uk/mediacentre/pressreleases/2007/july/july4.html.

Thianthai, C. (2004) Gender and class differences in young people's sexuality and HIV/AIDS risk-taking behaviours in Thailand. *Culture, Health and Sexuality* 6, 189–203.

Thirlaway, K.J. and Heggs, D. (2005) Interpreting risk messages: women's responses to a health story. *Health, Risk and Society* 7, 107–121.

Tholin, A., Rasmussen, F., Tynelius, P. and Karlson, J. (2005) Genetic and environmental influences on eating behaviour: the Swedish young male twins study. *American Journal of Clinical Nutrition* 81, 564–569.

Thomas, M.H. (2000) Abstinence-based programs for prevention of adolescent pregnancies: a review. *Journal of Adolescent Health* 26, 5–17.

Thomas, Y. (2006) The social epidemiology of drug abuse. *American Journal of Preventive Medicine* 32(6), S141–S146.

Thomas, Y.F. (2007) The social epidemiology of drug abuse. *American Journal of Preventive Medicine* 32(6S), S141–S146.

Thorndike, A.N., Biener, L. and Rigotti, N.A. (2002) Effect on smoking cessation of switching nicotine replacement therapy to over-the-counter status. *American Journal of Public Health* 92(3), 437–442.

Townsend, P. and Davidson, N. (1982) *Inequalities in Health: The Black Report.* Harmondsworth: Penguin.

Trafimow, D. (2000) Habit as both a direct cause of intention to use a condom and as a moderator of the attitude-intention and subjective norm-intention relations. *Psychology and Health* 15, 383–393.

Trandis, H.C. (1977) *Interpersonal Behaviour.* Montery, CA: Brooks/Cole.

Turner, B.S. (1987) *Medical Power and Social Knowledge.* London: Sage Publications.

Turner, R.J. (2003) The pursuit of socially modifiable contingencies in mental health. *Journal of Health and Social Behavior* 44(1), 1–17.

Tversky, A. and Kahneman, D. (1981) The framing of decisions and the rationality of choice. *Science* 221, 453–458.

UNAIDS (2006) UNAIDS/WHO AIDS Epidemic Update: December 2006. Accessed 1 November 2007 at: http://www.unaids.org/en/HIV_data/epi2006/default.asp.

Unal, B., Critchley, J. A. and Capewell, S. (2004) Explaining the decline in coronary heart disease mortality in England and Wales between 1981 and 2000. *Circulation* 109, 1101–1107.

Urberg, K.A., Shyu, S.J. and Liang, J. (1990) Peer influence in adolescent cigarette smoking. *Addictive Behaviour* 15(3), 247–255.

US Department of Health and Human Services (1999) *Physical Activity and Health: a Report of the Surgeon General.* Atlanta, GA: US Department of Health and Human Services, Centres for Disease Control and Prevention, National Center for Chronic Disease Prevention and Health Promotion.

Valante, T.M., Unger, J.B. and Johnson, C.A. (2005) Do popular students smoke? The association between popularity and smoking among middle school students. *Journal of Adolescent Health* 37, 23–329.

Van Empelen, P. and Kok, G. (2006) Condom use in steady and casual sexual relationships: planning, preparation and willingness to take risks among adolescents, *Psychology and Health* 21(2), 165–181.

Vanable, P.A., McKirnan, D.J., Buchbinder, S.P., Bartholow, B.N., Douglas, J.M., Judson, F. N. and MacQueen, K.M. (2004) Alcohol use and high-risk sexual behaviour among men who have sex with men: the effects of consumption level and partner type. *Health Psychology* 23, 525–532.

Vasilaki, E., Hosier, S.G. and Cox, W.M. (2006) The efficacy of motivational interviewing as a brief intervention for excessive drinking: a meta-analytic review. *Alcohol and Alcoholism* 41(3), 328–335.

Velicer, W.F., Prochaska, J.O., Rossi, J.S. and Snow, M.G. (1992) Assessing outcome in smoking cessation studies. *Psychological Bulletin* 111(1), 23–41.

Velicer, W.F., Prochaska, J.O., Bellis, J.B., DiClemente, C.C., Rossi, J.S., Fava, J.L. and Steiger, J.H. (1993) An expert system intervention for smoking cessation. *Addictive Behaviors* 18, 269–290.

Vellas, B., Conceicao, J., Lafont, C., Fontan, B., Garry, P.J., Adoue, D. and Albarede, J.L.(1990) Malnutrition and Falls. *Lancet* 336, 1147.

Velleman, D.B., Templeton, L.J. and Copello, A.G. (2005) The role of family in preventing and intervening with substance use and misuse: a comprehensive review of family interventions, with a focus on young people. *Drug and Alcohol Review* 24, 93–109.

Verma, R.K., Pulerwitz, J., Mahendra, V.S., Khandekar, S. and Barker, G. (2005) Promoting gender equity among young men to reduce HIV and violence risk: positive experiences of Yari Dosti in India. *Sexual Health Exch*ange 2, 5–6.

Verplanken, B. (2006) Beyond frequency: habit as a mental construct. *British Journal of Social Psychology* 45, 639–656.

Verplanken, B. and Orbell, S. (2003) Reflections of past behaviour: a self report index of habit strength. *Journal of Applied Social Psychology* 33, 1313–1330.

Vidrine, J.I., Cofta-Woerpel, L., Daza, P., Wright, K.L. and Wetter, D.W. (2006) Smoking cessation 2: behavioral treatments. *Behavioral Medicine* 32(3), 99–109.

Villarruel, A.M., Jemmott, J.B., Jemmott, L.S. and Ronis, D.L. (2004) Predictors of sexual intercourse and condom use intention among Spanish dominant Latino youth: a test of the planned behavior theory. *Nursing Research* 53(3), 172– 181.

von Sydow, K., Lieb, R., Pfister, H. et al. (2002) What predicts incident use of cannabis and progression to abuse and dependence? A 4-year prospective examination of risk factors in a community sample of adolescents and young adults. *Drug and Alcohol Dependence* 68, 49–64.

Wald, A., Langenberg, A.G.M., Krantz, E., Douglas, J.M., Handsfield, H.H., DiCarlo, R.P. (2005) The relationship between condom use and herpes simplex virus acquisition. *Annals of Internal Medicine* 143, 707–713.

Walker, J. (2001) Control and the psychology of health. Buckingham: Open University Press.

Wanless, D. (2004) *Securing Good Health for the Whole Population: Final Report*. London: Department of Health.

Warburton, D.E.R., Whitney Nicol, C. and Bredin, S.S.D. (2006) Health benefits of physical activity: the evidence. *Canadian Medical Association Journal* 174, 801–809.

Wardle, J. (2007) Eating behaviour and obesity. *Obesity Reviews* 8(1), 73–75.

Wardle, J. and Steptoe, A. (2003) Socioeconomic differences in attitudes and beliefs about healthy lifestyles. *Journal of Epidemiology and Community Health* 57, 440–443.

Wardle, J. and Steptoe, A. (2005) Public health psychology. *The Psychologist* 18, 672–675.

Wardle, J., Steptoe, A., Oliver, G. and Lipsey, Z. (2000) Stress, dietary restraint and food intake. *Journal of Psychosomatic Research* 48, 195–202.

Wardle, J., Herrera, M.L., Cooke, L. and Gibson, E.L. (2003) Modifying children's food preferences: the effects of exposure and reward on acceptance of an unfamiliar vegetable. *European Journal of Clinical Nutrition* 57, 341–348.

Warner, K.E. and Burns, D.M. (2003) Hardening and the hard-core smoker: concepts, evidence, and implications. *Nicotine and Tobacco Research* 5(1), 37–48.

Warner, L., Stone, K.M., Macaluso, M., Buehler, J.W. and Austin, H.D. (2006) Condom use and risk of gonorrhoea and chlamydia: a systematic review of design and measurement factors assessed in epidemiologic studies. *Sexually Transmitted Diseases* 33, 36–51.

Warwick, Z.S., Hall, W.G., Pappas, T.N. and Schiffman, S.S. (1993) Taste and smell sensations enhance the satiating effect of both a high carbohydrate and a high fat meal in humans. *Physiology and Behaviour* 53, 553–563.

Webb, E., Ashton, C.H., Kelly, P. and Kamali, F. (1996) Alcohol and drug use in UK university students. *Lancet* 348(9032), 922–925.

Webb, P., Bain, C. and Pirozzo, S. (2005) *Essential Epidemiology: An Introduction for Students and Health Professionals*. Cambridge: Cambridge University Press.

Webb, T.L. and Sheeran, P. (2006) Does changing behavioral intentions engender behavioral change? A meta-analysis of the experimental evidence. *Psychological Bulletin* 132, 249–268.

Wechsler, H., Nelson, T., Lee, J.E., Seibring, M., Lewis, C. and Keeling, R.P. (2003) Perceptions and reality: a national evaluation of social norms marketing interventions to reduce college students heavy alcohol use. *Journal of Studies of Alcohol* 64, 484–494.

Weinstein, N.D. (1984) Why it won't happen to me: perceptions of risk factors and susceptibility. *Health Psychology* 3, 431–457.

Weinstein, N.D. and Sandman,P.M. (1992) A model of the precaution adoption process: evidence from home radon testing. *Health Psychology* 11, 170–180.

Weinstein, N.D. and Klein, W.M. (1996) Unrealistic optimism: present and future. *Journal of Social and Clinical Psychology* 15(1), 1–8.

Weinstein, N.D., Rothman, A.J. and Sutton, S.R. (1998) Stage theories of behaviour: conceptual and methodological issues. *Health Psychology* 17, 290–299.

Weinstein, N.D., Marcus, S.E. and Moser, R.P. (2005) Smokers' unrealistic optimism about their risk. *Tobacco Control* 14, 55–59.

Weinstein, N.D., Kwitel, A., McCaul, K.D, and Magnan, R.E. (2007) Risk perceptions: assessment and relationship to influenza vaccination. *Health Psychology* 26, 146–151.

Weiser, S.D., Lieter, K., Heisler, M., McFarland, W., Percy-de Korte, F., DeMonner, S.M. et al. (2006) *Population-Based Study on Alcohol and High-Risk Sexual Behaviors in Botswana* 3, 10, e392. Accessed 15 December at: www.plosmedicine.org.

Wellings, K., Field, J., Johnson, A.M. and Wadsworth, J. (1994) *Sexual Behavior in Britain: The National Survey of Sexual Attitudes and Lifestyles*. Harmondsworth: Penguin.

Wellings, K., Collumbien, M., Slaymaker, E., Singh, S., Hodges, Z., Patel, D. and Bajos, N. (2006) Sexual and Reproductive Health 2 Sexual behaviour in context: a global perspective. *Lancet* 368, 1706–1728.

Welsh Assembly Government (2003) *Health and Active Lifestyles in Wales: A Framework for Action*. Cardiff: Welsh Assembly Government.

Welsh Assembly Government (2005) *Health Status Wales 2004–2005: Chief Medical Officer's Report Series*. Cardiff: Welsh Assembly Government.

Welsh Assembly Government (2007) *Welsh Health Survey 2005/2006*. Cardiff: Welsh Assembly Government.

Werch, C.E., Pappas, D.M., Carlson, J.M. and DiClemente, C.C. (1998) Short and long-term effects of a pilot prevention programme to reduce alcohol consumption. *Substance Use and Misuse* 33, 2303–2321.

West, R. (2005) Time for a change: putting the Transtheoretical (Stages of Change) Model to rest. *Addiction* 100(8), 1036–1039.

West, R. (2006) Smoking and smoking cessation in England: 2006. Retrieved 17/07/08 from www.smokinginengland.info/Ref/paper4.pdf.

West, R. (2007) *Theory of Addiction*. Oxford: Blackwell Publishing.

West, R., Hajek, P., Stead, L. and Stapleton, J. (2005) Outcome criteria in smoking cessation trials: proposal for a common standard. *Addiction* 100(3), 299–303.

Whitehead, M., Townsend, P., Davidson, N., Davidsen, N. (eds) (2002) *Inequalities in Health: The Black Report and the Health Divide* (Penguin Social Sciences) London: Penguin.

Whitelaw, S., Baldwin, S., Bunton, R. and Flynn, D. (2000) The status of evidence and outcomes in Stages of Change research. *Health Education Research* 15(6), 707–718.

WHO Expert Committee on Drug Dependence. (1969) *Sixteenth Report*. Geneva, World Health Organisation (WHO Technical Report Series, No.407).

Wiebe, G.D. (1951–1952) Merchandising commodities and citizenship on television. *Public Opinion Quarterly* 15, 679–691.

Willemsen, M.C., Wiebing, M., van Emst, A. and Zeeman, G. (2006) Helping smokers to decide on the use of efficacious smoking cessation methods: a randomized controlled trial of a decision aid. *Addiction* 101(3), 441–449.

Williams, E.C., Horton, N.J., Samet, J.H. and Saitz, R. (2007) Do brief measures of readiness to change predict alcohol consumption and consequences in primary care patients with unhealthy alcohol use? *Alcoholism: Clinical and Experimental Research* 31, 428–435.

Williamson, D.F., Madans, J., Anda, R.F., Kleinman, J.C., Giovino, G.A. and Byers, T. (1991) Smoking cessation and severity of weight gain in a national cohort. *New England Journal of Medicine* 324, 739–745.

Wilson, P. (1980) *Drinking in England and Wales*. London: HMSO.

Windschitl, P.D. and Wells, G.L. (1996) Measuring psychological uncertainty: verbal versus numeric methods. *Journal of Experimental Psychology: Applied* 2, 343–364.

Winer, R.L., Hughes, J.P., Feng, Q., O'Reilly, S., Kiviat, N.B., Holmes, K.K. and Koutsky, L.A. (2006) Condom use and the risk of genital human papillomavirus infection in young women. *New England Journal of Medicine* 354(25), 2645–2654.

Winger, G. (1992) *A Handbook on Drug and Alcohol Abuse: The Biomedical Aspects*. Oxford: Oxford University Press.

Wolitski, R.J., Parsons, J.T. and Gomez, C.A. (2004) Prevention with HIV-seropositive men who have sex with men: lessons from the Seropositive Urban Men's Study (SUMS) and the Seropositive Urban Men's Intervention Trial (SUMIT). *Journal of Acquired Immune Deficiency Syndrome* 37(S2), 101–109.

Wood, M.D., Read, J.P., Mitchell, R.E. and Brand, N.H. (2004) Do parents still matter? Parent and peer influences on alcohol involvement among recent high school graduates. *Psychology of Addictive Behaviours* 18(1), 19–30.

Wood, W., Quinn, J.M. and Kashy, D. (2002) Habits in everyday life: thought, emotion, and action. *Journal of Personality and Social Psychology* 83, 1281–1297.

World Cancer Research Fund (1997) *Food Nutrition, and the Prevention of Cancer: A Global Perspective*. Washington, DC: American Institute for Cancer Research.

World Health Organisation (WHO) (1992a) *The ICD-10 Classification of Mental and Behavioural Disorders: Clinical Descriptions and Diagnostic Guidelines*. Geneva: World Health Organisation.

World Health Organisation (WHO) (1992b) *International Classification of Diseases (ICD-10)* 10th edn. Geneva: World Health Organisation.

World Health Organisation (WHO) (2000). *International Guide for Monitoring Alcohol Consumption and Related Harm*. Geneva: World Health Organisation.

World Health Organisation (WHO) (2002) *World Health Report (2002): Reducing Risks, Promoting Healthy Life*. Geneva: World Health Organisation.

World Health Organisation (WHO) (2004a) *Report 916: Diet, Nutrition and the Prevention of Chronic Diseases*. Geneva: World Health Organisation.

World Health Organisation (WHO) (2004b) *The Tobacco Atlas*. Geneva: World Health Organisation.

World Health Organisation (WHO) *(2005) Multi-country Study on Women's Health and Domestic Violence Against Women*. Geneva: World Health Organisation.

World Health Organisation (WHO) (2007a) *The Global Burden*. Retrived 15/12/07 from: http://www.who.int/substance_abuse/facts/global_burden/en/index.html.

World Health Organisation (WHO) (2007b) *Tobacco*. Available at: http://www.who.int/topics/tobacco/en/.

World Health Organisation (Health Education Unit) 1986. Life-styles and Health. Social Science in Medicine 22 117–124.

Wrigley, N., Warm, D. and Margetts, B. (2003) Deprivation, diet and food retail access: findings from the Leeds 'Food Deserts' study. *Environment Planning* 35, 151–188.

Yang, M.U., Yang, M.S. and Kawachi, I. (2001) Work experience and drinking behaviour: alienation, occupational status, workplace drinking subculture and problem drinking. *Public Health* 115, 265–271.

Yeomans, M.R. (1996) Palatability and the microstructure of feeding in humans: the appetizer effect. *Appetite* 27, 119–133.

Yeomans, M.R. and Symes, T. (1999) Individual differences in the use of pleasantness and palatability ratings. *Appetite* 32, 383–394.

Yeomans, M.R., Gray, R.W., Mitchell, C.J. and True, S. (1997) Independent effects of palatability and within meal pauses on intake and appetite ratings in human volunteers. *Appetite* 29, 61–76.

Yoshikawa, H. (1994) Prevention as cumulative protection: effects of early family support and education on chronic delinquency and its risks. *Psychological Bulletin* 115(1), 28–54.

Young, S.E., Corley, R.P., Stallings, M.C. et al. (2002) Substance use, abuse and dependence in adolescence: prevalence, symptom profiles and correlates. *Drug and Alcohol Dependence* 68, 309–322.

Zaninotto, P., Wardle, H., Stamatakis, E., Mindell, J. and Head, J. (2006) *Forecasting Obesity to 2010*. Retrieved 2 December 2007 from: http://www.dh.gov.uk/en/Piblicationsandstatistics/Publications/PublicationsStatistics/DH_4138630.

Zeegers, T., Segaar, D. and Willemsen, M. (2005) *Roken: de Harde Feiten 2004 [Smoking: the Hard Facts 2004]*. The Hague: STIVORO.

Zhu, S., Melcer, T., Sun, J., Rosbrook, B. and Pierce, J.P. (2000) Smoking cessation with and without assistance: a population-based analysis. *American Journal of Preventive Medicine* 18(4), 305–311.

Zwar, N. and Richmond, R. (2002) Bupropion sustained release. A therapeutic review of Zyban. *Australian Family Physician* 31(5), 443–447.

Index

Page numbers in *italics* denotes a diagram/table